Toxic Turmoil

**Psychological and Societal
Consequences of Ecological Disasters**

The Plenum Series on Stress and Coping

Series Editor:
Donald Meichenbaum, *University of Waterloo, Waterloo, Ontario, Canada*

A Continuation Order Plan is available for this series. A continuation order will bring
delivery of each new volume immediately upon publication. Volumes are billed only upon
actual shipment. For further information please contact the publisher.

Toxic Turmoil
Psychological and Societal Consequences of Ecological Disasters

Edited by

Johan M. Havenaar
University Medical Center and
Altrecht Institute for Mental Health Care
Utrecht, The Netherlands

Julie G. Cwikel
Ben Gurion University of the Negev
Beer Sheva, Israel

and

Evelyn J. Bromet
State University of New York at Stony Brook
Stony Brook, New York

Kluwer Academic / Plenum Publishers
New York, Boston, Dordrecht, London, Moscow

Library of Congress Cataloging-in-Publication Data

Toxic turmoil: psychological and societal consequences of ecological disasters/edited
by Johan M. Havenaar, Julie G. Cwikel, and Evelyn J. Bromet.
    p.   cm — (Plenum series on stress and coping)
    Includes bibliographical references and index.
    ISBN 0-306-46784-4
    1. Ecological disasters—Psychological aspects.   2. Ecological disasters—Social aspects.   3.
Stress (Psychology)   I. Havenaar, Johan M., 1954–   II. Cwikel, Julie G.   III. Bromet, Evelyn
J.   IV. Series.

RA645.9 .T69 2002
616.89—dc21

                                                                                            2002067808

ISBN: 0-306-46784-4

©2002 Kluwer Academic / Plenum Publishers
233 Spring Street, New York, New York 10013

http://www.wkap.nl/

10 9 8 7 6 5 4 3 2 1

A C.I.P. record for this book is available from the Library of Congress

Printed in the United States of America

Contributors

Nozomu Asukai, Department of Stress Disorders Research, Tokyo Institute Psychiatry, Tokyo, 156-8585, Japan

Peter J. Baxter, University of Cambridge Clinical School, Addenbrooke's Hospital, Cambridge CB2 2QQ, United Kingdom

Steven M. Becker, School of Public Health and Medicine, Center for Disaster Preparedness, The University of Alabama at Birmingham, Birmingham, Alabama 35294-0022

Evelyn J. Bromet, Department of Psychiatry and Behavioral Science, State University of New York at Stony Brook, New York 11794-8790

Gary Coleman, WHO Collaborating Centre, University of Wales Institute, Cardiff, Wales

Eric J. Crighton, McMaster Institute of Environment and Health, Hamilton, Ontario, Canada

Julie G. Cwikel, the Charlotte and Jack Spitzer Department of Social Work and Director of the Center for Women's Health Studies and Promotion. Ben Gurion University of the Negev, Beer Sheva, Israel

Joop de Jong, Transcultural Psychosocial Organization (TPO), and Vrije Universiteit, 1016 EE Amsterdam, The Netherlands

Hilary M. P. Fielder, Department of Epidemiology and Public Health, University of Wales College of Medicine, Cardiff, Wales

Nathan Ford, Médécins sans Frontières, UK Office, United Kingdom

Berthold P. R. Gersons, Academic Medical Center, University of Amsterdam, de Meren, Department of Psychiatry, 1100 DD Amsterdam, The Netherlands

Johan M. Havenaar, University Medical Center and Altrecht Institute for Mental Health Care, 3512 PZ Utrecht, The Netherlands

Leighann Litcher-Kelly, Department of Psychiatry and Behavioral Science, State University of New York at Stony Brook, New York 11794-8790

Kazuhiko Maekawa, Department of Traumatology and Critical Care, University of Tokyo Faculty of Medicine, Tokyo, Japan

R. Srinivasa Murthy, Department of Psychiatry, National Institute of Mental Health and Neurosciences, P.O. Box 2900, Bangalore 560029, India

Stephen R. Palmer, Department of Epidemiology and Public Health, University of Wales College of Medicine, Cardiff, Wales

Ian B. Small, Médécins sans Frontières (Holland), Aral Sea Area Program, Uzbekistan

Anne Speckhard, Vesalius, Free University of Brussels, 1150 Brussels, Belgium

Joost B. W. van der Meer, Médécins sans Frontières (Holland), Aral Sea Area Program, Uzbekistan

Simon Wessely, Guy's King's and St. Thomas' School of Medicine, London, SE5 8AF, United Kingdom

Joris Yzermans, Academic Medical Center, University of Amsterdam, Division Public Health, Department of General Practice, 1100 DD Amsterdam, The Netherlands

Preface

When an accident involves many people and when its consequences are many and serious, we speak of a disaster. Disasters have the same causal factors as accidents: they differ from accidents by the gravity of consequences, not by causes. The action of a single individual may result in thousands of deaths and huge financial losses. The metal fatigue of a screw may, by a chain of events, cause an explosion killing hundreds or lead to a break in a dam and a devastating flood.

The fact that minor and unpredictable acts can lead to disasters is important because it allows us to predict that the years to come will bring with them more disasters with ever more severe consequences. The density of human populations is growing. By the year 2025 some four fifths of the world's population will be living in urban settings. An explosion or a gas leak in a densely populated area will cause incomparably more damage than a similar event in a rural area. Modern technology is immensely powerful (and its power is continuing to grow) and can be used in a disastrous manner. Aggression is just as possible now as it was in the past, but the tools of aggression are vastly more dangerous than ever before.

This book, edited by Johan M. Havenaar, Julie G. Cwikel, and Evelyn J. Bromet, is therefore very timely. It presents a series of descriptions of disasters—most caused by humans, some predictable and others not, some due to evil intent, and some due to ignorance and the still mysterious forces of nature. The disasters described did not only cause physical damage, human suffering, disability, and death; for a variety of reasons, their impact on the environment has been more lasting than is the case for most natural catastrophes. They also usually resulted in a painful series of legal and social consequences and in recriminations, accusations, and loss of trust and confidence among people and nations. The careful study of these examples provides valuable lessons about causes of disasters, about their consequences, and about ways of diminishing or preventing their consequences. This book does not deal with disasters due to forces of nature—volcano eruptions, earthquakes, floods, winds—nor with wars, although these usually produce huge damage, but most of the lessons learned from the study of disasters described in the volume will be useful in dealing with consequences of natural catastrophes and wars. Disaster preparedness referred to in the volume can and should help people when disaster strikes regardless of the reasons that produced them.

I hope that this book and its sequels will be read and studied not only by those dealing with public health and human welfare but also by the general public, politicians, and scientists worldwide because all of them have to work together if the consequences of disasters are to be averted and at least some of the disasters prevented.

NORMAN SARTORIUS

Contents

PART III: DEALING WITH ECOLOGICAL DISASTER

I

Introduction

1

Ecological Disaster

A Concern for the Future

JOHAN M. HAVENAAR

On September 11, 2001, as this book was on its way to press, disaster struck once again. Two hijacked airplanes, fully loaded with passengers and fuel crashed into the World Trade Center in New York and another into the Pentagon in Washington, D.C. A fourth airplane crashed into the country-side of Pennsylvania, apparently missing its intended target, but nevertheless killing all those on board. These unprecedented and brutal terrorist attacks hit the Western world at the core of its financial and military power. They left once-towering skyscrapers in piles of rubble, carrying to their deaths thousands of innocent civilians and hundreds of rescue workers. Many died in full view of bystanders who watched horrified as people jumped from the windows of the burning buildings. As undoubtedly planned, they dealt a re-sounding blow to the confidence of the most powerful nation in the world. People were caught in complete surprise as they went about their daily busi-ness. Around the world, people felt that the attacks had shaken the very foundations of their sense of security. They left us scared, vulnerable, and without adequate protection against the forces of terrorism. Coupled with repulsion and disbelief, various doomsday scenarios were beamed over news networks, phone lines, and electronic mail in a matter of hours.

JOHAN M. HAVENAAR • University Medical Center and Altrecht Institute for Mental Health Care, 3512 PZ Utrecht, the Netherlands.

Toxic Turmoil: Psychological and Societal Consequences of Ecological Disasters, edited by Johan M. Havenaar, Julie G. Cwikel, and Evelyn J. Bromet. New York, Kluwer Academic/Plenum Publishers, 2002.

As this nightmare experience will forever leave its mark on those who survived, and feelings of grief will live with those who have lost relatives or friends for years to come, so too the shock of faith will carry its momentum forward with as yet unforeseeable psychological consequences, which are nevertheless likely to affect people's lives all around the globe in a very direct and concrete way for decades.

This book is dedicated to victims of disasters all over the world. It focuses on a special type of disaster we term "ecological disasters." These disasters have in common with the events described that they are man-made and that they profoundly affect the sense of safety people need in order to continue their lives. They share these effects with wars and natural disasters. They also differ from these because in many cases they are determined by concerns for the future, anxiety about what might still happen rather that what has actually happened. The extent to which the bombing of the World Trade Center will turn out to be an ecological disaster will become clear as more information becomes available over the next months and years (e.g., questions as to whether people in the area were exposed to significant concentrations of toxic substances like asbestos from the cloud of dust and smoke that covered south Manhattan). The mail attacks with anthrax bacteria that have followed since certainly carry many elements typical for toxic disaster, especially because the fear these attacks evoke appears to be equally damaging to society as the attacks themselves. In both cases, much will depend on the way that information will be handled and whether there will be further terrorists attacks with biological or chemical weapons. The many questions these events evoke and the often partial answers to them that will circulate over time can themselves give their aftermath a "toxic" turn that cannot be directly linked to the toxic exposure itself. It is this type of information and its far-reaching societal consequences that are the focus of this book.

WHEN WORST COMES TO WORST

"Thousands of deaths and three and a half million people in Ukraine suffering from health damages." With this press release Reuter and Associated Press reminded us that the nuclear accident at Chernobyl (Ukraine), which occurred on April 26, 1986, continues to be relevant even in the next millennium. As a result of this disaster, which was the largest civil nuclear accident so far, several tons of radioactive material were dispersed over Europe and the rest of the world. Hundreds of thousands of people were relocated to less contaminated territories. In Belarus, the most seriously affected republic, about 20% of agricultural land was taken out of production (Shigematsu, 1991). To most people facts like these make "Chernobyl" the worst ecological nightmare one can imagine. Yearly press releases such as the one quoted above hardly raise doubts in the minds of most readers, even though every year the alleged death toll appears to show considerable variation. In May 1986 the *New York Post* reported: "15,000 dead in a mass grave." Ten years later the Russian press agency ITAR-TASS (April 23, 1992) claimed that over a hundred thousand people died as a result of the accident. In 1998 it was announced that 12,519 of the 350,000 Ukrainian firefighters and release workers involved in the cleanup after the accident had died (Reuters, April 23, 1998), and in 2000 a number of "about 4,000" was mentioned (Reuters, AP, April 26, 2000). The general picture remains: This was the most terrible ecological disaster ever, with mass casualties and unprecedented health consequences, which may last for generations to come.

Anyone who would take the trouble to compare what is reported in the popular press with the scientific literature about the health consequences of the Chernobyl disaster (e.g., the official health statistics published by the World Health Organization [WHO]), will fail to find any substantial support for these claims. According to official sources the death toll is below 30 (WHO, 1995). Direct deaths occurred primarily among the firefighters during the first hour. In later years a sharp increase of thyroid cancer among children has been observed, which was most probably caused by the fall out. Fortunately, almost all of these children survived the condition. The expected epidemic of leukemia or other cancers has not occurred (Alexander & Greaves, 1998), and an anticipated dramatic increase in the number of stillbirths and congenital malformation has not been substantiated (Castronovo, 1999; Dolk & Nichols, 1999).

The wide discrepancy between what is apparently common knowledge in the lay press and what is accepted scientific fact is by no means limited to the Chernobyl disaster. As we describe in this book, this information gap is typical for a type of disaster that has been in the focus of media attention during the past few decades. In this book we use the term "ecological disaster" to indicate the threat to the human environment they represent. Famous examples include Love Canal (1976), Seveso (Italy, 1976), Three Mile Island (Pennsylvania, USA, 1979), and Bhopal (India, 1984). All of these industrial incidents caused widespread contamination of adjacent areas with toxic chemicals or radioactive materials or have threatened to do so. One of the characteristics of these disasters appears to be their enormous psychological and societal impact regardless of the actual number of casualties they caused. They continue to confront us acutely with the fallibility of our technological systems.

By far the most deadly of these accidents was the Bhopal accident, vividly described by Srinivasa Murthy in this volume (Chapter 7). As a result of this accident at a pesticide factory in central India, several thousand people were killed and many more were seriously injured. Even though the Bhopal disaster resulted in far more victims than Chernobyl, it received far less attention. Perhaps this is because it is far removed from the epicenters of Western society, or perhaps because methylisocyanate, the deadly substance released at the time of this accident, does not have the same portentous reputation as radioactivity or dioxin.

Clearly remembered also is the near-accident at Three Mile Island (TMI) in Harrisburg, Pennsylvania, in 1979. There was no substantial release of radioactive material during this incident and there were no casualties. Yet this incident has become one of the most infamous examples of failing human technology. At the time, people living near the reactor were very anxious, and this continued to influence their sense of health and well-being for more than a decade. It is now the best-studied example of the widespread psychological impact this type of accident may have. What all of these events have in common, beyond their overriding psychological impact, is the enormous societal conflict they create. As the chapters in this book will demonstrate, these conflicts between lay people and experts, and, more important, between authorities and the general public, tend to be a toxic factor in their own right.

Judging from the dates of these events one might get the impression that most of these incidents occurred in the 1980s. However, as Baxter's and Fielder et al.'s contributions in this volume will demonstrate (Chapters 2 and 10), numerous similar but smaller events occur each year, with ecological implications quite similar to their large-scale counterparts. The airplane crash in Amsterdam in 1992, described by Yzermans and Gersons in Chapter 5, the recent nuclear accident in Japan, and yet another explosion in a chemical factory in south France in recent months are good examples of this.

The focus on these events should be interpreted against the background of contemporary concerns that man-made environmental factors may threaten the human ecosystem and thereby human health and survival. For most of the previous century average life expectancy has gradually increased, particularly in countries with high levels of industrial development. But in Central and Eastern Europe life expectancy started to decline steadily since the 1970s (WHO, 1999). Environmental pollution is believed to contribute to a great extent to this deterioration. However, recent research shows that the impact of environmental pollution at the population level is limited. There is now some evidence that ambient air pollution plays a small but statistically significant role in the etiology of respiratory disease (WHO, 1999). In addition, radioactive radon present in buildings is estimated to be responsible for 2 to 5% of lung cancers. But apart from these two examples the overall health statistics don't give rise to realistic concerns about health problems, which can be attributed to environmental changes in our ecosystem. Also, according to the same report, accidental releases of chemicals or other industrial hazards account for only a minority of work-related health problems (WHO, 1999). In fact, as Baxter argues in Chapter 2, a large-scale chemical disaster may also result from natural causes (e.g., a volcanic eruption of Vesuvius looming over the Italian city of Naples will threaten the lives of about a million inhabitants).

Yet according to the same source the influence of industrial pollution on health raises far more concern than lifestyle-related health hazards such as smoking or being overweight. Similarly, industrial disasters, especially if they pose a threat to our ecosystem, arouse much more fear and dread than their natural counterparts. The chapters brought together in this volume will make clear that the importance of these man-made events lies, at least thus far, not in their actual impact on physical health, but in their psychological and societal impacts. Incidents involving the release of toxic chemicals or radionuclides give rise to large-scale reactions among the public in unprecedented ways. Not only are the events themselves relatively new, the public's reaction is quite different from the ones that emergency workers and health authorities are familiar in dealing with. This is particularly the case for the widespread, unexplained health complaints that so often characterize their wake and that usually appear only months or years later. This book documents the public health consequences of these events and explores the ways health professionals and authorities cope with them.

In this chapter I give a working definition of ecological disasters and describe the theoretical mechanisms through which they can endanger health. I then introduce some of the central themes and controversies that surround these events and that will be discussed in the various chapters of this book.

WHAT ARE ECOLOGICAL DISASTERS?

The word "disaster" derives from the Latin roots "dis" meaning "bad" and "aster" meaning "star" (i.e., the word implies bad fate). Disasters are more easily recognized then defined (Green 1991). Many authors have tried to give a definition or make a classification of disasters (Berren, Beigel, & Ghertner, 1980; Quarantelli, 1984; van den Eynde & Veno, 1999). Usually these definitions contain terms such as "massive collective stress," "exceeding the systems ability to cope," and "causing wide-ranging disruption to human systems." Other recurrent elements are the fact that disasters occur suddenly, within a more or less circumscribed geographical area, involve some degree of loss, and are subject to human management. Berren et al. (1980)

mention five factors that can be used conceptually to distinguish one disaster from another:

- type of disaster: man-made versus natural
- duration
- degree of personal impact
- potential of recurrence
- control over future impact

One can easily recognize that these characteristics, however relevant, are hardly useful to build a classification system of mutually exclusive categories of disaster. Ecological disasters are usually man made, but not necessarily so. Their duration and degree of personal impact, chance of recurrence, and future control may vary. More important, these aspects may be subject to considerable debate.

Throughout the book we will use a broad definitition of ecological disaster, based on the general definition of disaster by Noji (1997; cf. Chapter 2), the definition of the UK National Surveillance for Chemical Incidents (cf. Chapter 10), and the definition by the United Nations Environmental Program (UNEP; cf. Chapter 10). The latter two are much more strictly formulated definitions of chemical exposures in relation to the number of victims involved. Our book has a broader scope. It includes accounts of nuclear accidents and attacks with biological weapons, which would also qualify as ecological disasters. We realize that any major disaster has an ecological component because it disrupts the matrix of human existence that we depend on for our sustenance. In our definition we will reserve the term ecological to indicate that a real or perceived serious deterioration of our environment by chemicals radionuclides or other noxious agent is at hand. In any definition ultimately a certain amount of "fuzzy logic" is unavoidable when you combine sets of overlapping terms like *(near-)incident/accident/catastrophe/disaster* and *chemical/nuclear/toxicological/ecological/environmental*. For pragmatic reasons we will define an ecological disaster as an *unpredictable or sudden, real or perceived collective exposure of recognizable population groups to hazardous substances or agents on such a scale that the stricken community needs extraordinary efforts to cope with it.*

In other words, there should be an event with considerable societal impact in direct relation to an exposure, or threatened exposure to what the military call ABC-type substances (atomic, biological, chemical). This definition excludes smaller exposure events involving fewer people, which may nevertheless have common characteristics with ecological disasters. For this we will reserve the term "incident" rather than disaster. Also not included in this definition is massive exposure of the population to ambient air pollution or electromagnetic fields from cell phones, broadcast antennas, and radar stations (Matthes, Bernhardt, & Repacholi, 1998) or exposure to seemingly omnipresent endocrine disrupters, which are alleged to endanger human and animal fertility (European Commission, 1997). Even so, as some of the examples in this book show, such smaller or diffuse events may be catastrophe to the people who are directly involved. Their consequences may be quite similar to those occurring in ecological disasters.

An extensive review by Rubonis and Bickman (1991) showed that the main predictor of distress after a disaster is the number of (immediate) deaths. These authors were unable to show a difference between natural and man-made disasters in terms of stress-related health outcomes. Despite this, there is reason to assume that ecological or toxicological disasters nevertheless constitute a distinct type of disaster. The individual and community response to accidents where hazardous substances are released is quite different from the response to nontoxic events, whether natural or technological (Havenaar & van den Brink, 1997). The main difference is the amount of social unrest they tend to create. Natural disasters usually have positive as well as negative effects. Ecologically "clean" technological disasters, such as a collapsing dam or a major train crash, where no dangerous substances are released, are similar in this respect. However devastating they may be, in some cases they also have a tendency to strengthen social ties and natural healing tendencies in the community (Quarantelli, 1985; Salzer & Bickman, 1999). The public's reaction to the recent terrorist attacks on America demonstrates this quite clearly. Ecological disasters, by contrast, appear to have a greater propensity to bring about negative psychological and societal effects: public discord and relentless debates, for example about the nature and extent of the damage or about who is to blame.

PATHOGENIC MECHANISMS IN ECOLOGICAL DISASTERS

In the aftermath of ecological disasters usually a complex set of factors is present, each of which may have an impact on the health of exposed individuals. (These are discussed in Chapter 3 in the social epidemiological approach to understanding ecological disasters by Julie Cwikel et al.) Table 1.1 lists the possible mechanisms by which health problems among the population may be linked to an ecological accident. The most straightforward and feared link is a direct negative influence of the toxic substance on human physiology. Short-term examples are radiation sickness after a nuclear accident or the typical skin lesion of chloracne after dioxin exposure. Long-term examples are the increased risk of cancer or birth defects after exposure to ionizing radiation.

Table 1.1   Possible Links between Health Problems and Ecological Disasters

- Physical effects of the exposure
- Psychological effects of the exposure ("stress")
- Physical and psychological effects of the response measures
- Interactions between these effects
- Chance (attribution)

The event may also induce a stress reaction because the event itself is a psychological traumatic life event. Typical for the psychological impact of ecological disasters is the stress-related response to a perceived direct threat to one's own health or, as will be described in Chapter 4 by Bromet and Litcher on mothers from TMI and Chernobyl, to the health of their children. Other factors that contribute to the psychological impact are the feeling of loss of control over one's life and the uncertainty of what will follow.

As important as the direct physical or psychological impact of these events are, there are also secondary health consequences that occur in the disaster response period. These may be physical effects, such as traffic accidents during evacuation or nutritional deficiencies resulting from dietary restrictions in contaminated areas, as well as psychological effects. A common example of the latter is the negative psychological consequences of evacuation, a fact that is unfortunately rarely taken into account in evacuation decisions. The loss of jobs or property and the uncertainty if one can ever return safely leave deep scars in the human soul. They can be felt and demonstrated for many years after an event (Bromet & Havenaar, 2002).

Another element of the countermeasures that can profoundly affect health outcomes is the way information is disseminated. In the immediate aftermath of an ecological disaster the authorities appear to be preoccupied with trying to prevent panic and social unrest. For this reason they tend to take a reassuring stance, trying to minimize the severity of the event, sometimes even falsely so. In the case of Chernobyl, attempts by the authorities to cover up the events probably aggravated the psychological damage. In some instances it has been reported that the authorities decided not to distribute protective iodine tables because they were afraid this would cause panic. Had they decided differently, later cases of thyroid cancer among children might have been prevented. The psychological and social mechanisms involved in the aftermath of ecological disasters will be dealt with in more detail in Cwikel et al.'s chapter, as well as in many of the case reports in part II.

Direct and indirect physical, psychological, and social mechanisms can interact in complicated ways. For example demoralization may lead to increased risk of exposure to radionuclides. Rumyantseva Drottz-Sjöberg,

Allen, Arkhangelskaya, Nyagu, Ageeva & Prilipko (1995) reported that people living in contaminated areas near Chernobyl were more likely to disregard precautionary measures if they had high levels of distress. People were sometimes convinced they would die from radiation anyway, so they felt no need to abstain from eating contaminated mushrooms or drinking milk from cows that had grazed in contaminated pastures (Mays, Avetova, Murphy, & Allen, 1998).

A final but nevertheless important way in which health problems may be linked to ecological disasters is chance. In this case health problems not causally related to the event are erroneously attributed to exposure to a hazardous substance. This type of association is likely to cause considerable debate and societal unrest.

COMMON CONTROVERSIES ABOUT THE HEALTH EFFECTS OF ECOLOGICAL DISASTERS

When trying to ascertain the nature and extent of the health damage caused by ecological disasters there is usually considerable scientific and public debate around a number of themes.

Is There a Health Problem?

Apart from acute intoxication syndromes or radiation sickness it may take months or years before health effects become apparent. Usually after these events one of the following scenarios develops, often in combination with one another. In one typical chain of events slowly more and more people will come forward with various health problems, which they attribute to the exposure. Often a local doctor or advocacy group backs them up. In many cases this is the beginning of a long struggle between patients, physicians, and health authorities to determine whether these complaints can be meaningfully attributed to the exposure.

In another typical case a cluster of a rare disease is discovered (e.g. leukemia or Down's syndrome), which is brought to the attention of the authorities. Usually it is practically impossible to rule out alternative explanations, including chance, because there are no data available on the health status of the exposed population prior to the accident and valid control groups are hard to assemble. A complicating factor is the fact that exposure tends to occur in selected groups or settings (e.g., economically deprived people already at risk for health problems related to poverty and detrimental lifestyles). As Hilary Fielder et al. discuss in chapter 10, methodological problems such as these are abundant in this research area. They make it extremely difficult, if not impossible, to ascertain whether there is a link between a cluster of health problems and an exposure. On the other hand it is at least as difficult to rule out such a link completely. Debates on whether there is a health effect therefore tend to extend for protracted periods of time.

Are the Health Problems Physical or Psychological in Origin?

If there are many people with health complaints attributed to the exposure, and especially if these complaints are of a rather nonspecific nature, the debate will move from the question of whether there is a health problem toward a second controversy. The question then arises whether these ailments are more likely to be caused by psychological mechanisms rather than physical ones. The victims themselves tend to cling to physical explanations with considerable vigor, but scientists find it difficult to give a firm answer to this question for a number of reasons.

More often than not there is uncertainty about the exposure itself, sometimes even about the substances involved. The El Al airplane crash in 1992, described by Yzermans and Gersons in Chapter 5, provides a good example. After an air freighter crashed into a densely populated residential area of Amsterdam, it took six years to discover the exact composition of the cargo onboard, which turned out to be harmless in the end. As the years went by, rumors abated that poisonous war gasses or radioactive materials had been onboard. With the ongoing uncertainty and with each report in the press, the number of people with health complaints attributed to the crash rose steadily.

A related problem is the fact that quite often the substances that have been released are underresearched. Sometimes relatively unknown substances or mixtures of substances are actually formed by chemical reactions at the time of the accident. But even if the substance is known, the actual levels of exposure may still be hard to determine. A second problem is the issue of long-term versus short-term effects. Many chemicals and radionuclides are known to have long-term effects, which are practically impossible to rule out in the short-term research. This means that people cannot easily or truthfully be reassured that there will be no danger in the future.

In addition there is no way to ascertain a psychological origin of the complaints other than to rule out a physical cause. Taken together all these factors tend to complicate the already difficult problem of differentiating between "real" physical health problems and psychological problems. One of the more interesting examples of this phenomena is the copycat syndrome. In the Goiania incident in Brazil (Petterson, 1988) children found a piece of radioactive cesium from a demolished hospital. Eventually 4 people died and about 250 people were investigated for symptoms of radiation sickness. It turned out that the majority of alleged "victims" of radiation sickness showed no signs of actual exposure, yet they presented with many of the same complaints as real victims. In India, a similar phenomenon was observed after an accident involving the release of sulfur dioxide (cf. Chapter 7). Recently in Belgium many young people suffered from gastrointestinal problems and dizziness after drinking Coca-Cola, believed to be contaminated. Later it turned out there was no evidence of actual contamination of the beverage, and it is now believed that mass psychogenic illness is the most likely explanation for this epidemic (Nemery, Fischler, Boogaerts, & Lison, 1999).

Are Stress-Related Health Problems Precursors of Future Disease?

Research on the aftermath of the TMI incident in 1979 has provided convincing evidence that this event caused changes in the excretion of stress hormones, blood pressure, and immune function (Davidson & Baum, 1992). Many researchers believe that the psychological or stress-related health complaints that occurred in the aftermath of ecological disasters are related to these neuroendocrine changes. They consider these changes themselves to be potential risk factors for the development of physical disorders later in life. In the case of the Amsterdam airplane crash this issue became part of the public debate about the consequences of the disaster. This was debated in the discussion of a cluster of autoimmune diseases to exposure to contaminants aboard the crashed airplane (see Chapter 5). Even though there is now considerable evidence that stress related to ecological disasters can have a long-term impact on human physiology, especially on neuroendocrine, immune, and cardiovascular function, as yet there is no solid evidence that these are actually linked to adverse clinical outcomes (Havenaar & van den Brink, 1997). Recent developments in the field of psychosomatics, however, provide compelling evidence from both animal and human studies that this may indeed be the case (McEwen, 2000). The most powerful example is probably the excess morbidity and mortality that was observed in two independent long-term follow-up studies among U.S. combatants from the Second World War (Elders, Shnahan, & Clipp, 1997; Lee, Vaillant, Torrey, & Elder, 1995). Whether such physical health consequences of stress also occur after ecological and other disasters is unknown. Cwikel, Goldsmith, Kordysh, Quastel, and Abdelgani (1997) report a higher systolic blood pressure among immigrants from the Chernobyl area to Israel. Bertazzi (1989) found a slightly increased mortality rate among victims of the Seveso dioxin accident in Italy in 1976, which he tentatively attributed to the effects of stress. Apart from these two examples there is no convincing evidence for a substantial stress-mediated effect on physical health among people exposed to ecological disasters.

What is the Role of "Reporting Bias"?

In the case of psychotraumatic and somatoform illnesses there has always been considerable debate on the role of reporting bias (Watson & Pennebaker, 1989). It is generally accepted among stress researchers that people who are in an endangered situation may be more likely to report physical complaints and symptoms than other people. There is some evidence that this may also play a role in the aftermath of an ecological disaster. Exposed persons may be more focused on their health and more likely to attribute health problems to the exposure (Havenaar & van den Brink, 1997; Roht et al., 1985). In these cases, people who suffer from physical diseases such as cancer or nonspecific "psychosomatic" complaints, which are apparently unrelated to the exposure, attribute their ill-health to the exposure. Similarly, people who believe they are entitled to financial compensations (e.g., because their houses or land have lost their value because of real or feared contamination) may be biased in their response. Even though terms such as "accident neurosis" or "compensation neurosis" never have been completely accepted in psychiatry, as opposed to widely accepted and well-researched clinical syndromes such as post-traumatic stress or somatoform disorders, the role of compensation in causing or maintaining these conditions never has been ruled out sufficiently (Mayou, 1996).

Finally, the term "reporting bias" may also be applied to the preference some news agencies show for sensational and negative consequences of disasters. This is an area of social psychology, which has thus far received only anecdotal attention.

CAN THE PSYCHOLOGICAL AND SOCIETAL HEALTH EFFECTS OF ECOLOGICAL DISASTERS BE PREVENTED?

One the most important reasons for compiling this book is to learn from events in the past and to draw lessons for the future. In the post-traumatic stress and disaster literature in general there is an ongoing debate about the possibility of preventing psychotraumatic stress disorders and other disaster-related stress disorders by providing immediate psychological help (e.g., through critical incident stress debriefing [CISD] or related techniques) (Gist, Lubin, & Redburn, 1999). An increasing number of studies show that the effects of such interventions are probably limited (e.g., Conlon, Fahy, & Conroy, 1999; Rose, Brewin, Andrews, & Kirk, 1999). One study even showed that police officers, who received debriefing one week after a shooting incident, exhibited significantly more post-traumatic stress disorder symptomatology than nondebriefed subjects (Carlier, Voerman, & Gersons, 2000). In addition, a number of studies seem to indicate that seeking help for psychological problems is actually diminished immediately following disasters (Lebedev 1990; Yates, Axsom, Bickman, & Howe, 1989). Providing immediate psychological support is therefore probably not the most advantageous action to take in the aftermath of ecological disasters.

More promising, albeit not yet systematically studied, are attempts to establish an open communication with the public. In a number of examples described in this book miscommunications appear to have made things worse. Information attributes are known to be important mediators of risk perception and subsequent health outcomes (Prince-Emburry 1992; Prince-Emburry & Rooney 1987; Sjöberg 1998). One important question that arises in this respect is the optimal level of openness in light of the many uncertainties. After the Kyshtym incident in the southern Urals in 1957, where a supply of weapons-grade plutonium exploded, the authorities kept the incident secret until 1989. There is no information on whether this course of action was able to prevent psychological distress among the population at the time. It seems unlikely, because rumors about the event circulated for years before it was reported publicly (Monroe, 1992). After the Chernobyl accident the authorities at first attempted to apply the same policy, but later the policy of glasnost (openness) made it impossible to keep the lid on the event. Attempts to cover up the incident are believed to have backfired, as later official announcements about the consequences of the accident were met with deep-seated mistrust.

Keeping nuclear accidents a secret is, however, not limited to the former Soviet Union. This was especially true during the period of the cold war as information surrounding a country's nuclear activity was veiled with secrecy due to its military implications. In ways quite similar to the Soviet approach, in the United States the dumping of nuclear waste from military nuclear facilities into the Columbia River near Hanford, California, was denied for many years.

Whatever information policy is adopted health authorities, media, medical personnel, and advocacy groups each have their own sources of information and standards to judge its quality. It is an open question if it will be possible in future events to develop productive ways for these different groups to cooperate in spreading information in a way that is least pathogenic. One key element in the information network is the press. One may wonder if the press should develop behavioral codes to prevent or control the "bad news syndrome."

OUTLINE OF THE BOOK

In this book we have brought together accounts of some of the world's most infamous ecological disasters to date in order to integrate what is known about these events and learn from them. The book is organized into three sections. The first section will give an overview of the extent of the threat to our environment by chemical and other toxic releases and will describe a model for understanding the mechanisms underlying their psychological impact. The second section is a compilation of case studies describing the events as they unfolded, the key players involved, the affected population, and the interventions that were initiated to mitigate their consequences. These case reports originate from all over the world and include many of the major accidents that have occurred thus far. Most of these chapters center around results of research projects carried out in the aftermath of the event. The third section will bring together some of the lines initiated in the case studies on a more general level. What are the possibilities and pitfalls for research on ecological disasters, what do we know so far about the effects of interventions, and how should these disasters be approached from a public health point of view? Because, as we will see throughout the book, public concern plays such a major role in the chain of events following an accident, a chapter is included in this section describing the experiences of those who are in the epicenter of these catastrophes. Finally, the lessons learned from previous ecological disasters will be summed up, and an attempt will be made to place them into a wider context of understanding.

REFERENCES

Alexander, F. E., & Greaves, M. F. (1998). Ionising radiation and leukaemia potential risks: Review based on the workshop held during the 10th symposium on molecular biology of hematopoiesis and treatment of leukemia and lymphomas at Hamburg, Germany on 5 July 1997. *Leukemia, 12,* 1319–1323.

Berren, M. R., Beigel, A., & Ghertner, S. (1980). A typology for the classification of disasters. *Community Mental Health Journal, 16,* 103–111.

Bertazzi, P. A. (1989). Industrial disasters and epidemiology. A review of recent experiences. *Scandinavian Journal of Work Environmental Health, 15,* 85–100.

Bromet, E. J., & Havenaar, J. M. (2002). Recent perspectives on the Psychiatric epidemiology of disasters. In M. Maj (Ed.), *The changing social contexts of psychiatry.* London: John Wiley & Sons.

Carlier, I. V., Voerman, A. E., & Gersons, B. P. (2000). The influence of occupational debriefing on post-traumatic stress symptomatology in traumatized police officers. *British Journal of Medical Psychology, 73,* 87–98.

Castronovo, F. P. Jr. (1999). Teratogen update: Radiation and Chernobyl. *Teratology, 60,* 100–106.

Conlon, L., Fahy, T. J., & Conroy, R. (1999). PTSD in ambulant RTA victims: A randomized controlled trial of debriefing. *Journal of Psychosomatic Research, 46,* 37–44.

Davidson, L., & Baum, A. (1992). Research findings after a nuclear accident: Three Mile Island. In J. H. Gold (Ed.), *Clinical Practice Number 24, American Psychiatric Press, 14,* 231–245.

Dolk, H., & Nichols, R. (1999). Evaluation of the impact of Chernobyl on the prevalence of congenital anomalies in 16 regions of Europe. EUROCAT Working Group. *International Journal of Epidemiology, 28,* 941–948.

Elder, G. H., Shnahan, M. J., & Clipp, E. C. (1997). Linking combat and physical health: The legacy of World War II in men's lives. *American Journal of Psychiatry, 154,* 330–336.

European Commission. (1997). *European workshop on the impact of endocrine disruptors on human health and wildlife.* Report of the proceedings 2–4 December 1996. Report EUR 17549.

Gist, R., Lubin, B., & Redburn, B. G. (1999). Psychosocial, ecological and community perspectives on disaster response. In R. Gist & B. Lubin (Eds.), *Response to disaster. Psychosocial, community and ecological approaches* (pp. 1–24). Philadelphia: Brunner Mazel.

Green, B. L. (1991). Evaluating the effects of disaster. *Psychological Assessment, 3*(4), 538–546.

Havenaar, J. M., & van den Brink, W. (1997). Psychological factors affecting health after toxic disasters. *Clinical Psychology Review, 17,* 359–374.

Lebedev, I. A. (1990). A judgment on the incidence of mental disorders in the Chernobyl disaster area. *Aktualnye Voprosy Obshchei i Subebnoi sikhiatrii,* Moscow, 69–72.

Lee, K. A., Vaillant, G. E., Torrey, W. C., & Elder G. H. (1995). A 50-year prospective study of the psychological sequelae of World War II combat. *American Journal of Psychiatry, 152,* 516–522.

Matthes, R., Bernhardt, J. H., & Repacholi M. H. (Eds.). (1998). *Risk perception, risk communication and its application to EMF exposure.* Proceedings of the international seminar on risk perception, risk communication and its application to EMF exposure. International Commission on Non-Ionizing Radiation Protection. Vienna, Austria.

Mayou, R. (1996). Accident neurosis revisited. *British Journal of Psychiatry, 168,* 399–403.

Mays, C., Avetova, E., Murphy, M., & Allen P. (1998). The weeping cow: Impact of countermeasures on daily life in Chernobyl-contamiated areas. *Proceedings of the 1998 annual conference Risk Analysis: Opening the Process* IPSN. Paris.

McEwen, B. S. (2000). Allostasis and allostatic load: Implication for neuropsychopharmacology. *Neuropsychopharmacology,* (2), 108–124.

Monroe, S. D. (1992). Chelyabinsk: The evolution of disaster. *Post-Soviet Geography,* (3), 533–545.

Nemery, B., Fischler, B., Boogaerts, M., & Lison, D. (1999). Dioxins, Coca-Cola, and mass sociogenic illness in Belgium. *Lancet, 354,* 77.

Noji, E. K. (1997). The nature of disaster: General characteristics and public health effects. In Noji, E. K. (Ed.), *The public health consequences of disasters* (pp. 3–20). New York: Oxford University Press.

Petterson, J. S. (1988). Perception vs reality of radiological impact: The Goiânia model. *Nuclear News* (31), 84–90.

Prince-Embury, S. (1992). Information attributes as related to psychological symptoms and perceived control among information seekers in the aftermath of technological disaster. *Journal of Applied Social Psychology, 22,* 1148–1159.

Prince-Embury, S., & Rooney, J. F. (1997). Perception of control and faith in experts among residents in the vicinity of Three Mile Island. *Journal of Applied Social Psychology, 17,* 953–968.

Quarantelli, E. L. (1985). An assesment of conflicting views on mental health: The consequences of traumatic events. In C. R. Figley, (Ed.), *Trauma and its wake* (pp. 173–218). New York: Brunnel Mazzel.

Quarantelli, E. L. (1994). What is disaster? The need for clarification in definition and conceptualization in research. In B. J. Sowder (Ed.), *Disasters and mental health selected contemporay perspectives* (pp. 41–73). Rockville: NIMH.

Roht, L. H., Vernon, S. W., Weir, F. W., Pier, S. M., Sullivan, P., & Reed, L. J. (1985). Community exposure to hazardous waste disposal sites. Assessing reporting bias. *American Journal of Epidemiology, 125,* 418–433.

Rose, S., Brewin, C. R., Andrews, B., & Kirk, M. (1999). A randomized controlled trial of individual psychological debriefing for victims of violent crime. *Psychological Medicine, 29,* 793–799.

Rubonis, A. V., & Bickman, L. (1991). Psychological impairment in the wake of disaster: The disaster-psychopathology relationship. *Psychological Bulletin, 109,* 384–399.

Rumyantseva, G. M., Drottz-Sjöberg, B-M., Allen, P. T., Arkhangelskaya, H. V., Nyagu, A. I., Ageeva, L. A. et al. (1995). The influence of social and psychological factors in the management of contaminated territories. In A. Karaoglou, G. Desmet, G. N. Kelly, & H. G. Menzel (Eds.), *The radiological consequences of the Chernobyl accident. Proceedings of the first international conference.* Minsk, Belarus, Luxembourg: Office for Official Publications of the European Communities.

Salzer, M. S., & Bickman, L. (1999). The short- and long-term psychological impact of disasters: Implications for mental health intervention and policy. In R. Gist, B. Lubin (Eds.), *Response to disaster. Psychosocial and ecological approaches* (pp. 63–82). New York: Brunner Mazel.

Shigematsu, I. (1991). The International Chernobyl Project. An overview. Assessment of the radiological consequences and evaluation of protective measures. Report by an international advisory committee. International Atomic Energy Agency. Vienna 1991.

Sjöberg, L. (1998). Worry and risk perception. *Risk Analysis, 18,* 85–93.

van den Eynde, J., & Veno, A. (1999). Coping with disastrous events: An empowerment model of community healing. In R. Gist & B. Lubin (Eds.), *Response to disaster. Psychosocial, community and ecological approaches* (pp. 167–190). Philadelphia: Brunner Mazel.

Watson, D., & Pennebaker, J. W. (1989). Health complaints, stress, and distress: Exploring the central role of negative affectivity. *Psychological Review, 96,* 234–254.

WHO (1995). Health consequences of the Chernobyl accident: Results of the IPHECA pilot projects and related national programmes. Geneva: author.

WHO (1999). *Overview of the environment in Europe in the 1990s.* Geneva: Author.

Yates, S., Axsom, D., Bickman, L., & Howe, G. (1989). Factors influencing help seeking for mental health problems after disasters. In R. Gist & B. Lubin (Eds.), *Psychosocial aspects of disaster* (pp. 163–189). New York: Wiley.

2

Public Health Aspects of Chemical Catastrophes

PETER J. BAXTER

The manufacture and distribution of chemicals by pipeline, water, rail, or road are inevitably associated with the risk of occupational and environmental exposure to toxic substances. Minor chemical incidents, such as accidents during road transport or fires involving chemicals, are not uncommon and on the whole are well dealt with by emergency services in most advanced industrialized societies. Any morbidity and mortality associated with these events is usually quite small. In contrast, a series of industrial disasters in the 1970s and early 1980s led to new legislation and international initiatives to prevent wide-scale chemical and radiological releases. The world's worst chemical disaster occurred in Bhopal, India, in 1984, a year that also saw the explosion of a liquid petroleum gas plant in Mexico City when over 500 people died. The fire in the Chernobyl reactor in 1986 was the worst incident in the history of the nuclear industry. In recent years higher awareness and tighter controls have been effective in preventing recurrences elsewhere of these extreme kinds of events.

Releases of chemical and radioactive substances outside the workplace, if large enough, can result in major incidents and even in what may be described as disasters. It is necessary to distinguish the two, as the term

PETER J. BAXTER • University of Cambridge Clinical School, Addenbrooke's Hospital, Cambridge CB2 2QQ, England.

Toxic Turmoil: Psychological and Societal Consequences of Ecological Disasters, edited by Johan M. Havenaar, Julie Cwikel, and Evelyn J. Bromet. New York, Kluwer Academic/Plenum Publishers, 2002.

disaster has many different connotations. It is not only a matter of semantics, as the planning and response measures to mitigate the different scales of these types of events are different. Over the past 30 years substantial interest has developed in our understanding of the impacts of natural disasters, and similar approaches have been applied to technological disasters over about the same time period. Indeed, the public health consequences of natural and technological disasters should be viewed from a multihazard perspective—for example, an earthquake may damage a chemical plant, or floodwaters may contain waste chemicals. An all-embracing definition of disaster applicable to the health sector (Noji, 1997) has gained acceptance:

> A disaster is the result of a vast ecological breakdown in the relation between humans and their environment, a serious and sudden event (or slow, as in drought) on such a scale that the stricken community needs extraordinary efforts to cope with it, often with outside help or international aid.

Under this definition there is a qualitative difference between a disaster and a major incident, and not necessarily a distinction based on numbers of casualties, for example. The key aspect of a disaster is a breakdown of the normal functioning of a society, so that reliance cannot be placed on the usual responses by emergency services or individuals to deal with the crisis. Disasters are characterized by a state of chaos to some degree or other, as well as the actual or perceived threat of death or injury. In a major incident, on the other hand, the emergency services can cope by rapidly extending what they are routinely doing. A good example is the emergency planning for major incidents in UK National Health Service (NHS) hospital services— the local hospitals respond by bringing in off-duty staff to cope with a sudden influx of casualties from a train crash or highway accident, but there is no actual failure of transport, communications, or the hospitals themselves:

> Major incident planning is the special mobilisation and organisation of NHS emergency services for the rescue and transport of large numbers of casualties and to cater for the threat of death or serious injury or homelessness to a large number of people. (Department of Health, 1998)

In a disaster such as an earthquake or flood the widespread destruction of structures and infrastructural links (e.g., transport and communications) can occur, so that planning should focus on responding to chaotic events. Doctors and nurses should be aware that this may even include field triage and treatment that are more akin to military medicine than what they learn in conventional training. Clearly, a disaster under this definition can be much more psychologically and physically traumatizing for larger numbers of people than a major incident, yet planning for disaster is still mistakenly regarded by many as merely an extension of major incident planning. Disaster medicine is a specialty in its own right (de Boer & Dubouloz, 2000; Lumley, Ryan, Baxter, & Kirby, 1996).

Until the last decade of the 20th century there were few systematic attempts anywhere to monitor the overall numbers of chemical incidents and evaluate their public health impacts. Between 1970 and 1998, 87 large-scale chemical incidents were recorded in the United States, with a total of 372 deaths, which is around the average figure for deaths in the United States from natural disasters (Lillibridge, 1997; Noji, 1997). In the United Kingdom over the same period there were 9 incidents and 167 deaths (IPCS, 1999). Worldwide during this 28-year period there were 350 such incidents involving 13,000 deaths, with tens of thousands more affected (Lillibridge, 1997). This is not a large mortality in comparison with other preventable causes of premature death, but the political, psychological, and social consequences of the disaster-scale events extend far wider than tolls of dead and injured. Thus at the Seveso incident in Italy in 1976, there were no serious casualties at the time of the chemical release, but the realization that up to 30,000 people living around the factory and their home environments had been contaminated by dioxin, the most toxic synthetic substance known, was in itself a reason for it to be classified a disaster, as the long-term effects on health were suspected to include adverse reproductive outcomes and cancer.

Much better information is needed on the incidence of chemical incidents and their public health impacts. In Europe a population-based surveillance system has been established in Wales, and a surveillance system in the United States has existed since 1990. In Wales in 1993–1995 there were 402 identified incidents with potential for exposure in 200,000 members of the public. The incidents involved smoke, organic chemicals, and toxic and flammable gases. Most strikingly, the involvement of health authorities, and therefore skilled health professionals, in the management of incidents arose only in less than 10% of those recorded (Bowen et al., 2000).

In this chapter the nature of chemical disasters and their potential for psychological and societal consequences will be outlined with reference to actual examples. A more complete review of chemical disasters is available elsewhere (Baxter, 1990), as is a detailed account of the clinical effects of exposure from chemical releases (Baxter, Adams, Aw, Cockroft, & Harrington, 2000). Gas bursts from deep lakes and hydrothermal systems in volcanic areas are a unique cause of disaster involving carbon dioxide (Baxter, 1997).

MEDICAL CONSEQUENCES OF CHEMICAL DISASTERS

Chemical releases are usually thought of as accidental escapes of chemicals into the air from a factory in a populated area, when exposure is by inhalation and possibly skin contact. The escape of a gas stored under pressure at a chemical plant, such as chlorine or hydrogen fluoride, is a prime example. Certainly most major chemical incident legislation and planning is directed toward such events, but some of the worst disasters have occurred from chemicals contaminating food or water, or beverages, when ingestion is the main route of exposure. Food poisoning can be of acute onset, within minutes or hours, just as with infectious causes, and the two causes can be impossible to distinguish clinically. But chronic exposure through ingestion can be the most insidious in that it can continue undetected until large numbers of people are exposed and develop catastrophic illness. The existence of a *latent period* between ingestion of the chemical and the development of the illness may last several months, during which large sectors of the population can continue to be exposed unaware that there is a health risk. An analogous example of an infectious disease agent is the prion disease bovine spongiform encephalopathy (BSE), which has a latent period of years and is transmitted in meat.

As already indicated, chemical disasters have special features that require quite specific consideration by emergency planners and responders. Very similar principles apply whatever the exposure route. *Exposure* to a chemical or mixture of chemicals may or may not result in immediate illness requiring the treatment of large numbers of people—in fact, there may be no casualties at the scene at all. Concern over the long-term effects of the exposure may be the most important consideration if there are no acute consequences. Any body organ system may suffer acute or long-term toxic insult capable of inducing a range of disease processes depending upon the agent involved, but fear of cancer and adverse reproductive outcomes may easily dominate the list of health concerns. *Evacuation* from the area of a toxic release contaminating the air or ground is usually a prime consideration, and a decision on this by the emergency services may need to be made immediately after a release has occurred or while it is occurring, as in a chemical fire that may burn for hours or days. Unfortunately, the information needed on which to base evacuation decisions may be missing or not available in the time frame, such as the level of exposure or contamination that may have occurred, or sufficient knowledge on the toxicology and human effects of the substance or substances involved. Even worse, the chemical or mixture of chemicals may not be readily identified at the time or even following intensive investigations after the event. When the identity of the chemical is known the amount of information available on its acute and chronic human health effects may be insufficient on which to base recommendations on the risk of exposure, even if the numbers of people exposed and the level of exposure can actually be ascertained. This is because for the vast majority of the 80,000 chemicals in regular commercial usage there are insufficient data on the hazards they present to human health. *Health risk assessment* may therefore have to be taken to decide on evacuation at the time of the incident without the officials being able to fully evaluate the risk, and even after the event it may be impossible to predict the longer-term health consequences. *Treatment* is symptomatic in the vast majority of chemical exposures: There are less than a dozen types of chemicals for which specific chemical antidotes are available.

INCIDENT INVESTIGATION

The only way to reduce the scientific uncertainties involved in major chemical incidents is to ensure that a multidisciplinary team with the necessary skills is part of the emergency response, so that health effects and exposure data are collected as soon as possible during or after the event. Epidemiological methods should form the basis of the investigation (Ackerman, Baxter, Bertazzi, Campbell, & Kryzanowski, 1997). A frequent source of renewed anxiety is the reassurances officials normally give when they are faced by the media, only to find subsequently that they may have misjudged the response of the community or the severity of the incident. The public can then lose trust in officialdom, when a disaster of a different kind arises as the emergency ceases to be manageable. This is often the outcome if an incident investigation is delayed or has to be set up under political pressure, where it may be too late to obtain the necessary exposure measurements or clinical data.

Chemical incidents, therefore, provide fertile ground for *toxic turmoil,* the title of this book, and the potential for profound psychological and societal responses in the face of uncertainties over exposure and health risks.

CHEMICAL SYNDROMES

As well as the known clinico-pathological effects of specific chemicals encountered in occupational settings, certain nonspecific symptomatology may arise as the focus of a known or suspected incident. These symptom complexes can also arise in the course of daily living or working in individuals who perceive they may have been exposed to a chemical and be suffering from its effects. Owing to the lack of specificity of the symptoms and the absence of evidence of harm according to clinical tests, it may be very difficult if not impossible for investigators to determine the attribution of the health complaints. These syndromes are:

- Multiple chemical sensitivity
- Nonspecific syndromes
- Mass hysteria or "copycat"

Multiple chemical sensitivity is a condition in which exposure to chemicals can initiate in certain individuals a clinical response to subsequent exposures to very low doses of that chemical and structurally unrelated chemicals. There is no objective evidence for this response, and the condition does not fit established disease processes. Various psychological and physical theories have been propounded by the syndrome's advocates, but no experimental evidence for these has been forthcoming (Graveling, Pilkington, George, Butler, & Tannahill, 1999).

Many occupational and environmental health hazards present as an increased reporting of *nonspecific syndromes* such as headache, backache, eye and respiratory irritation, tiredness, memory problems, and poor concentration (Spurgeon, Gompertz, & Harrington, 1996). Examples include sick building syndrome, exposure to electromagnetic fields and organophosphates, and recovery from acute and chronic gas exposures. A syndrome in this category arose at Camelford, Cornwall, in 1988, when the water supply to the community of 20,000 people became accidentally overloaded with aluminium sulphate at the supply plant. The outbreak of symptoms of fatigue, skin rashes, gastrointestinal problems, and joint pains immediately after the event was ascribed to drinking the water, and in some people anxiety/depression and memory and concentration problems persisted. Two separate government inquiries failed to confirm a toxic illness. Possibly the outcome would have been very different if the initial reassurances had been based upon actual evidence from a rapid field investigation. Wessely (Chapter 6, this volume) has reported in this volume on a comparable syndrome in Gulf War veterans.

Mass psychogenic or sociogenic illness, or mass hysteria, are terms given to acute outbreaks of so-called chemical illness, which is eventually shown to have no basis in chemical exposure. Hyperventilation, syncope, and rashes may feature strongly in the clinical presentation. The "condition" is of psychological origin and is spread in a copycat way. The detection of an unusual odor has sometimes preceded the onset of symptoms, where there is likely to be a background of stress. Newspaper and radio reports may facilitate the spread. An example is the Arjenyattah epidemic on the West Bank in March and April 1983, which took the form of 949 cases of acute nonfatal illness consisting of headache, dizziness, blurred vision, abdominal pain, myalgia, and fainting. There was a marked preponderance of female patients, particularly adolescent girls, but few older adults. All the clinical and biochemical tests were normal. The illness had possibly been triggered by the smell of hydrogen sulphide from a latrine (Landrigan & Miller, 1983). A similar outbreak was reported at a school in Georgia, in the United States in 1988, when the parents reported symptoms in their children that they thought were attributable to natural gas leaks at the school. The epidemic was stemmed by conducting a thorough investigation and taking the complaints seriously from the outset (Philen, McKinley, Kilbourne, & Parish, 1989). A full investigation was performed at a school in Tennessee in 1995 after the rapid spread of symptoms through a school after a teacher became ill in class (Jones et al., 2000). Unfortunately, the confirmation of the diagnosis can never be made with certainty and will not necessarily be well received by those affected and their families.

ROUTES OF EXPOSURE

Acute Chemical Incidents Involving Water, Food, and Drink

Acute poisoning caused by accidental chemical contamination of food and drink has been commonplace, particularly in developing countries. At one end of the scale disused chemical drums can be used to store household food and drink before they have been adequately decontaminated, or indiscriminate use of pesticides can easily lead to household food becoming tainted (Chaudry, Lall, Baijayantimala, Dhawan, 1998). At the other end of the scale, the international transport of foodstuffs can lead to inadvertent contamination in ship's holds or in trucks. Flour has been the medium for exposure in some notable incidents, a famous example being the Epping jaundice incident in England in 1965. An outbreak of 84 cases of jaundice occurred weeks after bread had been consumed from a bakery that had taken delivery of a sack of flour that had been in contact with methylene dianiline in a delivery van (Kopelman, Robertson, & Sanders, 1966). The deliberate addition of chemicals as adulterants has been widely practiced around the world. One of the most interesting has been the use of triorthocresylphosphate (TOCP) for the purpose in extending edible oils during times of food shortages (a clear oily liquid that is used by industry as a lubricant and hydraulic fluid). It was also used in the production of illicit liquor during the time of prohibition in the United States in the 1930s. It produces a characteristic outbreak of polyneuropathy with a characeristic inability to raise the hand or foot (wrist and foot drop). Epidemics have occurred at some time in every country of the world, including England during the Second World War. The latent period before the onset of symptoms is 3–28 days, so it is usually easy to identify the dietary source (Senayake & Jeyeratnam, 1981). An extraordinary epidemic of cardiomyopathy in Quebec in 1965–1966 was eventually tracked down to a cobalt additive that had been legitimately added in the production of beer (Morin, Foley, Martineau, & Roussel, 1967).

Chronic Incidents Involving Food

The cause of the acute outbreaks of poisoning can usually be identified with the appropriate medical detective work, even when they present as mysterious cardiac, hepatic, or neurological illnesses. Disastrous epidemics of toxic disease have occurred when the latent period was months, or exposure was long term and insidious. In these types of incidents the disease was not initially perceived as due to a chemical cause, and intensive investigation was required to identify the source of the problem.

Minamata disease is a classic example of this type of chemical outbreak that can have devastating consequences to the individuals and communities involved. In the 1960s and 1970s the disease became a symbol for the environmental movement in Japan and a warning to Western industrial countries of the perils of pollution. It stood for a state of lost innocence in Japan as expressed by Ishimuro Michiko (1990) in her book on the fishermen of Minamata Bay, *Paradise in the Sea of Sorrow:* " The characters are . . . also projections of ourselves in the past, that is, manifestations of our ancestors who believed in, and acted according to, certain values and a way of life that we have long lost" (Michiko, 1990, p. 373).

In 1956 the first cases of the disease appeared in poor fishermen and their families who lived almost solely on a diet of fish. They had moved to live in Minamata Bay from outer islands after the Second World War and their problem was largely ignored by the local citizens who were unwittingly eating the contaminated fish but were more protected by their better diet. Initially the disease was thought to be of an infectious origin, and only 3 years later did suspicion fall on mercury as the causal agent—when neurologists realized that the manifestations were the same as organic mercury poisoning that has as its main manifestations speech disturbance, unsteady gait and coordination, and blindness. Investigations eventually showed that the local chemical factory was discharging mercury into the bay. It was not until 1968 that a fishing ban was introduced and the bay was eventually dredged of contaminated mud over a 10-year period ending in 1987. Over 2,000 persons developed Minamata disease (2,252 were eventually officially recognized) and 28 individuals were born with cerebral palsy due to the organic mercury exposure of their mothers. The extensive lesions in the brain in adults and infants were irreversible (Tsubaki & Irukayama, 1977). The settlement of the claims of the victims has only happened in recent years.

The latent period of Minamata disease was probably over 10 years, but in another outbreak of methyl mercury poisoning in Iraq in 1971–1972 the latency was only 32 days with a maximum of 3 months. This was probably the largest outbreak of its kind ever, though official figures limited the number of deaths to 459, and there were 6,530 hospital admissions (Al-Tikriti & Al-Mufti, 1976). The victims and their families had run short of food and decided to eat bread made from the imported seed grain treated with methyl mercury as a fungicide. They had washed the grain of its warning marker dye and fed trial amounts to chickens, which did not show signs of acute intoxication. Legislation has eliminated this form of seed treatment in the European Community.

Another very characteristic disease of chemical contamination is yusho, or "oil disease," which first occurred in epidemic form affecting about 10,000 people in Japan in 1968 (Kuratsane, 1996; Kuratsane, Yoshimura, Matsazuka, & Yamaguchi, 1972). The main manifestation was the sudden onset of severe chloracne, a condition not unlike teenage acne of the face but severer and all over the body. Once again, there was considerable diagnostic confusion at the outset, with slowness to appreciate the epidemic nature of the affected patients, even though some had reported that they believed the rice oil was responsible. An unusual chemical was eventually identified in fat biopsies that was also present in the oil, a polychlorinated biphenyl used as an inert liquid in heat exchange equipment in the plant that manufactured the oil. A defect in a pipe had led to the cross-contamination. The average latency period was around 70 days. A more or less identical outbreak, referred to as yucheng, occurred in central Taiwan in 1979 when 2,000 people were affected. Yusho and yucheng victims developed abnormalities in liver function, and concerns arose over the possible risk of later developing liver cancer. In the Taiwan epidemic, developmental abnormalities were identified in the offspring of some of the mothers exposed to the contaminated oil (Rogan et al., 1988).

These incidents should not be viewed as isolated events. Organic mercury incidents have occurred on a smaller scale in Japan and in other countries. The risks of consuming fish contaminated by organic mercury or PCBs has become a worldwide public health issue. Mercury and PCB contamination of fish is especially prevalent in the Great Lakes region of the United States and Canada. Other incidents of contamination of the food chain by PCBs have occurred (Drotman, Baxter, Liddle, Brokopp & Skinner, 1983), despite discontinuation of the manufacture of PCBs in the 1970s, the last publicized one being in Belgium in 1999 (Bernard et al., 1999). In the latter, the pattern of the polychlorodibenzofurans and polychlorodibenzodioxins found in contaminated foodstuffs and poultry products was the same as that in the contaminated rice oil in the yusho epidemic. Within weeks in Belgium an outbreak of mass sociogenic illness, which was linked to the consumption of "contaminated" Coca-Cola, occurred on a background of the dioxin scare (Nemery, Fischler, Boogaerts, & Lison, 1999). These events led to a political crisis in Belgium and the resignation of two government ministers.

The last great chemical, food-borne epidemic was the toxic oil syndrome in Spain in 1981 (WHO, 1992). There was an explosive outbreak of what appeared to be an atypical pneumonia in Madrid and provinces northwest of Madrid, with 11,000 acute hospital admissions, which at the height of the outbreak were running at 600 per day. Over 20,000 cases and 330 deaths were reported. An infectious agent was at first believed to be the cause, but clinical and laboratory investigations were all negative. As the outbreak of pneumonia began to wane, a more sinister chronic disease eventually began to develop in 30% of those who had recovered from the pneumonia. This was a previously unrecognized syndrome of peripheral neuropathy, muscle damage, and collagen disease-like manifestations such as dry eye syndrome and scleroderma. An ascending type of nerve and muscle paralysis led to deaths in some hospitalized victims. Clinicians treating the patients began to identify a common dietary link, first in the children affected, which led to the identification of rape-seed oil sold on the streets as the vehicle of a possible chemical contaminant. Investigations showed that rape-seed oil was widely sold on streets as a cheap substitute for olive oil, and on this occasion had been illicitly refined from an industrial type of rape-seed oil containing aniline as a chemical marker. The disease became chronic and debilitating in survivors.

However, a follow-up study covering the years 1981–1994 did not find a raised mortality in this group compared to the general Spanish population (Borda et al., 1998). Changes in food safety legislation were passed in Spain as a result of this tragedy. The chemical contaminants responsible for the toxic oil syndrome have never been satisfactorily identified. A curious sequel was the sudden emergence of patients with an identical syndrome in the United States in 1989, with numerous additional cases reported in several other countries worldwide. This disease was called eosinophilic myalgia syndrome and was caused by the consumption of an over-the-counter medication containing contaminated L-trytophan, an amino acid (Martin et al., 1990). Despite the realization that the two conditions could have a common chemical cause, no likely candidate among the contaminants has been identified. An additional problem has been the absence of an animal model for the syndromes that could be used to confirm experimentally the etiological basis for the outbreaks.

Airborne Releases

Two notable industrial accidents resulting in the airborne release of chemicals into populated areas have occurred on a disaster scale. At Seveso, Italy, on July 10, 1976, a chemical cloud containing dioxin (TCDD, 2,3,7,8—tetrachlorodibenzodioxin) was released as a result of an accident in a plant manufacturing 245-trichlorophenol. Dioxin is the most toxic synthetic substance known, a suspected human teratogen, and is now a recognized human carcinogen. The chemical was produced in an exothermic reaction that went out of control, but its presence as a contaminant in the normal industrial process was already well known before the accident. Nevertheless, the seriousness of the release went unrecognized until July 17, when the presence of dioxin was suspected and then confirmed on July 23. The contaminated areas were not evacuated until July 26, despite earlier evidence of birds, animals, and vegetation dying there. About 700 people were rapidly evacuated. That significant exposure had occurred in this incident was eventually confirmed in 1988 when laboratory tests of serum collected from residents in Zone A, the worst affected area, showed the highest levels of dioxin ever recorded in human studies (Landi et al., 1997).

The only acute clinical finding was chloracne in 187 children who were exposed by playing outside at the time the chemical cloud passed over. Epidemiological studies were set up in 1979 to establish the long-term health risk of the exposure, given the worldwide concerns over the health effects of dioxin pollution. To date there is some evidence for slight increases in cancer deaths, which could be related to the exposure; a slight increase in mortality from ischemic heart disease is also present (Bertazzi, Bernucci, Brambilla, Consonni & Pesatori, 1998). It will be yet some years of follow-up before the full consequences of this incident can be assessed, but it had a profound impact on legislation, especially in the form of the EC Seveso Directive, and the chemical industry worldwide.

Another factory accident with an impact far wider than the country in which it occurred was the world's worst industrial disaster at Bhopal, India, in 1984 (see Chapter 7, this volume). About 40 tons of the highly irritant gas methyl isocyanate flowed in a cloud over the city of Bhopal in the early hours of December 3. About 4,000 people died from the acute effects of inhaling the gas, with over 100,000 others affected. Long-term lung damage (persistent small airways obstruction) has been confirmed as one of the sequelae in many of the survivors (Cullinan, Acquilla, & Ramana, 1997). The U.S.-based Union Carbide plant used methyl isocyanate to manufacture carbaryl pesticides. Information on the human health effects of this chemical was virtually nonexistent before this incident. This event illustrated well the potential hazard for populations around plants storing highly toxic gases such as chlorine, ammonia, phosgene, and so forth. Even in low concentration many of these gases can cause death and serious acute lung injury for great distances downwind (Baxter, Davies, & Murray, 1989). Fortunately, major accidental releases of these gases have been rare. Legislation now applies in all major industrialized countries during manufacture, storage, and shipping to ensure that such major hazards are controlled.

Fires

An early example of a chemical fire occurred in a mercury mine in Austria in 1804 when mercury vapor escaped into the air and spread over the countryside: 900 people in the vacinity developed signs of mercury poisoning, such as mercurial tremor, and many cows suffered from salivation, cachexia, and spontaneous abortion. Generally speaking, releases of chemicals from fixed installations or from containment during their distribution last for a duration of minutes rather than hours. Toxic incidents lasting days or weeks can, however, arise from fires. In the Gulf War in February 1991 about 600 naturally pressurized oil wells were set afire in Kuwait. They were not extinguished until the following November, during which time concern developed over the potential health consequences of the chemical particle fall out, but none were confirmed. Formidable fires can occur from the combustion of stored plastic PVC. These fires may take days to put out, and the plumes contain irritant gases, combustion products, and dioxin (Baxter, Heap, Rowland, & Murray, 1995). The combustion of tire dumps can last for weeks, and the smoke plumes present hazards to populations downwind. Planned evacuation of nearby populations as a precautionary measure has to be a consideration in the management of such crises.

Hazardous Waste

Public awareness of the environmental consequences of indiscriminate use and disposal of chemicals began with the publication of Rachel Carson's book *Silent Spring* in 1962. A decade later public health departments in heavily industrialized parts of the United States became inundated with reports of ill-health effects from people living near sites of toxic waste disposal—legal and illegal. Chemicals include persistent organic pollutants (POPs) such as PCBs, dioxins, and the pesticides DDT and dieldrin, as well as chlorinated solvents. Two notable sites were Love Canal, New York State, and Woburn, Massachusetts. Love Canal had been a waste disposal site used for municipal and chemical waste for 30 years since 1953, but homes were built over the site during the 1960s and leachates began to be detected in the late 1960s. A limited follow-up of residents identified low birthweight in the offspring of Love Canal residents (Vianna & Polan, 1984), but no causal link for other diseases including cancer. Investigations at these and other sites have documented a variety of symptoms of ill-health in exposed persons, such as headache, fatigue, and neurobehavioral problems (Miller, 1996). The psychological and social consequences of these incidents may outweigh the toxic effects of chemical exposure. Billions of dollars have been spent in the United States managing these sites under the Superfund program, the total number of which may exceed 400,000 sites. Hazardous waste, including the cleanup of disused industrial sites, is now a well-recognized problem throughout the world.

Terrorism

Sarin, an organophosphorous compound developed as a nerve gas after the Second World War, was used in a terrorist attack on the Tokyo subway on March 20, 1995. The planned release caused 12 deaths and more than 5,000 people were hospitalized (Okumura et al., 1996). The same agent had been used in an incident in a residential area in the city of Matsumoto in 1994, when 7 people died and about 600 residents and rescue staff were poisoned (Morita et al., 1995). These incidents in Japan have led to a new worldwide awareness of the threat of planned chemical and biological releases by terrorist groups.

EVACUATION INCIDENTS

An overview of the public health impact of chemical incidents should not overlook those types of events where major evacuations occur without a major chemical release, or widespread death and injury, occurring. At Bhopal, up to half a million people temporarily self-evacuated from the city as a result of the acute episode, but two weeks later during the official deactivation of chemicals on the plant, a quarter of the population of the city of around a million self-evacuated. A large-scale official evacuation was ordered following a train derailment and a fire in a tanker car containing 90 tons of chlorine at Mississauga, Canada, on November 10, 1979. Within 24 hours, 90% of the population at risk had obliged—about 220,000 people—without death or injury. Three hospitals and a nursing home were included (Zelinskey & Kosinski, 1992). Rapid evacuation of such a large number of people to relative safety is impressive, but it may not necessarily be possible in congested cities in other parts of the world.

EPIDEMICS SUSPECTED OF HAVING A CHEMICAL ORIGIN

In any unusual outbreak of disease a chemical cause should be considered at the outset. Delays in investigating potential routes of exposure, such as water and beverages, fish, edible oil, flour, and dairy products, may result in the cause never being found, as in the toxic oil syndrome in Spain. Fortunately, such events today seem to have become a rarity. However, an outbreak of neurological disease affecting 45,000 people in Cuba in 1992–1993 appeared to have the hallmarks of a food-borne chemical epidemic, though subsequent investigation ruled this out. Affected patients showed bilateral optic neuropathy or a distal predominantly sensory neuropathy sometimes associated with deafness, or a combination of both optic and peripheral sensory neuropathy. The illness was probably related to a nutritional deficiency, itself brought about in a society under ecological stress in the presence of chronic food shortages (Cuba Neuropathy Field Investigation Team, 1995).

Indeed, a very substantial proportion of the cases were psychogenic on a background of social stress (Thomas, Plant, Baxter, Bates, & Santiago Luis, 1995).

In 2000 an outbreak of paralysis in children in the Dominican Republic was at first attributed to pesticide poisoning, but it was found to be polio from a mutant form of a live virus from the oral polio vaccine (polio was previously thought to have been eradicated from this country) (Clarke, 2001). The mysterious emergence of the prion disease BSE in the United Kingdom is another example of an infectious disease manifesting as a chronic neurological condition.

PSYCHOLOGICAL AND SOCIETAL IMPACTS

Some authors (e.g., Bertazzi, 1989) have identified specific causes of stress in communities and individuals following a major chemical incident:

1. *Acute Stress Reaction.* Acute exposure to a toxic gas can induce terror, especially if it starts to affect breathing. Asthma sufferers in particular may fear they are dying. Posttraumatic stress disorder may be a consequence of gassing or inhalation accidents. In a major incident, fear may be compounded by having to evacuate from homes at short notice.

2. *Uncertainty about Long-Term Effects.* After taking stock of any immediate health reactions in a chemical disaster, the long-term effects of most concern to the general population are cancer and birth defects. Medical scientists will also be anxious about other effects on organ systems that may come to light when the toxicological knowledge base for most substances in industrial usage is so limited. The setting up of epidemiological studies to investigate the health effects of accidental exposures is usually an essential consideration, especially if as is hoped the population can be eventually assured that their fears are ungrounded.

3. *Housing and Job Security.* The Seveso incident was an example where an area became temporarily uninhabitable because of the concerns over ground contamination, as dioxin is extremely resistant to degradation. House values in the affected area might fall following a major incident as a result of the publicity and fears of future accidents. Interestingly, concerns that planning measures around major hazard sites, as required in the Seveso Directive, including involvement of local communities in emergency response, would result in declines in property values were unfounded in the United Kingdom.

4. *Media Siege.* The attention of the media after a major incident may reinforce negative aspects of the event and add to concerns over who is to blame and the long-term risks of exposure. Scientists from many different backgrounds will be consulted for their opinions, some of these

unfortunately will play up to the worst fears of exposure to substances such as dioxin, as occurred after a plastics fire (Baxter et al., 1995). Relatively few pundits temper their views with the appropriate caution and awareness of the alarm they can cause, which may be more devastating to the individual and his or her family than the effects of the chemical exposure. As with many environmental hazards, society has to come to terms with scientific uncertainty and appreciate that no one can ever give complete reassurance over risk. Increasingly governments and officials accept the need for a precautionary approach when giving opinions rather than issuing bland assurances that are then contradicted by independent "experts."

5. *Social Rejection.* Stigma may be attached to survivors. Certain major incidents can arouse the same fears of having been tainted as has marked the survivors of the atomic bomb explosions (the "hibakusha") in Japan in the Second World War, who feared to register for medical support. They worry that their children will not get married because of widespread and unfounded fears that the effects of radiation may be passed on to future generations. Young female victims in the yusho incident found it difficult to find marriage partners for similar reasons. The poor are frequently at the brunt of chemical disasters, as was the case in the toxic oil syndrome, and they may be blamed or their concerns ignored by other strata of society.

6. *Cultural Pressures.* Women pregnant at the time of the exposure in a major incident will have particular concerns about any risk to reproductive outcome. In the Seveso incident no clear guidance could be given, but many women sought abortions anyway, in conflict with Italian and Roman Catholic religious beliefs.

7. *Inadequate Medical Follow-up and Compensation.* Inadequate treatment and delay in compensation are continuing to dog the lives of survivors of the Bhopal incident. Critics state that there has been no systematic attempt to document the medical and social consequences of the disaster. Disasters can undoubtedly bring the latent tensions of a society to the surface. At Bhopal, the eruption of these forces sustained a chronic disaster making the recovery and rehabilitation of the half a million people involved near impossible (Rajan, 1999). Delays and arguments over settling litigation issues present additional difficulties.

DISASTER MITIGATION AND HEALTH-RISK ASSESSMENT

Disaster management should address the four main phases of disasters: planning, preparedness, emergency response, and rehabilitation. The health sector is a key partner in what is a multisector activity at national and local levels. The official involvement of health professionals in chemical emergency planning has been only recent (OECD, 1994), despite legislative requirements for on-site and off-site planning in the European Community since the Seveso Directive came into force in 1984. Public health and hospital preparedness for dealing with the casualties of mass chemical incidents has also lagged well behind, including the management of mental health aspects, which in many incidents may be the only related health effects. The key to limiting the health consequences of chemical incidents and preventing them becoming disasters is adequate planning and the rapid response in an actual event. Recently in the United Kingdom rapid health sector responses were able to successfully establish the health risk in two major oil tanker spills—the *Braer* in Shetland (Campbell, Cox, Crum, Foster, & Riley, 1994) and the *Sea Empress* off the Pembrokeshire coast in Wales (Lyons, Temple, Evans, Fone, & Palmer, 1999).

The adequate measurement of exposure in a community in major chemical incidents is hardly ever achieved (the Braer incident is an exception), and this is a continuing limitation of the health-risk assessment. The other serious limitation is the inadequate knowledge of the toxicity of chemicals, especially their long-term consequences. The best example is dioxin. Even before the Seveso incident in 1976, the extreme toxicity and the persistence of the chemical in the environment, as well as previous industrial accidents involving the substance, have led to debate over its carcinogenic risk to humans. Few chemicals have engendered over recent decades as much political and public controversy as dioxin. The issue was not resolved until 1997, when a working group for the International Agency for Research on Cancer (IARC), sifting all the animal, laboratory, and human evidence, concluded that it was a human carcinogen. Even so, it appears to be atypical in causing an increased risk of all cancers combined and not at a specific site such as the liver (Hoover, 1999). And controversy continues on the risk at very low-level exposures for informing the regulatory process and for advising on individual exposures. Dioxin is not unique in presenting these uncertainties—it is just one of the best publicized. Failure to adequately manage and communicate risk and scientific uncertainty is a common and potent cause of psychosocial stress in chemical disasters.

REFERENCES

Ackerman, U., Baxter, P., Bertazzi, P. A., Campbell, D., & Kryzanowski, M. (Eds.). (1997). *Assessing the health consequences of major chemical incidents—Epidemiological processes.* Copenhagen: WHO.

Al-Tikriti, K., & Al-Mufti, A. W. (1976). An outbreak of organomercury poisoning among Iraqui farmers. *Bulletin WHO, 53 (suppl.),* 23–36.

Baxter, P. J. (1990). Review of major chemical accidents and their medical management. In V. Murray (Ed.), *Major chemical disasters—Medical aspects of management* (pp. 7–20). London: Royal Society of Medicine.

Baxter, P. J. (1997). Volcanoes. In E. K. Noji (Ed.), *The public health consequences of disaster* (pp. 179–204). New York: Oxford University Press.

Baxter, P. J., Davies, P. C., & Murray, V. (1989). Medical planning for toxic releases into the community: The example of chlorine gas. *British Journal of Industrial Medicine, 46,* 277–285.

Baxter, P. J., Heap, B. J., Rowland, M. G. M., & Murray, V. S. G. (1995). Thetford plastics fire, October 1991: The role of a preventive medical team in chemical incidents. *Occupational & Environmental Medicine,* 694–698.

Baxter, P. J., Adams, P. H., Aw, T.-C., Cockroft, A., & Harrington, J. M. (Eds.). (2000). *Hunter's diseases of occupations.* 9th ed. London: Arnold.

Bernard, A., Hermans, C., Broeckhaert, F., De Poorter, G., De Cock, A., & Houins, G. (1999). Food contamination by PCB's and dioxins. *Nature, 401,* 231–232.

Bertazzi, P. A. (1989). Industrial disasters and epidemiology. *Scandinavian Journal of Work Environment Health, 15,* 85–100.

Bertazzi, P. A., Bernucci, I., Brambilla, G., Consonni, D., & Pesatori, A. C. (1998). The Seveso studies on early and long-term effects of dioxin exposure: A review. *Environmental Health Perspectives, 106,* 625–633.

Borda, I. A., Philen, R. M., Posada de la Paz, M., Gomez de la Camera, A., Ruiz-Navarro, M. D., Ribota, O. G. et al. (1998). Toxic oil syndrome mortality: The first 13 years. *International Journal of Epidemiology, 27,* 1057–1063.

Bowen, H., Palmer, S. R., Fielder, H. M. P., Coleman, G., Routledge, P. A., & Fone, D. L. (2000). Community exposures to chemical incidents: Development and evaluation of the first environmental public health surveillance system in Europe. *Journal of Epidemiology & Community Health, 54,* 870–873.

Campbell, D., Cox, D., Crum, J., Foster, K., & Riley, A. (1994). Late effects of grounding of tanker Braer on health in Shetland. *British Medical Journal, 309,* 773–774.

Carson, R. (1962). *Silent spring.* New York: Houghton Mifflin.

Chaudry, R., Lall, S. B., Baijayantimala, M., & Dhawan, B. (1998). A foodborne outbreak of organophosphate poisoning. *British Medical Journal, 317,* 268–269.

Clarke, T. (2001). Polio's last stand. *Nature, 409,* 278–280.

Cuba Neuropathy Field Investigation Team. (1995). Epidemic neuropathy in Cuba—Clinical characterisation and risk factors. *New England Journal of Medicine, 333,* 1176–1182.

Cullinan, P., Acquilla, S., & Ramana, D. V. (1997). Respiratory morbidity 10 years after the Union Carbide gas leak at Bhopal: A cross-sectional survey. *British Medical Journal, 314,* 338–342.

de Boer, J., & Dubouloz, M. Handbook of disaster medicine. (1998). Utrecht: van der Wees. 2000.

Department of Health (1998). *Planning for Major Incidents.* London: Department of Health.

Drotman, D. P., Baxter, P. J., Liddle, J. A., Brokopp, C. D., & Skinner, M. D. (1983). Contamination of the food chain by polychlorinated biphenyls from a broken transformer. *American Journal of Public Health, 73:* 290–292.

Graveling, R. A., Pilkington, A., George, J. P. K., Butler, M. P., & Tannahill, S. N. (1999). A review of multiple chemical sensitivity. *Occupational & Environmental Medicine, 56,* 73–85.

Hoover, R. N. (1999). Dioxin dilemmas. *Journal of the National Cancer Institute, 91,* 745–746.

International Programme on Chemical Safety (IPCS). (1999). *Public health and chemical incidents.* Cardiff: International Clearing House for Chemical Incidents.

Jones, T. F., Craig, A. S., Hoy, D., Gunter, E. W., Ashley, D. L., Barr, D. B. et al. (2000). Mass psychogenic illness attributed to toxic exposure at a high school. *New England Journal of Medicine, 342,* 96–130.

Kopelman, H., Robertson, M. H., & Sanders, P. G. (1966). The Epping jaundice. *British Medical Journal, 1,* 514–516.

Kuratsane, M. (1996). *Yusho: A human disaster caused by PCBs and related compounds.* Fukuoka: Kyushu University Press.

Kuratsane, M., Yoshimura, T., Matsazuka, J., & Yamaguchi, A. (1972). Epidemiological study on yusho, a poisoning caused by ingestion of rice oil contaminated with a commercial brand of polychlorinated biphenyls. *Environmental Health Perspecives, 1,* 119–28.

Landi, M. T., Needham, L. L., Lucier, G., Mocarelli, P., Bertazzi, P. A., & Caporaso, N. (1997). Concentrations of dioxin 20 years after Seveso. *Lancet, 349,* 1811.

Landrigan, P. J., & Miller, B. (1983). The Arjenyattah epidemic. *Lancet 2,* 1474–1476.

Lillibridge, S. R. (1997). Industrial disasters. In E. K. Noji (Ed.), *The public health consequences of disasters* (pp. 354–372). New York: Oxford University Press.

Lumley, J. S. P., Ryan, J. M., Baxter, P. J., & Kirby, N. (1996). *Handbook of the medical care of catatrophes.* London: Royal Society of Medicine.

Lyons, R. A., Temple, J. M., Evans, D., Fone, D. L., & Palmer, S. R. (1999). Acute health effects of the Sea Empress oil spill. *Journal of Epidemiology & Community Health, 53,* 306–310.

Martin, R. W., Duffy, J., Engel, A. G., Lie, J. T., Bowles, C. A., Moyer, T. P. et al. (1990). The clinical spectrum of the eosinophilia myalgia syndrome associated with L-trytophan ingestion. Clinical features in 20 patients and aspects of pathophysiology. *Annals of International Medecine, 113,* 124–134.

Michiko, I. (1990). *Paradise in the sea of sorrow.* Kyoto: Yamaguchi.

Miller, A. B. (1996). Evaluation of risks associated with hazardous waste. In R. Bertollini, M. D. Lebowitz, R. Saracci, & D. A. Savitz (Eds.), *Environmental epidemiology* (pp. 49–62). Boca Raton, FL: CRC Press.

Morin, Y. L., Foley, A. R., Martineau, G., & Roussel, J. (1967). Quebec beer-drinkers' cardiomyopathy: Forty eight cases. *Canadian Medical Association Journal, 97,* 881–883.

Morita, H., Yanagisawa, N., Nakajima, T., Shimizu, M., Hirabayashi, H., Okudera et al. (1995). Sarin poisoning in Matsumoto, Japan. *Lancet, 346,* 290–293.

Nemery, B., Fischler, B., Boogaerts, M., & Lison, D. (1999). Dioxins, Coca Cola, and mass sociogenic illness in Belgium. *Lancet, 354,* 77.

Noji, E. K. (1997). The nature of disaster: General characteristics and public health effects. In E. K. Noji, (Ed.), *The public health consequences of disasters* (pp. 3–20) . New York: Oxford University Press.

Okumura, T., Takasu, N., Ishimatsu, S., Miyanoki, S., Mitsuhashi, A., Kumada, K. et al. (1996). Report on 640 victims of the Tokyo subway Sarin attack. *Annals of Emergency Medicine, 28*(2), 129–135.

Organisation for Economic Cooperation and Development (OECD). (1994). *Health aspects of chemical accidents.* Paris: Author.

Philen, R. M., McKinley, T. W., Kilbourne, E. M., & Parish, R. G. (1989). Mass sociogenic illness by proxy: Parentally reported epidemic in an elementary school. *Lancet, 2,* 1372–1376.

Rogan, W. J., Gladen, B. C., Hung, K-L., Koong S. L., Taylor, J. S., Wu, Y. C. et al. (1988). Congenital poisoning by polychlorinated biphenyls and their contaminants in Taiwan. *Science, 241,* 334–336.

Senayake, N., & Jeyaratnam, J. (1981). Toxic polyneuropathy due to gingli oil contaminated with tri-cresyl phosphate affecting adolescent girls in Sri Lanka. *Lancet, 1,* 88–89.

Spurgeon, A., Gompertz, D., & Harrington, J. M. (1996). Modifiers of non-specific symptoms in occupational and environmental syndromes. *Occupational & Environmental Medicine, 53,* 361–366.

Thomas, P. K., Plant, G. T., Baxter, P., Bates, C., & Santiago Luis, R. (1995). An epidemic of optic neuropathy and painful sensory neuropathy in Cuba: Clinical aspects. *Journal of Neurology, 242*, 629–638.

Tsubaki, T., & Irukayama, K. (Eds.). (1977). *Minamata disease.* Amsterdam: Elsevier.

Vianna N. J., & Polan, A. K. (1984). Incidence of low birth weight among Love Canal residents. *Science, 226,* 1217–1219.

World Health Organization. (1992). *Toxic oil syndrome: Current knowledge and future perspectives.* Copenhagen: World Health Organization.

Zelinsky, W., & Kosinski, L. A. (1992). *The emergency evacuation of cities.* Lanham, MD: Rowman & Littlefield.

3

Understanding the Psychological and Societal Response of Individuals, Groups, Authorities, and Media to Toxic Hazards

JULIE G. CWIKEL, JOHAN M. HAVENAAR,
and EVELYN J. BROMET

INTRODUCTION

Ecological disasters are breaches of public safety and environmental security caused by natural or human processes due to ignorance, accident, mismanagement, or design. Despite the apparent increase in ecological disasters in recent decades, environmental breaches have been recorded as far back as antiquity. The earliest recorded example occurred in Mesopotamia over four thousand years ago when agricultural lands were damaged from inadequate drainage systems, which led to high levels of salt in the soil

JULIE G. CWIKEL • Department of Social Work and Center for Women's Health Studies and Promotion, Ben Gurion University of the Negev, Beer Sheva, Israel. JOHAN M. HAVENAAR • University Medical Center and Altrecht Institute for Mental Health Care, The Netherlands. EVELYN J. BROMET • Department of Psychiatry and Behavioral Science State University of New York at Stony Brook, New York 11794-8790.

Toxic Turmoil: Psychological and Societal Consequences of Ecological Disasters, edited by Johan M. Havenaar, Julie G. Cwikel, and Evelyn J. Bromet. New York, Kluwer Academic/Plenum Publishers, 2002.

(*Environmental Disasters*, 1998). Some ecological disasters, such as nuclear power plant accidents, oil spills, or industrial accidents occur suddenly. Others develop insidiously, as occurred in Minimata, Japan, when mercury from industry waste contaminated fish consumed by local residents. The ecological erosion in the area around the Aral Sea represents another example of "creeping environmental disaster" (see Chapter 9). Yet another example of chronic environmental damage with disastrous proportions was caused by massive burning of forests, in the Borneo and Sumatra slash and burn fires in 1997–1998 (*Environmental Disasters*, 1998).

As the world becomes more crowded, more heavily industrialized, and more energy needy, it seems inevitable that more ecological disasters will happen. Chapter 2 and each chapter in Part II of this book describes in detail recent sentinel ecological events out of the many hundreds of ecological incidents and disasters. The importance of these disasters is being recognized increasingly, both by the public and by policymakers. Some of these disasters became a focal point for the development of new protective policy and awareness of the importance of assessing these types of hazards. For example, following the Seveso and Bhopal accidents, countries across Europe classified hundreds of sites that produce or store potentially toxic materials as high-risk or "Seveso" sites, meaning that extra precautions are required. The aims of the Seveso Directives include prevention of environmental accidents and limiting their damage to affected populations and the environment in the future (Wettig & Faure, 1999).

The health effects of exposure following industrial disasters can vary along two major axes: a biological axis and psychological axis. This chapter focuses on the latter. In many cases interactions occur between the biological and psychological, or stress-related health effects. The disaster literature shows that the greater the physical damage and loss of human lives, the more likely the psychological toll will be high as well (Rubonis & Bickman, 1991). Also some psychological manifestations, such as depression, may be accompanied by biological changes such as changes in eating and sleeping patterns. Finally, exposure to certain compounds such as organophosphates and other pesticides may cause neurological damage that may present primarily with psychological symptoms (Bazylewicz-Walczak, Majczakowa, & Szymczak, 1999; Mearns, Dunn, & Lees-Haley, 1994).

While the numbers of dead, injured, or hospitalized can be counted, the psychological and social sequelae are harder to quantify—there is no universal unit for indicating the amount of anxiety, depression, social disruption, or family hardship that these events produce. Despite the enormous psychological and social costs of these disasters, until recently there has been a tendency not to take into account this axis in assessing the adverse effects of these disasters. Today, with a greater understanding of how stress affects human health, we are able to trace some of the health effects of ecological disasters to acute and chronic psychological and physiological stress reactions.

STRESS-RELATED HEALTH EFFECTS OF ECOLOGICAL DISASTERS

The effects of disasters on mental health have been well documented (Bromet & Havenaar, 2002). Stress-reactions described after disasters typically include emotional manifestations of depression, grief, anxiety, Post-traumatic stress disorder (PTSD), and somatization, and behavioral expressions of stress, including changes in illness behavior, domestic violence, substance abuse, and problems in work or role functioning (Bromet & Dew, 1995; Havenaar & van den Brink, 1997). As noted above, it is only recently that the psychological component of the health effects of ecological disasters has been the subject of systematic research. In a pioneer qualitative study using in-depth interviews, the American psychiatrist Lifton (1967) described the psychological toll of the atomic bombs on Hiroshima survivors 17 years after the event. The first study of the psychological impact of disasters that used an epidemiologic approach was conducted after the 1979 accident in Three Mile Island. This study examined the psychological distress of a representative population sample living in the vicinity of the reactor as part of the overall evaluation of the impact of the accident (Bromet, Parkinson, Schulberg, Dunn, & Gondek, 1982). Following the Chernobyl accident in 1986, several mental health studies were conducted to assess psychological sequelae, such as PTSD. Some were initiated by researchers from outside the former Soviet Union (FSU), for example, studies led by Dutch, French, and Finnish teams (Havenaar, Rumyantseva et al., 1997; Viel et al., 1997; Viinamaki et al., 1995). Local research groups, who had started in the early 1990s to incorporate PTSD and other psychiatric symptom scales into their research, conducted other studies. Despite considerable variation in the classification systems and in the methods of assessment used in various countries and cultures (Yevelson, Abdelgani, Cwikel, & Yevelson, 1997), the common core of findings clearly indicates the size and importance of the stress-related health consequences of this ecological disaster (Lee, 1996).

Psychological effects following ecological disaster may be either a direct effect of exposure to the stressful event itself, for example, being a witness to the destruction caused to a pristine environment by an oil spill (see Chapter 12 for the distress reflected in personal accounts from eyewitnesses), or maybe a reaction to the countermeasures that were taken to combat the physical effects of the exposure. For example, people exposed to an ecological disaster may be advised to leave the area or may even relocate voluntarily, such has been the case for many Ukrainian and Belarussian citizens who migrated to Israel, the United States, and Europe after the Chernobyl disaster. The loss of social support and status that emigration entails may create other stressors, which could then lead to increased alcoholism, depression, or hypertension (Cwikel, Abdelgani, Goldsmith, Quastel, & Yevelson, 1997; Cwikel, Goldsmith, Kordysh, Quastel, & Abdelgani, 1997; Lerner, Mirsky, & Barasch, 1994).

One of the problems that arises in the psychiatric epidemiology of ecological disasters is the need to differentiate between physical consequences of exposure to toxic agents and the effects of stress. Physical health problems can be related to stress in at least three different ways. First, the stress response can manifest itself as physical complaints, for example, through the physical manifestations of anxiety and depression. Second, some indications can be found in the literature that stress related to ecological disasters can lead to physical morbidity, such as increased hypertension, reported cardiac problems, and adverse reproductive events (Cwikel, Goldsmith et al., 1997; Davidson & Baum, 1986; Pesatori et al., 1998). Such physical consequences may be either a direct result of the stressful experience by altering host neuroendocrine function, such as has been demonstrated in PTSD (Yehuda et al., 2000), and/or by an increase in health damaging behaviors such as substance abuse, family violence, and risk taking (Krieger, 2001).

In some cases it is not entirely clear whether observed outcomes are caused by physical effects of the exposures or by psychological effects (Cwikel, 1997). For example, a follow-up of the Seveso industrial accident in which dioxin or TCDD (2,3,7,8-tetrachlorodibenzodioxin) was released during production showed that those exposed had evidence of increased mortality from cardiopulmonary and endocrine diseases (Pesatori et al., 1998). The authors of this study commented that the findings could reflect either a biological response to exposure or an effect of stress. Indeed, many questions are yet unanswered about how toxic materials affect the body's stress response system, which then get expressed as symptoms similar to those that are directly attributable to the physical effects of exposure.

A third way health problems can be linked to the psychological impact of an ecological disaster is through changes in health perception following the disaster, and the attribution of previously existing or newly occurring yet unrelated health problems to the exposure. These are some of the most difficult problems for clinicians, families, and the public health community to assess and treat. For example, if a child develops leukemia in the years following an ecological disaster, the family may attribute this to the disaster, without having any scientific basis for this assumption.

The best way to assess the estimated burden of distress and disease specifically attributable to the exposure is to conduct epidemiological research that includes comparison populations that were not exposed to the toxic stressor. However, even when these research findings are available, individuals may still feel resentment and helplessness if their particular health problem has not received the adequate scientific and medical attention it deserves. While in a strict sense these health effects should be considered as spurious, they may at the same time be the most prominent ones. They may have considerable significance from a public health perspective, because they express the concern people have about their health as a result of the exposure to chemicals, radiation, or other harmful agents, a concern that will drive the demand for further investigations of interventions. Chapter 5 describes how such a situation occurred after an airplane crash that was thought to have toxic substances on board. The firmly established belief that the Chernobyl disaster caused widespread disease among the effected populations is another example.

In this chapter we present a social epidemiological model as an integrated framework for understanding the social and psychological impact of ecological disasters. Social epidemiology combines classical epidemiological concepts such as host-agent-environmental interactions with concepts from the behavioral sciences, such as coping, stress, and community resources, with those typically used in public health, such as risk assessment (Cwikel, 1994a, 1994b; Krieger, 2001, p. 696). This model is presented with an emphasis on what makes ecological disasters particularly distressing (Havenaar & van den Brink, 1997). Two other theoretical approaches are discussed that can be applied in conjunction with the social epidemiological framework. One, the conservation of resources model (Hobfoll, 1988) describes the stressfulness of an event in objective terms that help to predict which individuals are likely to develop psychological distress. The other, the amplification of risk model (Kasperson et al., 1988), provides concepts that can facilitate our understanding of the role of information and risk communication in these events. After these models have been discussed in relation to ecological disasters, an example will be provided on the basis of the experience of the first author who used a social epidemiological approach in a health care program for immigrants to Israel from areas affected by the Chernobyl disaster.

THE SOCIAL EPIDEMIOLOGICAL MODEL FOR UNDERSTANDING HEALTH EFFECTS OF ECOLOGICAL DISASTERS

The hallmark of the social epidemiological model is its multifactorial approach to understanding the health effects due to noxious environmental agents. The model incorporates social and psychological considerations into what was formerly a strictly biomedical approach to public health. The conceptual and research tools draw on methods from behavioral science, such as ethnography, focus groups, and qualitative research, and those from classical epidemiology, such as accident investigation, toxicology, and physical measurements of health. The social epidemiological model uses the classical epidemiological triangle of *agent, host, and environment factors* as its central organizing principle for data collection and intervention design (Last, 1995; Mausner & Bahn, 1974). For the conceptualization of the psychological response to toxic exposure at the level of the individual, the stress paradigm is used, either alone or in conjunction with more recent theoretical formulations from stress research (Hobfoll, 1989, 1998; Lazarus & Folkman, 1984). These concepts are particularly useful to understand the psychological response of the host (see below). Other useful concepts, which may help us to understand public reactions at the societal level, may be found in the risk perception and risk communication literature and are reviewed below in the section on "Amplification and Risk" (Kasperson et al., 1988; Slovic, 1987).

Host, agent, and environmental factors can interact in complicated patterns codetermining health outcomes. Figure 3.1 shows the complex interplay among these factors. The elements in the schema may interact over all the phases of a disaster situation, including the immediate warning stage (if indeed such a stage exists), the immediate postimpact stage, and the

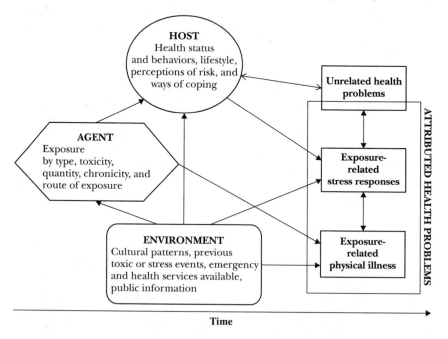

Figure 3.1. A Social Epidemiological Schema for the Interaction between Social and Individual Responses to Ecological Disasters.

long-term follow-up stage. Components in the schema, such as information, knowledge, and community sentiments may evolve over time and interact.

Host or environmental factors that increase the risk or probability of psychological distress or other types of morbidity are called *risk factors*. For example, the presence of an underlying chronic illness or recent personal loss can increase the vulnerability of the host. Some risk factors, such age or ethnic background, are immutable descriptors, while others, such as attitudes, behaviors, or public policy, can be modified over time due to circumstance or from a public health intervention.

Host or environmental factors that decrease the likelihood of an adverse health effect are called *protective factors*. For example, the presence of health services or trained emergency personnel or other societal resources can significantly moderate how the agent is diffused in the physical environment and among population groups. Protective factors that decrease the vulnerability or increase the host's resistance to the noxious agent may include education, supportive social networks, the accumulation of community resources and health services, and prior, positive coping experiences.

The range of data collection methods mentioned to evaluate community concern in relation to potential health risks and available resources is described in Chapter 13. The social epidemiological approach combines a direct evaluation of the debilitating aspects of the environmental disaster with an assessment of the available protective resources at the personal and community levels. It is therefore primarily a pragmatic, action-oriented approach that guides the actions of health care authorities and other actors confronted with this type of disaster. Once relevant data are collected, the approach lends itself to the development of appropriate public health policies, programs, and interventions. For example, the European Commission initiated project ETHOS in 1996 to help improve the quality of life among residents of Belarus (in the Brest region) contaminated by the Chernobyl accident. Using an interdisciplinary team (e.g., experts on radiation protection, economics, agronomy, industrial safety, sociology, and risk management), and working with the local inhabitants, the project integrated social and technological aspects of environmental rehabilitation. An emphasis was placed at working through the mistrust that local residents had for scientists and government officials to improve communication (Dubreuil et al., 1999).

AGENT FACTORS

The agent is defined as the noxious environmental exposure. It may vary by type, quantity, level of toxicity, and duration of exposure. In ecological disasters, the agent can be a chemical substance such as lead, dioxin, mercury, ionizing radiation, or an infectious organism. In some cases an agent will only become toxic after interaction with another agent in the environment (e.g., in a reaction with oxygen during an explosion or uncontrolled fire). In the social epidemiological model, the actual physical presence of a toxic agent in significant quantity is neither a necessary nor a sufficient etiological factor. It is not sufficient because in any given population, not all persons exposed develop an illness even if the substance is present in significant concentrations. Neither is it a necessary factor because distress can develop even in the absence of personal exposure of the host to the toxic agent. From a psychological or societal point of view, it is rather the information about the presence of an agent and the credibility of that presence that act as the pathogenic factors. Stress-related health effects can occur if a potentially harmful agent is believed to be there, or, to paraphrase the sociologist W. I. Thomas, if a situation is believed to be real, it is real in its consequences (1966).

There are a number of agent characteristics that make them particularly liable to be perceived as psychologically stressful. Toxic exposure, particularly radiation, is associated in the public mind with cancer, neurological damage, and congenital anomalies. These health effects may manifest themselves in the present or in the future, or even in a next generation, and may be subject to scientific controversy. The substances are perceived as being not controllable, confinable, discernible, or clearly measurable and thus very frightening.

Another factor determining the stressfulness of these events is that most exposure events are the result of human failure. Technological failures are seen as a result of human actions, a loss of control over something that is thought to be under control (Baum, Fleming, & Davidson, 1983). Often there is a public perception that a particular agency, a private or public body, should have been able to prevent or mitigate the damage of the ecological disaster. This is particularly important when early warning or protective systems fail to prevent the disaster and it explains community resentment and dissatisfaction that appears in the aftermath of most ecological disasters. As the disaster unfolds, the sense of lack of control may be further strengthened when the authorities appear unable to provide an adequate technological answer to the original technical failure. In terms of conservation of resource models (see below), this may be interpreted as a failure to adequately gain expected coping returns following significant resource investment. For example, following the Chernobyl disaster, there were many attempts to extinguish the fire that was burning inside the reactor. However, the cleanup phase was also hindered by technological failures. After initial attempts to use robots to clean the reactor roof of radioactive debris failed, human beings, cynically referred to as "robotniki" were deployed, with significant risk to these people. Still later attempts to contain the highly radioactive plant in a colossal concrete structure called the sarcophagus turned out to be partially unsuccessful as stories about leakage and corrosion started to appear within a few years after the event (Mould, 1988; Park, 1989).

HOST FACTORS

The host is defined as the person who has experienced exposure to a noxious agent. In classical epidemiology, which usually focuses primarily on the physical effects of exposure, important host factors that will affect the susceptibility of a person to toxic substances are sex, age, and pre-exposure health status. For example, young children are more likely to develop cancer after exposure to ionizing radiation than adults; smog mainly affects persons with pre-existing pulmonary problems (Ministry of Health, 1952; Stewart, 1997).

The Stress Paradigm

For understanding of the psychological response of individuals to these events, the stress paradigm is usually applied, using concepts such as stressor, appraisal, coping, and distress. One central concept to explain whether an exposure event will lead to psychological impairment or social disability in a given individual is *appraisal* (Lazarus & Folkman, 1984). Appraisal is the evaluation a person makes of a threat, weighed against his or her ability to cope with it. The perception of present and future risk in a disaster (i.e., a situation that exceeds a persons or a community's accumulated coping resources) is a central element in the production of psychological dysfunction, both as a short-term reaction and as a long-term health outcome. Appraisal can be conceptualized as taking place in two distinct phases, *primary appraisal,* when information is being assessed of the harmfulness of the event, and *secondary appraisal,* when a person tries to make a reasonable judgment about how to respond effectively to the exposure. The importance of appraisal, or the risk and hazard perception associated with an exposure, points to the importance of information in determining the outcomes of these disasters. Adequate information about the potential harmfulness of the exposure is often lacking, for example, whether the toxic substance released in the accident is only harmful if breathed or also after skin contact. In such situations, people also find it hard to judge how to protect themselves, their loved ones, and their community from this threat.

Another important host factor that will shape health outcomes is the process of *attribution.* Stress syndromes and other health problems that develop over time are frequently attributed to the exposure in situations involving toxic substances. Some unrelated health problems might for many reasons also be erroneously attributed to the exposure. For example, there can be misinformation about the health problems caused by an exposure, or there may be an exaggeration of the chance that such an effect is expected to occur. The possibility of compensation can also provoke some individuals to misattribute their health problems to the exposure. This is indicated in Figure 3.1 by the box that includes a portion of the unrelated health problems.

Perception of risk and attribution may be partly determined by other host factors, such as intelligence and education, and partly by environmental factors, such as the available information and the public perception of the event. Other important psychological host factors are coping styles. An example of how susceptibility to negative health outcomes can be influenced by coping and other risk-related behavior was given by Mays, Avetova, Murphy, and Allen (1998) who describe that a perceived inability to avoid exposure to radionuclides among certain inhabitants living in areas contaminated by Chernobyl led them to ignore advice to abstain from drinking milk from cows grazing in contaminated pastures or not to eat mushrooms from forests in these areas.

A Conservation of Resources Model of Stress

One of the shortcomings of the stress paradigm has been that it relies heavily on appraisal, which is an internal cognitive process largely independent of the agent (Hobfoll, 1989). To arrive at a more objective way to quantify the psychological impact of negative life events Hobfoll (1988) formulated the conservation of resources (COR) model. The COR is a stress-response model that describes how individuals and communities react over the short term and try to cope over the long haul with the stress following exposure to disasters (for an update see Hobfoll, 1998). In the recent past the model has been successfully applied to predict mental health consequences of both natural and environmental disasters (Arata, Picou, Johnson, & McNally, 2000; Hegstad, 2000; Smith & Freedy, 2000). The COR model stipulates that affected populations try to enhance and retain resources and build a resource reservoir to protect themselves and their loved ones against destructive and painful losses. According to this model, stress occurs when (1) resources are threatened with loss, (2) resources are actually lost, or (3) there is a failure to adequately gain resources following significant resource "investment" (Hobfoll, 1998, p. 55). Resources may be objects (e.g., house, land), personal characteristics (e.g., health, self-esteem, sense of mastery), conditions (e.g., spouse, job, friends), or energies (e.g., credits, money).

Ecological disasters seriously tax these resources for a number of obvious reasons. First, these disasters pose a serious threat to one's health, which is one of the most highly valued resources by most people (e.g., Arata et al., 2000). There may be actual health damage, however; in many of the examples given in this book, the threat is future oriented and has not yet materialized. The widespread anxiety that the attacks with anthrax have caused demonstrates this point. Despite the fact that the yearly death toll by influenza, car accidents, or hand guns each exceeds by far the risk from these sinister envelopes, the perceived threat they pose to future health and well-being is undoubtedly far greater in the eyes of most people than these more commonplace health hazards.

Ecological events also have a profound effect on people's sense of mastery. Many of the health impacts of ecological disasters are uncertain and beyond one's control. They may affect the entire community, and in the worst-case scenario endanger human existence itself, illustrating the profound threat to human resources these disasters represent. Other tangible resources that may be adversely affected by ecological disasters have been mentioned by Bertazzi (1989) (and mentioned in Chapter 2, this volume). They include housing and job insecurity, which arise as areas are being evacuated, plants are shut down, or products from contaminated regions are no longer valued in the market place. After the Exxon *Valdez* oil spill, resource-loss variables (e.g., selling off possessions, deterioration in health and personal relations, changes at work) accounted for between 30–39% of the variance in symptoms of anxiety, PTSD, and depression among fishermen from the affected area (Arata et al., 2000).

ENVIRONMENTAL FACTORS

Whether a susceptible host will become ill as a result of exposure to a harmful agent further depends on the presence of environmental factors that either facilitate or hinder the agent. Some physical conditions may prevent the transmission of the agent, while others can interact with the agent to cause more deaths or injuries. For example, the weather conditions, the location, and the timing of the Bhopal disaster interacted with the methyl isocyanate gas that was released. At the time of the accident, weather conditions caused an atmospheric inversion of the chemical cloud that stayed close to the ground instead of dissipating. Also behavioral factors played a role in creating an environment where so many casualties could occur. The release occurred at night and because most people were fast asleep at the time the poisonous vapors were allowed to creep through residential neighborhoods unnoticed and killed thousands of people (Lillibridge, 1997).

The way society at large responds to a disaster can either be instrumental in helping affected individuals and communities to respond in an effective way to meet their psychological needs, or the controversies and conflicts in a community can be so virulent that they impede the organization and delivery of mental health services. Freudenberg (1997) coined the term "corrosive community" to describe this situation, which is quite typical for the aftermath of an ecological disaster. Chapter 5 on how the community of Amsterdam coped with 1992 Bijlmer plane crash shows how difficult it can be to meet the information and psychological needs of an affected community in the case of uncertainty about the toxicity of the event, even in the presence of adequate community resources. The expressed need for a "caring government" can be felt so deeply, that the lack of this can lead to statements to the extent that "governmental mismanagement can make us sick" (Boin, van Duin, & Heyse, 2001).

Since typically some health services are already functioning, the first step after a disaster is to designate one central information center and additional centers, clinics, or telephone lines as available for those needing help to cope with the disaster. The assumption is that at least some professionals have previously received training in risk communication, crisis intervention, and short-term therapy protocols in disaster situations. One of the most important skills required is to be able to interface with existing nonclinical community services, including churches, community agencies such as teacher-parent groups, the Red Cross, local lay leaders who are well recognized and respected, and other informal social networks. This is because most people affected by disaster situations are more likely to represent a normal-functioning community-dwelling population and not a cluster of persons at high risk for adverse mental health outcomes. A project designed to offer crisis counseling following the Mississippi River flood readied a large group of mental health professionals only to find that most of the affected population preferred to go to nonmental health personnel such as clergy and police officers for advice (North & Hong, 2000).

From a societal point of view public information is probably the single most important factor influencing the stress response. It will be discussed in more detail below. Public information is the result of a complex interaction, partly guided by planned communications by authorities and experts, and partly by media and informal networks. Cultural patterns and other contextual factors (e.g., the question whether the exposure occurred as a result of a willful act as during a war or terrorist attack or as a result of neglect during peace time) may have a strong impact on the public evaluation of an event and therefore may act as important modifiers of a the stress response. Previous toxic or stress events may also color public opinion.

Finally, the availability of emergency and health services to susceptible or affected hosts can have a critical effect on health status. Unfortunately, populations with inadequate access to health care services are more likely to be located closer to sites with possible environmental hazards (Soliman, Derosa, Mielke, & Bota, 1993). Ecological disasters often strike hardest among populations who have the lowest levels of accumulated coping resources such as education, political connections, and professional training, both in underdeveloped countries and among socially disadvantaged communities in developed countries. In these countries basic infrastructure in emergency services, health, and communication can be so lacking that all the effort aimed at helping the affected population has to be created ad hoc (compare with Chapters 7 and 13).

IDENTIFYING HIGH-RISK GROUPS

One of the important elements of using the social epidemiological model is that it may help to identify high-risk groups for psychological health effects. High-risk groups may include specific age groups or combinations of host factors (e.g., older persons living alone), occupational groups, and persons with concomitant morbidity. For example, older immigrants from around Chernobyl sustained psychological distress for longer periods than younger ones, which was expressed in increased somatic complaints (Cwikel & Rozovski, 1998). Usually in the immediate post-impact stage, mental health and research personnel try to target specific geographical areas and high-risk individuals where help is most needed. Epidemiological research may be initiated at this stage (see, for example, Chapter 7 in this volume on the Bhopal experience). The populations at risk, once identified using field observations by those involved in postdisaster management, may become the target of outreach efforts by the public health community. Cultural sensitivity at this initial stage is particularly important, not only to avoid alienating the affected populations, but more important, to ensure that clinically meaningful material is collected. Moreover, the opportunity to provide effective services may be lost if professionals fail to comprehend the survivors' perceptions of what makes the situation so stressful. Examples of this point of view can be found in Chapter 12, and Criterion 6 in Chapter 13 (both in this volume).

An important risk group is mothers with young children. Several risk factors are present among this group. First of all, the health of their children is often jeopardized in a very serious way. This is also true for unborn children. Prenatal exposure to ionizing radiation is harmful to the fetus, particularly during the 8–25–week window of gestation, increasing the risk of mental retardation (Shigematsu, Chikako, Kamada, Akiyama, & Sasaki, 1995). The disaster therefore represents the loss of one of the most valuable things a mother has, her child. Furthermore, women are more likely than men to have low status, low self-esteem, and a higher prevalence of mental health problems, particularly depression (Collins et al., 1999). The resources available to them to cope with the threat of ecological disaster are therefore fewer. Studies by Bromet and Shulberg (1986) of residents living in the vicinity of the TMI nuclear power plant in 1979, and by Havenaar, van den Brink, et. al. (1996) confirme the importance of this risk group. The mental health of mothers may have indirect effect on the health and well-being of their children because mothers may worry excessively over minor health problems they may have. Chapter 4 provides a detailed analysis of the mental health of mothers and children following two nuclear disasters.

A second risk group is evacuees. For example, residents of Pripyat, the company town on the edge of Chernobyl, who were evacuated and thereafter not allowed to return to their homes suffered significant losses not only of property but also of their familiar social environment. Havenaar, van den Brink, et. al. (1996) have shown that persons who had been evacuated from contaminated areas in Belarus to cleaner territories had a higher risk of developing a psychiatric disorder than other inhabitants from the same region.

A third high-risk group is persons with previous mental disorders. Several studies have shown that a personal history of psychopathology is a risk factor for poor mental health after a disaster (e.g., Bromet & Schulberg, 1986). However, findings in this area are not entirely consistent (for a review see Bromet & Havenaar, 2002). A related group of high-risk individuals consists of those who have had recent life events that entail loss (e.g., separation, divorce, unemployment) (Cwikel et al., 2000; Gerrity & Flynn, 1997; Sattler, Kaiser, & Hittner, 2000). For example, in the first author's study of immigrants to Israel from areas exposed to Chernobyl 8 years after the accident, she found that those who reported stressful life events, such as marital discord or illness in the family, in addition to exposure, had additive stress effects. The highest stress groups were those with both Chernobyl exposure and reported stressful life events (Cwikel et al., 2000).

THE ROLE OF PUBLIC INFORMATION

In the description of the social epidemiological model, the central position of risk perception is evident. The degree to which a person will perceive an event as stressful depends upon how it is being appraised in light of the resources a person has to cope with the event (Lazarus & Folkman, 1984). An example of this is provided in the first author's study of the long-term psychological functioning of immigrants to Israel exposed to the Chernobyl. In this study she examined the influence of a retrospective cognitive assessment of the negative impact of the Chernobyl disaster on psychological distress. The questionnaire included items such as "the events caused serious difficulties to close family members" and "I thought it might harm me or my family sometime in the future," which combined elements of primary and secondary appraisal. This negative retrospective assessment was found to be a major determinant of long-term psychological stress reactions (Cwikel et al., 2000). Similar results were reported by Bromet and Litcher among mothers affected by both TMI and Chernobyl (Chapter 4 in this volume). They found that perceptions of perceived risk (the accident affected their health and the health of their children) predicted increases in anxiety scores 10–11 years following the disasters, irrespective of the actual health impact of the disaster. In another study, by Havenaar, de Wilde, van den Bout, Drottz-Sjöberg, and van de Brink (in press) it was shown that risk perception plays an important role as a mediating factor in explaining differences in subjective health between a population exposed to the Chernobyl disaster and an unexposed population. These studies support the hypothesis, also voiced by Yzermans and Gersons in Chapter 5, that public information management is one of the key factors in mitigating population stress reactions.

However, as will be apparent in several chapters throughout the book, it is not a simple task to communicate information about an event involving risk, particularly in ecological disasters affecting large numbers of people.

Amplification of Risk

The literature on the "perception of risk" (Slovic, 1987) provides a conceptual framework within which the differential appraisal of the risks of events or technologies by different members of society may be understood. Kasperson et al. (1988) use the term "social amplification of risk" to describe the situation where laymen judge the amount of risk ascribed to a certain hazard to be far greater than experts say it is. He uses a signal amplification metaphor to describe this phenomenon. Risks are primarily conveyed by risk messages. This situation is typical for ecological disasters where all but a few people who actually witnessed the exposure event know about it exclusively through official or informal risk messages.

Risk messages may contain factual, inferential, value-related, and symbolic meanings. The factual information refers to the content of the message (e.g., a radiation reading in the area of residence), while the inferential meaning relates to the conclusions that can be drawn from the presented evidence (e.g., the emission poses a serious health threat). Value-related and symbolic meanings are related to cultural values and symbols that may evoke specific images (e.g., "global terrorism," "Hiroshima," "the nuclear energy lobby," and so forth). There are several characteristics of the risk messages that will influence the way they will be communicated and whether amplification will occur. Some of these are: the volume of the information, the degree to which there is dispute about the contents of the message, and whether the messages carry strong symbolic connotations, like the ones mentioned above.

In the case of the Chernobyl disaster, initially, the "volume" of the messages was low. This seems to have kindled all kinds of rumors. In later stages the volume of the information grew to proportions larger then life: extensive media coverage with wide display of alleged victims suffering from leukemia, loss of hair, congenital malformation, without offering any proof that these were in fact caused by the Chernobyl disaster (van den Bout, Havenaar, & Meijler-Iljina, 1995). In an analysis of media coverage of the Love Canal and Three Mile Island incidents, Mazur (1981) argues that the massive quantity of media coverage not only reported the events but also defined and shaped the issues. Dispute about the factual information and its implications is also a very common feature as demonstrated, for example, by the ongoing debates about exposure of soldiers in the Gulf War to chemical or biological weapons (see Chapter 6 for a detailed account). The third factor, the extent to which the event activated symbolic and cultural heuristic schemes, is illustrated by a citation from a Ukrainian newspaper, quoted in Bertazzi's (1989) seminal article on ecological disasters, that symbolized the anxious premonitions that "Chernobyl" evoked in many people. According to the book of Revelation "Chernobila" (the Russian word used for the star 'Wormwood') fell after the third of seven angels had blown its trumpet as a warning against great plagues that will befall mankind (Revelation 8:10–11). The fact this citation emerges in a Russian newspaper and even in a scientific text demonstrates the mythical atmosphere and the sense of dread that surrounds the Chernobyl accident.

Another important concept that has emerged from risk-perception research is *signal value*. Signal value is a heuristic concept that describes the propensity of an event to induce a significant medical response or political response. It is based on the observation that the information value an event has is systematically related to the amount of hazard a certain event reflects. Events have a "high signal value" if they suggest that a new risk has appeared, or that the risk is different or more serious than previously understood. A good example of this is the recent anthrax threat. Even though the number of people killed is relatively low, it has been clear from the start that these deaths had a far greater significance than mortality from other, more common causes. The term signal value does not necessarily have a negative connotation; it implies that an event is taken very seriously and that action should be taken, such as the Seveso Directives, mentioned in the beginning of the chapter. The names of other incidents thought to herald future danger now have a certain ominous ring, e.g. names like Hiroshima, Bikini beach, Three Mile Island, Bhopal, Chernobyl, and now World Trade Center.

According to the signal value of an event, it will induce all kinds of social activities, which may be seen as secondary events, and secondary risk messages that will influence appraisal may in turn induce anxiety. In fact the anxiety expressed by the affected population may itself be interpreted as a secondary risk message, a "crying out" that something terrible has happened. The secondary risk messages carry the impact of the event further throughout society, "as ripples in a pond after a stone has been thrown in," to use Kasperson's metaphor (Kasperson et al., 1988).

The Role of Authorities and Media in Risk Communication Following Ecological Disasters

From the study of risk perception and risk communication in controversial environmental problems, the following findings have relevance (Aldrich, 2000; Allman, 1985; Fischhoff, Bostrom, & Quadrel, 1993; Havenaar & van den Brink, 1997; Levi, 1994):

- Lay persons and experts disagree about the health risks from any given toxic source such as radiation or toxic chemicals.
- Experts tend to base their opinions on mortality statistics that are often country- or state-wide, when data for small areas and specific population groups are more appropriate for environmental epidemiology and the public health surveillance required after ecological disasters.
- The nonscientific public is likely to formulate its assessment of risk on personal experience or shared stories or sensationalist media sources.
- Affected persons tend to think of all toxic substances as one group and do not differentiate by source and extent of exposure.

These observations emphasize that communicating to the lay public requires a thorough understanding of the scientific issues in order to be able to present them succinctly. This includes clear differentiation between types of toxic exposures and explanations about the knowledge base for the assumption of risk or lack of risk both in the general population and among high-risk groups (Goldman, Hedetniemi, Hebert, Sassaman, & Walker, 2000; Ng & Hamby, 1997). If, however, those in authority are perceived as not being reliable, having a political agenda, or presenting the interests of interested parties aside from the affected population, this will seriously undermine the effectiveness of risk communication. Once the public has lost its belief in the credibility of the source of information, it will be unlikely to trust others whom it associates with the same source (e.g., scientists working for the government or for industry) (Byrd, VanDerslice, & Peterson, 2001; Peters, 1996).

The literature provides several documented examples of failure in risk communication, the Chernobyl disaster with all its initial secrecy and later misinformation being the most well known. Chapter 5 by Yzermans and Gersons also provides a clear example. Churchill (1997) mentions two mistakes commonly made in many other disaster situations: (1) a failure to respond quickly with reliable and specific information—generally, the first 24 hours are considered the critical window, and (2) failure to designate a primary spokesperson who is credible and reassuring to the public.

Unfortunately to date, to the best of our knowledge, there are hardly any examples of successful risk communication following ecological disasters, let alone experimental or quasi-experimental studies to test the effectiveness of alternative communication styles. What is available is anecdotal or based on conventional wisdom acquired from either expert panels (e.g., Goldman et al., 2000), post hoc assessment from staff members from the Agency for Toxic Substances and Disease Registry (ATSDR) involved in risk communication (e.g., Tinker, Collins, King, & Hoover, 2000), accumulated expertise from analyzing communication problems in past disaster situations (e.g., Ng & Hamby, 1997), or social science expertise gained from simulation experiments and community assessments of how people perceive health risks (e.g., Fischhoff et al., 1993). In Chapter 9 in this volume on human service responses to toxic disaster, a creative example of developing special communication materials following the St. Basile-le-Grand incident is presented. However, like other initiatives reported, it lacks an empirical evaluation of its effectiveness in reducing anxiety and allaying misplaced fears. Outside the domain of ecological disaster reaction, yet probably relevant for this subject as well, comes communications in response to community concerns about biomedical research facilities. In this field there is a consensus among professionals that it is critical to involve community members in the design, implementation, and analysis of risk communication activities (Goldman et al., 2000; Ng & Hamby, 1997).

Ideally, following an ecological disaster, there should be a clear public body responsible for communication with the affected public, either the Environmental Protection Agency, the Ministry of Health, or some other governmental body. For example, during the Israeli Gulf War, the public was faced with the threat of SCUD missiles and biological warheads. The Israeli army spokesperson, Nachman Shai, appeared to be exceptionally good at transmitting reassuring information and advice over national television about stress management that helped the public cope with the stress of the war. Professionals who took part in stress management consultations during the Gulf War mentioned his calm demeanor repeatedly as a coping asset (Cwikel, Kacen, & Slonim-Nevo, 1993).

More often than not, however, there are multiple actors on the scene, each with their own political agenda. For example, when an ecological disaster happens at a privately owned factory, such as the Bhopal disaster in the Union Carbide plant, industry spokespersons are likely to be interested in limiting the liability of their employer rather than delivering concise, factual material. When a coalition of actors is involved in information delivery to the public, there is a greater likelihood that the public's right to know will be protected. The drawback of this situation is the emergence of contradictory information, as some of the case examples in the book will amply illustrate.

When many sectors are involved, it is critical to coordinate media contact and information release. When information is accurate and provides specific guidelines on how to avoid exposure and manage environmental hazards, this can decrease stress reactions. Unfortunately, too often authorities summarily dismiss or downplay the adverse health effects and delegitimize complaints from affected populations with the suggestion that they are trying to increase their chances of compensation.

The media can play a pivotal role in either providing responsible information on the situation or inflating rumors that increase anxiety. Churchill's chapter on "Effective Media Relations" in the book *The Public Health Consequences of Disasters* is highly recommended for the essentials of media communication. He states that "one must determine the primary target audience for every public health message to ensure that the message is crafted appropriately, timed for the greatest impact, and conveyed through the medium most likely to reach that audience" (1997, p. 124). Unfortunately our experience with disasters is that those involved have not taken his advice. As Havenaar and van den Brink state, "More often than not, media coverage tends to focus on information supporting the public fear that something terrible has happened and that the worst is yet to come" (1997, p. 360). Recently, fueled by the commotion anthrax has created, there have been a slew of articles, television debates, and features about what is right and wrong about the public information campaign.

The Role of Advocacy Groups

Over time, immediate news releases may give way to information released to the media by advocacy groups, self-help, and volunteer organizations or collaborations between concerned scientists and people within

58   JULIE G. CWIKEL ET AL.

the establishment and representatives of the exposed population. These groups are often very effective in making sure that the problems affecting the exposed population are not forgotten and taken off the public agenda.

For example, those people who may have been exposed to radiation released from the Hanford nuclear facility located in eastern Washington state from 1944 to 1972 formed a lobbying group called the Hanford Downwinders. They initially tried to interest the government in seriously monitoring their health effects and were met with disinterest. They then joined forces with physicians from the Oregon chapter of the Physicians for Social Responsibility, public health and environmental activists, and Native American tribal leaders from the exposed areas to form a public lobby. They then succeeded in activating the government into assessing the long-term impact of this exposure on the health of the affected population (Goldsmith et al., 1999). This group now runs the Hanford Health Information Archives, which contains medical records and information on the impact of the radiation exposure, the Hanford Health Information Network, and a Web site: *http://www.hhia.org*. Other examples of advocacy groups are described by Speckhard in Chapter 12.

APPLIED SOCIAL EPIDEMIOLOGY—COMMUNITY INTERVENTIONS WITH IMMIGRANTS TO ISRAEL FROM THE AREAS AROUND CHERNOBYL

Starting in 1989, a large-scale emigration began from the areas surrounding the damaged Chernobyl reactor to countries of the West, but particularly Israel and the United States. The largest concentration of exposed persons outside the FSU now lives in Israel. Many were motivated to both distance themselves from the contamination and to gain access to a health care system that would treat their perceived radiation exposure. A total of around 150,000–200,000 exposed persons arrived, and many were disappointed when the health establishment had no services set up to answer their perceived physical health needs (Lerner et al., 1994). Initially, researchers at Ben Gurion University studied current health problems such as the thyroid function of immigrants (Quastel et al., 1997) before conducting a longitudinal study of the psychological functioning of immigrants from these exposed regions based on the principles of social epidemiology. These principles included a focus on both physical and mental health status, using culturally sensitive research tools, incorporating qualitative findings from open-ended preliminary interviews into the research, and at a later stage developing support programs, policies, and ways for dissemination of the information gathered in the research. In the study of the psychological impact, two waves of data were collected. The first was obtained in 1994, or 6 years after the event (Cwikel et al., 1997). The sample included 137 adults from the most exposed regions, 240 from less-exposed regions, and 331 from comparison, nonexposed republics, with the exposure region classified using International Atomic Energy Agency (IAEA) maps of ground cesium in the last place of residence before immigration. "More exposed" communities were defined as those in which levels of ground cesium were more than 1 ci/km^2 (>37 GBq/km^2), and "less exposed" were places with contamination less than 1 ci/km^2 (<37 GBq/km^2). The response rate was 91%. The follow-up survey took place 1 year later and included 73% of the baseline respondents.

Some of the previously published findings based on this research have been referred to in previous sections. Other important findings included:

- Proximity to the accident and levels of exposure were related to increasing levels of long-term psychological distress, even 8 years after the accident (Cwikel et al., 2000).
- Over time, psychological stress reactions decreased except for somatization (Cwikel, Abdelgani et al., 1997).

Starting in 1996, the research team conducted a series of seminars for health and absorption workers to educate and sensitize them to the difficulties that Chernobyl-exposed immigrants face. We reviewed the events leading up to and following the accident, the scientifically documented health effects, and potential sources of psychological stress. In addition, we produced two educational pamphlets, one in Hebrew for health care workers and one in Russian for the lay population. These pamphlets summarized what is known about the scientific literature, including stress effects, and where concerned individuals could go for consultation. In addition, we taught two undergraduate university courses on the psychosocial aspects of technological disasters in order to educate those in the social and behavioral sciences.

For the immigrants themselves, we conducted both support groups of 10 sessions and focus groups, each having both a Russian speaking and a Hebrew speaking coleader. In these seminars, we tried to reinforce the use of active coping strategies while providing reliable resources and information to counteract anxieties.

One example of a coping method for dealing with anxiety was the recurrent initial unwillingness to talk about the accident and denial that it had any psychological impact, followed by a barrage of concerns and anxieties. We termed this phenomenon "encapsulated anxiety," since unlike repressed anxiety, the person is well aware of the concerns but keeps them isolated to prevent their intrusion on daily functioning. For example, in an interview with a young woman about to be married, she commented, "No, I never think about Chernobyl, that's in the past and there is no need to dwell on it." Later in the interview, when asked about her feelings concerning pregnancy, she replied, "Yes, if I get pregnant, I will do every medical check-up there is, since you never know how I have been affected by the Chernobyl accident and if my child will be normal." Another manifestation recurred in interviews with liquidators. Initially, they would dismiss the accident and its impact on them and then later in the interview proceed to explain in detail how their health was adversely affected by their work around the reactor. Thus, we found that for some of the immigrants, who were exposed, Chernobyl-related anxiety emerged only when there was something salient in the present that rekindled their worries. Otherwise, the anxiety was "encapsulated" in order to facilitate current day-to-day functioning (Cwikel & Hare, 1998).

Another example of a coping strategy was apparent in the social stigma associated with exposure to radiation from Chernobyl that was evident within the population that originated in the Commonwealth of Independent States (CIS). Those who were unmarried were less willing to marry a person who came from the area around Chernobyl than someone who originated in FSU without exposure. A similar stigmatic differential was found among older respondents when asked if they would want their child to marry someone who had been exposed to Chernobyl compared with other immigrants. Stigma against those who had been exposed was apparent both among the exposed groups and the comparison group (Cwikel, 2000). These findings are similar to the social stigma that was attached to being a Hiroshima survivor (Lifton, 1967). The stigma reflects the fear of genetic damage from radiation exposure, whether justified scientifically or not. Open discussion of these issues provided a way to lessen anxieties about them.

CONCLUSION

The handling of risk communication by governmental and nongovernmental authorities and health care professionals in a responsible fashion can mitigate the long-term psychological fall out when ecological disasters strike. Even today, there is too little attention paid in the official emergency response plans to the psychological aspects of these situations. Nuclear power plant emergency directives simply state, "If you are advised to evacuate the area, stay calm and do not rush." To their credit, they encourage the public to stay informed (FEMA, 1997). On the other hand, some places have developed mental health guidelines for natural and other disasters (e.g., New York State Psychological Association) (Carll, 1996), but these lack the psychosocial knowledge of what we have learned from ecological disasters, specifically. There is a need to bring these two bodies of knowledge together.

It is also important to recognize that personal and professional experience gained from work after ecological disasters provides a framework for understanding community responses. In the next disaster, many of those who will be working are likely to be young people who have not experienced many of the major disasters of the past century. It is very important to create accessible bodies of knowledge about how to manage the physical and mental health needs that arise, and this volume is an important addition. The Internet has also been shown to be an important source of accumulated professional practice wisdom. Each community needs to examine its own ecological risks and develop proactive disaster planning so that the infrastructure exists when the need arises. The importance of working proactively is that when disasters do strike, there will be well-trained personnel who have gained knowledge, expertise, and collaborative experience on how to successfully weather this crisis. This can make a big difference.

REFERENCES

Aldrich, T. E. (2000). Environmental epidemiology forward. *Chemosphere, 41*(1–2), 59–67.

Allman, W. (1985). Staying alive in the 20th century. *Science, 85,* 31–41.

Arata, C. M., Picou, J. S., Johnson, G. D., McNally, T. S. (2000). Coping with technological disaster: An application of the conservation of resources model to the Exxon *Valdez* oil spill. *Journal of Traumatic Stress, 13*(1), 23–39.

Baum, A., Fleming, R., & Davidson, L. M. (1983). Natural disaster and technological catastrophe. *Environment and Behavior, 15*(3), 333–353.

Bazylewicz-Walczak, B., Majczakowa, W., & Szymczak, M. (1999). Behavioral effects of occupational exposure tot organophosphorours pesticides in female greenhouse planting workers. *Neurotoxicology, 20*(5), 819–826.

Bertazzi, P. A. (1989). Industrial disasters and epidemiology. A review of recent experiences. *Scandinavian Journal of Work, Environment and Health, 15,* 85–100.

Boin, A., van Duin, M., & Heyse, L. (2001). Toxic fear: The management of uncertainty in the wake of the Amsterdam air crash. *Journal of Hazardous Materials, 88,* 213–234.

Bromet, E. J., & Dew, M. A. (1995). Review of psychiatric epidemiologic research on disasters. *Epidemiologic Reviews, 17*(1), 113–119.

Bromet, E. J., & Havenaar, J. M. (2002). Mental health consequences of disasters. In Santorius, N., Gaebel, W., Lopez-Ibor, J. J., and Maj, M. (Eds.), *Psychiatry in society.* Chichester, UK: Wiley.

Bromet, E. J., Parkinson, D., Schulberg, H., Dunn, L., & Gondek, P. (1982). Mental health of residents near the Three Mile Island reactor: A comparative study of selected groups. *Journal of Preventive Psychiatry, 1,* 255–276.

Bromet, E. J., & Schulberg, H. C. (1986). The Three Mile Island disaster: A search for high-risk groups. In J. H. Shore (Ed.), *Disaster stress studies: New methods and findings* (pp. 1–19). Washington, DC: American Psychiatric Press.

Byrd, T. L., VanDerslice, J., & Peterson, S. K. (2001). Attitudes and beliefs about environmental hazards in three diverse communities in Texas on the border with Mexico. *Review Panama Salud Publica, 9*(3), 154–160.

Carll, E. K. (1996). *Developing a comprehensive disaster and crisis response program for mental health: Guidelines and procedures.* Albany, NY: New York State Psychological Association.

Churchill, R. E. (1997). Effective media relations. In E. K. Noji (Ed.), *The public health consequences of disasters* (pp. 122–132). New York: Oxford University Press.

Collins, K. S., Schoen, C., Joseph, S., Duchon, L., Simantov, E., & Yellowitz, M. (1999). *Health concerns across a women's lifespan: The Commonwealth Fund 1998 Survey of Women's Health.* Washington, DC: Commonwealth Fund.

Cwikel, J. (1994a). After epidemiological research: What next? Community action for health promotion. *Public Health Reviews, 22,* 375–394.

Cwikel, J. (1994b). Social epidemiology: An integrative research and practice strategy applied to homelessness. *Journal Social Service Research, 19*(1–2), 23–47.

Cwikel, J. (1997). Comments on the psychosocial aspects of the International Conference on Radiation and Health. *Environmental Health Perspectives, 105,* (Suppl.) 6, 1607–1608.

Cwikel, J. (2000). *Social stigma among immigrants to Israel from the area around Chernobyl.* Unpublished manuscript.

Cwikel, J., Abdelgani, A., Goldsmith, J. R., Quastel, M., & Yevelson, I. I. (1997). Two-year follow-up study of immigrants to Israel from the Chernobyl area. *Environmental Health Perspectives, 105,* (Suppl.) 6, 1545–1550.

Cwikel, J. G., Abdelgani, A., Rozovski, U., Kordysh, E., Goldsmith, J. R., & Quastel, M. R. (2000). Long-term stress reactions in new immigrants to Israel exposed to the Chernobyl accident. *Anxiety, Stress and Coping, 13,* 413–439.

Cwikel, J. G., Goldsmith, J. R., Kordysh, E., Quastel, M., & Abdelgani, A. (1997). Blood pressure among immigrants to Israel from areas affected by the Chernobyl disaster. *Public Health Reviews, 25*(3–4), 317–335.

Cwikel, J. G., & Hare, J. (1998, July 5–9). *Immigrants to Israel exposed to Chernobyl: Intervention models for promoting coping.* Paper presented at the Joint World Congress of the International Federation of Social Workers and the International Association of Schools of Social Work, Jerusalem, Israel.

Cwikel, J. G., Kacen, L., & Slonim-Nevo, V. (1993). Stress management consultation to Israeli social workers during the Gulf War. *Health and Social Work, 18*(3), 172–183.

Cwikel, J., & Rozovski, U. (1998). Coping with the stress of immigration among new immigrants to Israel from Commonwealth of Independent States (CIS) who were exposed to Chernobyl: The effect of age. *International Journal of Aging and Human Development, 46*(4), 305–319.

Davidson, L. M., & Baum, A. (1986). Chronic stress and posttraumatic stress disorders. *Journal Consult Clin Psychol, 54*(3), 303–308.

Dubreuil, G. H., Lochard, J., Girard, P., Guyonnet, J. F., Le Cardinal, G., Lepicard, S. et al. (1999). Chernobyl post-accident management: The ETHOS project. *Health Physics, 77*(4), 361–372.

Environmental Disasters. (1998). Retrieved on March 7, 2000, from http://www. umweltbundesamt.de/uba-info-daten-e/daten-e/environmental-disasters.htm

Federal Emercency Management Agency (FEMA), (1997). Fact Sheet: Nuclear Power Plant Emergency, Retrieved on March 7, 2000, www.fema.gov

Fischhoff, B., Bostrom, A., & Quadrel, M. J. (1993). Risk perception and communication. *Annual Reviews Public Health, 14,* 183–203.

Freudenburg, W. R. (1997). Contamination, corrosion, and the social order: An overview. *Current Sociology, 45,* 19–39.

Gerrity, E. T., & Flynn, B. W. (1997). Mental health consequences of disasters. In E. K. Noji (Ed.), *The public health consequences of disasters* (pp. 101–121). New York: Oxford University Press.

Goldman, M., Hedetniemi, J. N., Hebert, E. R., Sassaman, J. S., & Walker, B. C., Jr. (2000). Community outreach at biomedical research facilities. *Environonmental Health Perspectives, 108* (Suppl.) *6,* 1009–1013.

Goldsmith, J. R., Grossman, C. M., Morton, W. E., Nussbaum, R. H., Kordysh, E. A., Quastel, M. R. et al. (1999). *Environmental Health Perspectives, 107*(4), 303–308.

Havenaar, J. M., de Wilde, E. J., van den Bout, J., Drottz-Sjöberg, B-M., & van de Brink, W. (in press). Perception of risk and subjective health among victims of the Chernobyl disaster. *Social Science and Medicine.*

Havenaar, J. M., Rumyantseva, G. M., van den Brink, W., Poelijoe, N. W., van den Bout, J., van Engeland, H. et al. (1997). Long-term mental health effects of the Chernobyl disaster: An epidemiological survey in two former Soviet Regions. *American Journal of Psychiatry, 154,* 1605–1607.

Havenaar, J. M., & van den Brink, W. (1997). Psychological factors affecting health after toxicological disasters. *Clinical Psychology Review, 17*(4), 359–374.

Havenaar, J. M., van den Brink, W., Kasyanenko, A. P., van den Bout, J., Meijler-Iljina, L. I., Poelijoe, N. W. (1996). Mental health problems in the Gomel Region (Belarus). An analysis of risk factors in an area affected by the Chernobyl disaster. *Psychological Medicine, 26,* 845–855.

Hegstad, H. J. (2000). *Predicting postdisaster adjustment after the Red River flood: An analysis of resource loss and pre-flood preventive behaviors.* University of North Dakota. Dissertation Abstracts International, Vol. 60 (12-13): 6365.

Hobfoll, S. E. (1988). *The ecology of stress.* Washington, DC: Hemisphere.

Hobfoll, S. E. (1989). Conservation of resources: A new attempt at conceptualizing stress. *Amercian Journal of Community Psychology, 9,* 91–103.

Hobfoll, S. (1998). *Stress, culture, and community: The psychology and philosophy of stress.* New York: Plenum.

Kasperson R. E., Renn, O., Slovic, P., Brown. H. S., Emel, J., Goble, R. et al. (1988). The social amplification of risk: A conceptual framework. *Risk Analyses, 3*(2), 177–191.

Krieger, N. (2001). A glossary for social epidemiology. *Journal of Epidemiology and Community Health, 55,* 693–700.

Last, J. M. (Ed). (1995). *A dictionary of epidemiology.* (3rd ed.) New York: Oxford University Press.

Lazarus, R. S., & Folkman, S. (1984). *Stress, appraisal, and coping.* New York: Springer.

Lee, T. T. (1996, April 8–12). *Environmental stress reactions following the Chernobyl accident.* Proceedings of EC/IAEA/WHO international conference One Decade After Chernobyl. Vienna.

Lerner, Y., Mirsky, J., & Barasch, M. (1994). *New beginnings in an old land.* In A. Marsella, T. Bornemann, S. Ekblad, & J. Orley (Eds.), *Amidst peril and pain: Understanding the mental health and well-being of the world refugees* (pp. 153–192). Washington, DC: American Psychological Association.

Levi, L. (1994). *The legacy of Chernobyl—Psychosocial aspects.* Presentation to the ministerial conference in Helsinki. Stockholm, Sweden: Karolinska Institute.

Lifton, R. J. (1967). *Death in life. Survivors of Hiroshima.* New York: Random House.

Lillibridge, S. R. (1997). Managing the environmental health aspects of disasters: Water, human excreta, and shelter. In E. K. Noji (Ed.), *The public health consequences of disasters,* (pp. 65–79). New York: Oxford University Press.

Mausner, J. S., & Bahn, A. K. (1974). *Epidemiology: An introductory text.* Philadelphia: W. B. Saunders.

Mays, C., Avetova, E., Murphy, M., & Allen, P. (1998). *The weeping cow: Impact of countermeasures on daily life in Chernobyl contaminated areas.* Proceedings of the 1998 annual conference Risk Analysis: Opening the Process IPSN, Paris.

Mazur, A. (1981). *The dynamics of technical controversies.* Washington DC: Communication Press.

Mearns, J., Dunn, J., & Lees-Haley, P. R. (1994). Psychological effects of organophosphate pesticides: A review and call for research by psychologists. *Journal of Clinical Psychology, 50*(2), 286–294.

Ministry of Health. (1954). *Mortality and morbidity during the London fog of December 1952.* London: HMSO.

Mould, R. F. (1988). *Chernobyl. The real story.* Oxford: Pergamon.

Ng, K. L., & Hamby, D. M. (1997). Fundamentals for establishing a risk communication program. *Health Physics, 73*(3), 473–482.

North, C. S., Hong, B. A. (2000). Project CREST: A new model for mental health intervention after a community disaster. *American Journal of Public Health, 90,* 1057–1058.

Park, C. C. (1989). *Chernobyl, the long shadow.* London: Routledge.

Pesatori, A. C., Zocchetti, C., Guercilena, S., Consonni, D., Turrini, D., & Bertazzi, P. A. (1998). Dioxin exposure and non-malignant health effects: A mortality study. *Occupational & Environental Medicine, 55*(2), 126–131.

Peters, R. G. (1996). A study of the factors determining perceptions of trust and credibility in environmental risk communication: The importance of overcoming negative stereotypes. *International Archives of Occupational & Environmental Health, 68*(6), 442–447.

Quastel, M. R., Goldsmith, J. R., Cwikel, J., Merkin, L., Wishkerman, V. Y., Poljak, S. et al. (1997). Commentary: Lessons learned from the study of immigrants to Israel from areas of Russia, Belarus, and Ukraine contaminated by the Chernobyl accident. *Environmental Health Perspectives* (Suppl.) *105*(6), 1523–1528.

Rubonis, A. V., & Bickman, L. (1991). Psychological impairment in the wake of disaster: The disaster-psychopathology relationship. *Psychological Bulletin 109,* 384–399.

Sattler, D. N., Kaiser, C. F., & Hittner, J. B. (2000). Disaster preparedness: Relationships among prior experience, personal characteristics, and distress. *Journal Applied Social Psychology, 30*(7), 1396–1420.

Shigematsu, I., Chikako, I., Kamada, N., Akiyama, M., & Sasaki, H. (1995). *Effects of A-bomb radiation on the human body.* Translated by B. Harrison. Tokyo: Harwood Academic Publishers.

Slovic, P. (1987). Perception of risk. *Science 236,* 280–285.

Smith, B. W., & Freedy, J. R. (2000). Psychosocial resource loss as a mediator of the effects of flood exposure on psychological distress and physical symptoms. *Journal of Traumatic Stress, 13*(2), 349–357.

Soliman, M. R., Derosa, C. T., Mielke, H. W., & Bota, K. (1993). Hazardous wastes, hazardous materials and environmental health inequity. *Toxicology and Industrial Health, 9*(5), 901–912.

Stewart, A. (1997). A bomb-data: Detection of bias in the life span study cohort. *Environmental Health Perspectives, 105* (Suppl.) *6,* 1519–1521.

Thomas, W. I. (1966). *Social organization and social personality.* Chicago: Phoenix Books/University of Chicago Press.

Tinker, T. L., Collins, C. M., King, H. S., Hoover, M. D. (2000). Assessing risk communication effectiveness: Perspectives of agency practitioners. *Journal of Hazardous Materials, 73*(2), 117–127.

van den Bout, J., Havenaar, J. M., & Meijler-Iljina, L. I. (1995). Health problems in areas contaminated by the Chernobyl disaster: Radiation, traumatic stress or chronic stress? In J. Kleber, C. Figley, & B. P. R. Gersons (Eds.), *Beyond trauma: Cultural and societal dynamics.* New York: Plenum.

Viel, J. F., Curbakova, E., Dzerve, B., Elgite, M., Zvagulre, T., & Vincent, C. (1997). Risk factors for long-term mental and psychosomatic distress in Latvian Chernobyl liquidators. *Environmental Health Perspectives, 105* (Suppl.) *6,* 1539–1544.

Viinamaki, H., Kumpusalo, E., Myllykangas, M., Salomaa, S., Kumpusalo, L., Kolmakov, S. et al. (1995). The Chernobyl accident and mental wellbeing—a population study. *Acta Psychiatrica Scandinavia, 91,* 396–401.

Wettig, J., & Faure, C. (1999). *Chemical accident prevention, preparedness and response. The European Commission.* Retrieved on September 24, 2001 from http://europa.eu.int/comm/environment/seveso

Yehuda, R., Bierer, L. M., Schmeidler, J., Aferiat, D. H., Breslau, I., & Dolan, S. (2000). Low cortisol and risk for PTSD in adult offspring of Holocaust survivors. *American Journal of Psychiatry, 157,* 1252–1259.

Yevelson, I. I., Abdelgani, A., Cwikel, J., & Yevelson, I. S. (1997). Bridging the gap in mental health approaches between East and West: The psychosocial consequences of radiation exposure. *Environmental Health Perspectives, 105* (Suppl.) *6,* 1551–1557.

II

Case Examples of Ecological Disasters

4

Psychological Response of Mothers of Young Children to the Three Mile Island and Chernobyl Nuclear Plant Accidents One Decade Later

EVELYN J. BROMET and LEIGHANN LITCHER-KELLY

INTRODUCTION

Over the past two decades, our research group investigated the psychological well-being of mothers of young children in the aftermath of the nuclear power plant accident at Three Mile Island (TMI) in central Pennsylvania and the melt down at the Chernobyl nuclear power plant in northwest Ukraine. In spite of differences in culture and magnitude, these two catastrophic events had a number of common characteristics, making the comparison in the psychological responses to these events extremely valuable. Common features included the intangible nature of exposure to radiation, the delay in the evacuation order, incomplete disclosure by the authorities about what occurred, contradictory reports in the news media as the events

EVELYN J. BROMET and LEIGHANN LITCHER-KELLY • Department of Psychiatry and Behavioral Science State University of New York at Stony Brook 11794-8790.

Toxic Turmoil: Psychological and Societal Consequences of Ecological Disasters, edited by Johan M. Havenaar, Julie G. Cwikel, and Evelyn J. Bromet. New York, Kluwer Academic/Plenum Publishers, 2002.

unfolded, widespread rumors about adverse or bizarre effects on plants and animals, ensuing distrust of government authorities, the tendency to attribute new health problems to radiation exposure, fears about health effects on future generations, health monitoring by government agencies, and most important, lack of resolution about potential risks to the population at large.

Clearly, notwithstanding these shared features, the events themselves were different in a number of respects. In particular, the magnitude of devastation caused by the TMI accident was far less than that ensuing from Chernobyl. Specifically, the malfunction at TMI began on March 28, 1979, leading to a partial melt down of the core and a small (0.4–1 terabecquerel) release of radioiodine (Whitcomb & Sage, 1997) primarily inside the reactor itself. The average exposure dose to the 2 million people within 50 miles of the plant was estimated to be 0.015 mSv. No increases were found in cancer morbidity or mortality that could be attributed to the TMI accident (Hatch, Beyea, Nieves, & Susser, 1990). On March 30, the governor of Pennsylvania (who was a nuclear engineer by profession) issued an advisory to pregnant women and preschool children to evacuate the 5-mile area surrounding the plant. In fact, 60% of the entire population in the 5-mile radius of the plant evacuated (Flynn, 1981; Houts, Cleary, & Hu, 1988). The evacuation was temporary, and almost all of the families returned to the area within 2 weeks (Houts et al., 1988).

The Chernobyl accident, which began on April 26, 1986, resulted in a melt down and extensive contamination of regions of Ukraine, Belarus, and Russia (Whitcomb & Sage, 1997). In all, about 50 million curies of radioactive material were released. The official count was 31 deaths from radiation sickness although the Chernobyl Union, a citizens' lobby, estimated that 256 cleanup workers died because of the accident (Feshbach & Friendly, 1992). There has also been a substantial increase in thyroid disease in exposed children, with the highest rates found in those who were in utero to age 2 when the event occurred (Bard, Verger, & Hubert, 1997; Nikiforov, Gnepp, & Fagin, 1996). Initially, 115,000 people were evacuated from the 10-kilometer zone surrounding the plant (Bard et al., 1997), and subsequently thousands more were relocated (Cardis, 1996). During the evacuation, women were strongly advised to have an abortion, although they were not given the true reason, and most reportedly complied. The cities and towns in which evacuees were resettled were at first unreceptive and even hostile. To complicate matters further, the Soviet Union collapsed in the early 1990s, and the socioeconomic chaos that followed added to the intense stress already imposed on the evacuee population.

In spite of vast differences in magnitude, both accidents created a situation of enduring uncertainty for the exposed populations. Research addressing the psychological impact of these adverse events documented that mental health effects occurred up to 10 years later (Baum &

Fleming, 1993; Bromet, Parkinson, Schulberg, Dunn, & Gondek, 1982; Cwikel, Abdelgani, Goldsmith, Quastel, & Yevelson, 1997; Davidson & Baum, 1986; Dew & Bromet, 1993; Dew, Bromet, Schulberg, Dunn, & Parkinson, 1987; Dohrenwend, 1983; Havenaar et al., 1997; Houts, et al., 1988; Viinamäki et al., 1995; Yevelson, Abdelgani, Cwikel, & Yevelson, 1997). Consistent with epidemiologic studies showing that mothers of young children are a high-risk group for psychological distress and clinical depression (e.g., Brown & Harris, 1978), this subgroup had particularly elevated rates of depression, demoralization, and post-traumatic stress disorder (PTSD) symptoms following both the TMI (Bromet, et al., 1982) and Chernobyl (Havenaar et al., 1997) disasters.

This chapter provides a direct comparison of the levels of distress reported by mothers of young children affected by TMI and Chernobyl 10–11 years after the events. Both the TMI and Chernobyl studies, funded by the National Institute of Mental Health (USA), sampled mothers of young children. The women, who were in their late 20s when the accidents occurred (late 30s when interviewed 10 years later), completed similar measures of psychological well-being (including three subscales from the Symptom Checklist-90 [SCL-90] and self-ratings of health), and answered similar questions about the perceived effects of the accident on their health and that of their children.

METHOD

Samples

TMI. A panel of 156 women living within 10 miles of TMI were mailed questionnaires in 1989 shortly after the 10th anniversary of the TMI accident (Dew & Bromet, 1993). They had all lived within 10 miles of TMI when the accident happened and had delivered a child between January 1978 and March 1979. The sample was originally drawn from newspaper birth announcements because Pennsylvania law prohibited access to vital statistics records. Fortunately, at the time the sample was assembled, hospitals routinely reported births to the local newspapers, thereby minimizing sample bias (Bromet & Schulberg, 1986).

Almost all of the women left the area at the time of the crisis, and most returned within 2 weeks. The women were interviewed in their homes 12, 30, and 42 months after the accident as part of our NIMH-funded study of high-risk groups. At the 10th anniversary in 1989, we did not have funding so we mailed a questionnaire to the members of the cohort. The 156 respondents who returned this questionnaire represented 38% (156/412) of the original sample. In a series of analyses comparing responders and nonresponders to the questionnaire, we found no significant differences on demographic, mental health, and attitudinal variables obtained at earlier waves (Dew & Bromet, 1993). The original sample included controls living near another nuclear power plant and near a coal-fired plant in western Pennsylvania. However, both comparison sites underwent massive unemployment in the early 1980s with the demise of the steel industry. They were thus dropped as comparison groups for the TMI follow-up study. Instead, we utilize data from a normative community sample of women living near Philadelphia described by Derogatis (1983).

Chernobyl. A total of 600 mothers of young children were interviewed in 1997. Three hundred of the mothers were evacuated to Kiev from the 10-kilometer zone around Chernobyl (Bromet, Goldgaber et al., 2000; Litcher et al., 2000). They were randomly selected from a sampling frame of 693 such families with children born between February 1, 1985, and January 31, 1987, who resided in Kiev in 1996 and were on one or more of the following lists: the Ukraine Ministry of Health's National Register of Persons Affected by Radiation as a Result of the Chernobyl Accident, Help for Families from Chernobyl, and Children of Chernobyl for Survival. The 300 women interviewed for the study represent 92% (300/326) of those originally approached. The majority (80.7%) of the women were evacuated from Pripyat, a city of approximately 50,000 people that was built for Chernobyl employees.

In addition, 300 mothers of gender-matched homeroom classmates of the evacuee children were interviewed. Most of the control families were in Kiev when the accident happened. None had lived in the contaminated regions. The response rate for this group was 85% (300/352).

Procedures

The TMI mothers completed a mailed questionnaire. The Kiev samples were interviewed face-to-face by trained lay interviewers employed by SOCIS-Gallop of Kiev, a sociological research institute (Bromet, Goldgaber et al., 2000). The interviews were closely monitored both by SOCIS supervisors and by the American investigators. All measures were translated and back-translated into Russian and Ukrainian using standard translation procedures.

Measures

Well-Being. Psychiatric symptoms were assessed with the anxiety, depression, and hostility subscales of the SCL-90 (English version—Derogatis, 1983; Russian version—Tarabrina et al., 1996). The items are rated on a 5-point scale (0 = not at all distressed, 4 = extremely distressed) and reflect symptoms in the past 2 weeks. The anxiety subscale contains 10 items; in a U.S. normative sample of women, one standard deviation above the mean was 0.74. The depression subscale contains 13 items (one standard deviation = 0.78), and the hostility subscale has 6 items (one standard deviation = 0.66). Because there are no normative data for the SCL-90 in Ukraine, we used one standard deviation from the American normative sample to compare the TMI and Chernobyl study groups.

The women also provided an overall rating of their health. For TMI sample, the response options were excellent, good, fair, or poor. For Kiev, the options were excellent, good, moderate, bad, and very bad. The low end of the response scale was expanded for the Chernobyl study to reflect known differences in response styles. The differences in response scales could have influenced the distribution for each group, however, and will be considered later in the chapter.

Risk Factors. Both studies included information on age, current marital status, number of children, education, and religion. In addition, in both sites, the mothers were asked whether they thought the accident affected their health, and whether they thought it affected their children's health. The response options for TMI mothers were "yes, unsure, and no," while for Chernobyl, they were "yes very, yes somewhat, and no."

Site-specific data included the following: In the TMI study, we categorized distance of residence from the plant in 1979 (0–5 vs. 6–10 miles). In addition, the mothers were asked questions about risks associated with TMI in the 1981 and 1982 interview waves, 2.5 and 3.5 years after the accident. In this chapter, we analyze the extent to which earlier TMI-health worries to self or child and perceptions of danger predicted the level of anxiety at the 10-year follow-up. The analysis also adjusted for mental health history in the year prior to the 1982 interview, defined as clinical episodes of anxiety and/or depression meeting Research Diagnostic Criteria (Spitzer, Endicott, & Robins, 1978).

Further analysis of the Chernobyl sample focused on two additional items: whether a physician ever diagnosed the mother with a Chernobyl-related disease, and whether the mother was ever diagnosed with vascular dystony. Also known as "vegetative dystonia," this diagnosis reflects symptoms such as headaches, fatigue, dizziness, changes in blood pressure, and abdominal pain. Vascular dystony was the "official" diagnosis in Ukraine for "Chernobyl-related conditions" based on tests not used in Western medicine (Stiehm, 1992). In addition, we selected a parsimonious set of epidemiologic risk factors for further multivariate analysis of the relationship of Chernobyl stress to anxiety. For the evacuees, five risk factors, significantly related to anxiety, were considered in the multivariate model: lifetime depression (based on a modified version of the Structured Clinical Interview for DSM-III-R [Phelan et al., 1991], (OR = 1.6, 95%, CI = 1.0–2.6, $p < 0.05$), current smoking (0 = no to 4 = more than 1 pack/day; OR = 1.5, CI = 1.0–2.1, $p < 0.05$), perceived standard of living = low (OR = 1.6, CI = 1.0–2.5, $p < 0.05$), number of life events in past year (out of 18, for example, not being paid for work, home being burglarized, husband unfaithful; OR = 1.1, CI = 1.0–1.3, $p < 0.05$), and social support (single item rated 0 = never to 4 = always assessing how often the respondents felt that they had someone to turn to in times of need; OR = 2.0, CI = 2.1–3.3, $p < 0.01$). For the Kiev controls, six epidemiologic risk factors were included: high education (OR = 1.4, 95%, CI = 1.1–1.9, $p < 0.05$), lifetime depression (OR = 2.2, CI = 1.4–3.6, $p < 0.001$), current smoking (OR = 1.4, CI = 1.1–1.9, $p < 0.01$), standard of living (OR = 1.6, CI = 1.0–2.6, $p < 0.05$), life events (OR = 1.4, CI = 1.2–1.6, $p < 0.001$), and perceived lack of goods and services (OR = 2.4, CI = 1.5–4.0, $p < 0.001$).

ANALYSIS

Differences in well-being among the TMI, Chernobyl evacuee, and Kiev comparison mothers were evaluated using one-way analysis of variance and chi square tests. The SCL-90 anxiety, depression, and hostility subscales were highly intercorrelated, ranging from $r = 0.73$ (anxiety and hostility) to 0.87 (anxiety and depression) for TMI; $r = 0.66$ (anxiety and hostility) to 0.81 (anxiety and depression) for evacuees; and $r = 0.67$ (depression and hostility) to 0.82 (anxiety and depression) for the Kiev controls. We thus selected a single subscale, anxiety, to explore the relationships of perceived risks from the accidents with current symptoms. The samples in each site were dichotomized into high (> 0.74) and low (≤ .74) anxiety groups, using one standard deviation above the mean for a normative U.S. sample as the cutpoint as noted above (Derogatis, 1983). The relationships of accident beliefs to anxiety were analyzed using bivariate and multivariate logistic regression analysis.

RESULTS

Background Characteristics

The TMI, evacuee, and Kiev comparison groups were similar in terms of age, marital status, and number of children (Table 4.1). Specifically, 10 years after the accident, most were in their late 30s, were currently married, and had an average of two children. The TMI sample had less education than

Table 4.1   Differences in Demographic Characteristics of TMI and Chernobyl
Samples 10–11 Years Post-Accident[a]

	TMI (n = 156)	Evacuees (n = 300)	Kiev controls (n = 300)
Age, median	~37	37	38
Current married	~95.0%	88.7%	89.4%
Children, median number	2	2	2
Education > high school	56.4%	60.3%	64.9%
Religion	Protestant, 71.0%	Orthodox 69.0%	Orthodox 64.9%
Currently employed	—	61.0%	79.8%
Husband employed	—	87.4%	92.1%

[a]None of the group comparisons was statistically significant with the exception employment of evacuees vs. Kiev controls (chi square = 25.3, $df = 1$, $p < 0.001$).

the Kiev women, although the differences were not statistically significant. The majority of the TMI sample were Protestant , while the majority of the women in Kiev were Russian Orthodox. We did not have current data on employment status of TMI mothers at the 10th anniversary, but earlier data suggest that about half of the TMI mothers were working outside the home and almost all of their husbands were employed. In the Kiev samples, compared to the controls, fewer evacuee mothers were gainfully employed (chi square = 25.3, $df = 1$, $p < 0.001$), and somewhat more of their husbands were unemployed (chi square = 3.06, $df = 1$, $p < 0.08$).

Well-Being

The evacuee mothers had the highest and the TMI sample the lowest symptom scores on all three subscales of the SCL-90 (Table 4.2). The proportion with high distress, using the American cut-point described above, ranged from 48% (depression) to 54% (anxiety) in the evacuees, 38% (depression) to 42% (hostility) in the Kiev controls, compared to 24% (anxiety) to 34% (hostility) in the TMI sample. The differences among the three groups were statistically significant. However, it is instructive to note that the scores of the TMI mothers were higher than expected based on the normative sample. In addition, for both the TMI and Kiev controls, the scale with the largest percentage scoring in the high-distress level was hostility, while for evacuees, the highest distress was found for anxiety.

Almost all of the TMI mothers rated their health as excellent or good (Figure 4.1). In contrast, in both Kiev samples, the modal self-rating of health was "moderate." In comparison with Kiev controls, the evacuee mothers were significantly more likely to rate their health as bad (2 [group] by 4 [rate health excellent/good, moderate, bad, very bad] chi square = 17.0; $df = 3$; $p < 0.001$).

**Table 4.2   SCL-90 Symptom Levels of TMI and Chernobyl Samples
10–11 Years Post-Accident**

	TMI ($n = 156$)	Evacuees ($n = 300$)	Kiev controls ($n = 300$)	$F_{2,756}$	p
Anxiety (10 items)					
Mean (SD)	.50 (.52)	.96 (.65)	.73 (.55)	32.8	.001
Median	.40	.90	.60		
Range	0–3.0	0–3.1	0–2.9		
> .74*	24%	54%	40%		
Depression (13 items)					
Mean (SD)	.68 (.65)	.88 (.57)	.76 (.54)	6.7	.001
Median	.54	.77	.69		
Range	0–3.5	0–2.6	0–2.9		
> .78*	31%	48%	38%		
Hostility (6 items)					
Mean (SD)	.54 (.56)	.67 (.48)	.59 (.46)	4.1	.05
Median	.33	.67	.50		
Range	0–2.5	0–2.5	0–2.5		
> .66*	34%	51%	42%		

*One standard deviation above of the mean of the Derogatis' U.S. normative sample (1983).

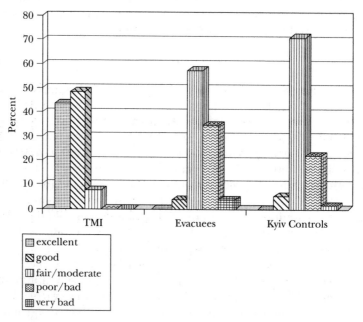

Figure 4.1. Self-Rating of Health by TMI and Chornobyl Mothers.

Table 4.3   Differences in Beliefs About the Health Impact of
TMI and Chernobyl[a,b]

	TMI (n = 156) %	Evacuees (n = 300) %	Kiev controls (n = 300) %
1. Worried about your health because of . . .?	Yes 42.9 Unsure 17.3 No 39.7	Very 44.7 Some 51.3 No 4.0	Very 15.2 Some 65.2 No 19.6
2. Worried about your child's health because of . . .?	Yes 51.9 Unsure 20.5 No 27.6	Very 58.3 Some 40.3 No 1.3	Very 29.8 Some 59.9 No 10.4

[a]The 3 (group) × 3 (level of worry) chi square tests were highly significant for both variables ($p < 0.001$).
[b]Evacuees were significantly more worried than controls ($p < 0.001$).
[b]Four Kiev controls did not answer question 1, and 1 control did not answer question 2.

Perceived Risk to Health

Only a minority of TMI mothers reported that they were *not* worried about their own health or their children's health because of TMI. However, fewer TMI mothers were unequivocally worried about the accident's health effects than was true for the Kiev samples. As expected, the evacuee mothers were significantly more likely to be very worried about their own health and their children's health than the Kiev comparison group (Table 4.3).

Figure 4.2 shows that in all three groups, those who believed that their health was affected by the accident had significantly higher anxiety scores than those who believed that their health was not affected (or somewhat affected in the Chernobyl samples).

In the TMI sample, we next examined whether distance of residence from the plant or perceptions of danger and worries about health reported at previous waves and at the 10-year point were significant predictors of anxiety at the 10-year follow-up (Table 4.4). Living within the 5-mile radius of the plant in 1979 (hence being subject to the governor's advisory about evacuation) was not a significant predictor of anxiety at the 10-year anniversary. In contrast, believing that TMI was dangerous in 1981 was strongly related with anxiety in 1989. Eight-two percent of the high-anxiety group had previously evaluated TMI as dangerous, compared to 55% of the low-anxiety group. As expected, the odds ratios were largest for the cross-sectional data obtained at the 10-year anniversary. In 1989, close to 90% of the high-anxiety group expressed concerns about TMI, compared to approximately 60% of the low-anxiety group. With two exceptions (worries about self/spouse health in 1981 and TMI perceived as dangerous in 1982), the significant bivariate odds ratios reported in Table 4.4 remained significant in the multivariate

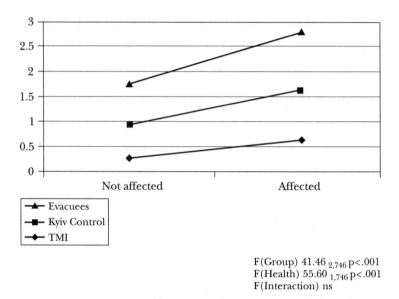

F(Group) 41.46 $_{2,746}$ p<.001
F(Health) 55.60 $_{1,746}$ p<.001
F(Interaction) ns

Figure 4.2. Relationship between Believing Health Affected by Accident and Anxiety score. *Note.* For the Chernobyl site, the "affected grioup" included mothers who believed that their health was "very" affected by Chernobyl; the "note affected group" believed that their health was "somewhat" or "not" affected. For the TMI site the "affected group" included mothers who believed their health was affected by TMI (answer = yes or unsure); the "not affected group" answered "no."

analysis that adjusted for earlier episodes of anxiety/depression (data not shown).

The relationship of Chernobyl-stress variables to anxiety were highly significantly in the evacuees (Table 4.5). Thus, 55% of evacuee mothers with high anxiety said that Chernobyl very much affected their health, compared with 33% of the low-anxiety mothers. Close to two thirds of high-anxiety mothers, compared to fewer than half of the low-anxiety mothers, believed that their children's health was very much affected by Chernobyl and reported that they had been diagnosed with Chernobyl-related disease or with vascular dystony. In addition, each variable remained significant in multivariate models that adjusted for epidemiologic risk factors (lifetime depression, current smoking, perceived standard of living, social support, and life events).

In the Kiev controls, all but one of the Chernobyl stress variables (being diagnosed with vascular dystony) was significantly associated with anxiety, although overall, fewer controls than evacuees believed that their health or their children's health was affected by the radiation exposure. The odds

Table 4.4   Predictors of High SCL-90 Anxiety Symptom Levels (> .74)
in TMI Sample

Variable	Low anxiety N (%)	High anxiety N (%)	OR (95% CI)
Distance of home from TMI			
More than 5 miles	74 (62.7)	24 (63.2)	1.0 (0.5–2.1)
0–5 miles	44 (37.3)	14 (36.8)	
TMI currently dangerous: 1981			
Yes/unsure	65 (55.1)	31 (81.6)	3.6 (1.5–8.9)^a
No	53 (44.9)	7 (18.4)	
Worried that children have special health problems due to TMI: 1981			
Yes	5 (4.2)	2 (5.3)	1.3 (0.2–6.8)
No	113 (95.8)	36 (94.7)	
Think self or spouse has physical or emotional problems due to TMI: 1981			
Yes	17 (14.4)	11 (28.9)	2.4 (1.0–5.8)^b
No	101 (85.6)	27 (71.1)	
TMI currently dangerous: 1982			
Yes/unsure	69 (58.5)	27 (77.1)	2.4 (1.0–5.7)^b
No	49 (41.5)	8 (22.9)	
Worried about health because of living near TMI: 1982			
Yes/unsure	43 (36.4)	15 (45.5)	1.5 (0.7–3.2)
No	75 (63.6)	18 (54.5)	
Worried about child's health because of living near TMI: 1982			
Yes/unsure	74 (62.7)	29 (85.3)	3.4 (1.2–9.6)^a
No	44 (37.3)	5 (14.7)	
TMI currently dangerous: 1989			
Yes/unsure	73 (61.9)	34 (89.5)	5.2 (1.7–15.8)^c
No	45 (38.1)	4 (10.5)	
Worried health affected by TMI: 1989			
Yes/unsure	60 (58.8)	34 (89.5)	8.2 (2.7–24.6)^c
No	58 (49.2)	4 (10.5)	
Worried child's health affected by TMI: 1989			
Yes/unsure	78 (66.1)	35 (92.1)	6.0 (1.7–20.7)^a
No	40 33.9)	3 (7.9)	

^{a} $p < .05$
^{b} $p < .01$
^{c} $p < .001$

Table 4.5 Relationship of Chernobyl Stress to High SCL-90 Anxiety Symptom Level (> .74) in Evacuees and Kiev Comparison Group

	Evacuee mothers			Comparison mothers		
	Low anxiety N (%)	High anxiety N (%)	OR (95% CI)	Low anxiety N (%)	High anxiety N (%)	OR (95% CI)
Chernobyl affected your health						
Yes very	45 (32.8)	89 (54.6)	2.5 (1.5–3.9)[c]	25 (14.1)	33 (27.7)	2.3 (1.3–4.2)[b]
Some/no	92 (67.2)	74 (45.4)		152 (85.9)	86 (72.3)	
Chernobyl affected child's health						
Yes very	67 (48.9)	108 (66.3)	2.1 (1.3–3.3)[b]	42 (23.3)	47 (39.5)	2.1 (1.3–3.6)[b]
Some/no	70 (51.1)	55 (33.7)		138 (76.7)	72 (60.5)	
Ever told by physician that you have a Chernobyl-related disease						
Yes	61 (44.5)	102 (63.0)	2.1 (1.3–3.4)[c]	27 (14.9)	29 (24.6)	1.9 (1.0–3.3)[a]
No	76 (55.5)	60 (37.0)		154 (85.1)	89 (75.4)	
Ever diagnosed with vascular dystony						
Yes	54 (42.5)	95 (64.2)	2.4 (1.5–3.9)[c]	43 (26.5)	32 (29.1)	1.1 (0.7–1.9)
No	73 (57.5)	53 (35.8)		119 (73.5)	78 (70.9)	

[a] $p < .05$
[b] $p < .01$
[c] $p < .001$

ratios remained significant after adjusting for selected epidemiologic risk factors (education, lifetime depression, current smoking, standard of living, lacking basic goods and services, and stressful life events).

Lastly, we note that in a separate multivariate logistic regression analysis that included evacuee versus comparison group status, each of the Chernobyl stress factors remained statistically significant (data not shown).

COMMENT AND CONCLUSION

The central issue addressed in this chapter is whether TMI and Chernobyl had long-term psychological sequelae. Our findings suggest that both events had an impact on the women a decade later. A larger than expected proportion of TMI mothers had SCL-90 scores above one standard deviation of an American normative sample, and there was a strong relationship between risk perceptions and anxiety. The Chernobyl evacuees in Kiev had significantly elevated scores over the control group, and there was also a strong relationship between perceptions of threat to health and anxiety in both the evacuees and controls. What was unanticipated was that the odds ratios describing the cross-sectional relationships between perceptions of accident risk and anxiety were much larger in size for the TMI sample than for either of the Kiev samples. That is, almost all of the TMI women with high anxiety reported being currently worried about TMI, whereas two thirds of the high-anxiety Chernobyl mothers and 25–40% of the Kiev comparison mothers in the high-anxiety group expressed accident-related concerns.

Overall, the Kiev women rated their health more poorly than did the TMI mothers, even though they were demographically similar in many respects. We note that in November 1998 a national survey of Ukraine was conducted by the Kiev International Institute of Sociology. In the sample of 1,600 adults, 276 were mothers in the same age range as the Chernobyl study samples (ages 28–55). Among this subsample of national survey respondents, 23.9% rated their health as bad or very bad, 58.7% rated their health as "moderate," and 17.3% rated their health as good or excellent (only 1.4% checked excellent). Thus, caution should be exercised in interpreting the differences between the TMI and Kiev women because they likely reflect both differences in actual morbidity and cross-national variations in response sets.

With a few exceptions (e.g., Green et al., 1990; McFarlane, Policansky, & Irwin, 1987), the vast majority of studies of natural and human-made disasters have been cross-sectional and reflect adjustment within 1–2 years of the events (Bromet & Dew, 1995). The one area where there have now been several long-term studies is radiation exposure. Thus, three English-language reports of survivors of Hiroshima and Nagasaki conducted 10–20 years later report elevated rates of anxiety, depression, fatigue, and post-traumatic stress type symptoms (Lifton, 1967; Misao et al., 1961; Yamada, Kodama, & Wong, 1987; for review, see also Bromet, 1998). Long-term follow-up studies of TMI also suggested sustained effects (Baum & Fleming, 1993; Dew & Bromet, 1993; Dew et al., 1987). Other research on Chernobyl described in this book (see Chapters 1 and 3, this volume), as well as a study of exposed and unexposed villagers in a contaminated area of Russia (Viinamaki et al., 1995) also consistently show long-term effects, particularly on somatic symptoms of distress (see also Havenaar & van den Brink, 1997; Havenaar et al., 1997). Indeed, in spite of methodological differences in design, measures, samples, and timing of data collection, the studies are consistent in demonstrating an intractable nature, or persistence, of distress-related symptomatology.

Thus, our data from mothers affected by both TMI and Chernobyl extend earlier findings by showing high levels of subclinical symptoms and a strong relationship between perceptions of danger and poorer mental health 10–11 years after the accident. In the TMI group, those with high levels of anxiety were particularly likely to express accident-related concerns about the plant. To date, public health surveillance programs are monitoring the rates of cancer in the affected population. In light of the apparent long-term psychological effects of these events, we believe that public health programs should monitor the mental health of the affected populations as well.

Finally, there have been very few studies of disasters occurring in non-Western settings even though many of the world's worst disasters occur in third world countries. More research is needed that includes both culture-specific measures and internationally used measures of psychological morbidity and risk factors. The adaptation of Western measures for the Kiev populations afforded us an unprecedented opportunity to compare the responses of similar-aged mothers of young children to these two nuclear power plant accidents. The findings underscore the practical and theoretical importance of understanding the very long-term effects of these technological disasters. As nuclear power plants continue to age and plans for disposal of radioactive waste and nuclear weapons disposal are enacted, the risk perceptions and their mental health consequences will become increasingly important to evaluate in other settings.

ACKNOWLEDGMENTS. The research described in this report was funded by National Institute of Mental Health grants MH35425: The Three Mile Island Accident: Psychiatric Sequelae (E. J. Bromet, principal investigator) and MH51947: Children's Mental Health after the Chernobyl Nuclear Plant Accident (E. J. Bromet, principal investigator).

REFERENCES

Bard, D., Verger, P., & Hubert, P. (1997). Chernobyl, 10 years after: Health consequences. *Epidemiologic Reviews, 19,* 187–204.

Baum, A., & Fleming, I. (1993). Implications of psychological research on stress and technological accidents. *American Psychologist, 48,* 665–672.

Bromet, E. (1998). Psychological effects of radiation catastrophes. In L. E. Peterson & S. Abrahamson (Eds.), *Effects of ionizing radiation: Atomic bomb survivors and their children (1945–1995)* (pp. 283–294). Washington DC: Joseph Henry Press.

Bromet, E. J., & Dew, M. A. (1995). Review of psychiatric epidemiologic research on disasters. *Epidemiologic Reviews, 17,* 113–119.

Bromet, E. J., Goldgaber, D., Carlson, G., Panina, N., Golovakha, E., Gluzman, S. F. et al. (2000). Children's well-being 11 years after the Chernobyl catastrophe. *Archives of General Psychiatry, 57,* 563–571.

Bromet, E. J., Parkinson, D. K., Schulberg, H. C., Dunn, L. O., & Gondek, P. C. (1982). Mental health of residents near the Three Mile Island reactor: A comparative study of selected groups. *Journal of Preventive Psychiatry, 1,* 225–275.

Bromet, E. J., & Schulberg, H. C. (1986). The TMI disaster: A search for high risk groups. In J. H. Shore (Ed.), *Disaster stress studies: New methods and findings* (pp. 2–19). Washington DC: American Psychiatric Press.

Brown, G., & Harris, T. (1978). *Social origins of depression.* New York: Free Press.

Cardis, E. (1996). Epidemiology of accidental radiation exposures. *Environmental Health Perspectives, 104(suppl.)* (3), 643–649.

Cwikel, J., Abdelgani, A., Goldsmith, J. R., Quastel, M., & Yevelson, I. I. (1997). Two-year follow-up study of stress-related disorders among immigrants to Israel from the Chernobyl area. *Environmental Health Perspectives, 105,* 1545–1550.

Davidson, L. M., & Baum, A. (1986). Chronic stress and posttraumatic stress disorders. *Journal of Consulting and Clinical Psychology, 54,* 303–308.

Derogatis, L. R. (1983). *SCL-90-R: Administration, scoring & procedures manual-II.* Towson, MD: Psychometric Research.

Dew, M. A., & Bromet, E. J. (1993). Predictors of temporal patterns of psychiatric distress during 10 years following the nuclear accident at Three Mile Island. *Social Psychiatry and Psychiatric Epidemiology, 28,* 49–55.

Dew, M. A., Bromet, E. J., Schulberg, H. C., Dunn, L. O., & Parkinson, D. K. (1987). Mental health effects of the Three Mile Island nuclear reactor restart. *American Journal of Psychiatry, 144,* 1074–1077.

Dohrenwend, B. P. (1983). Psychological implications of nuclear accidents: The case of Three Mile Island. *Bulletin of the New York Academy of Medicine, 59,* 1060–1076.

Endicott, J., & Spitzer, R. (1978). A diagnostic interview: The Schedule for affective disorders and schizophrenia. *Archives of General Psychiatry, 33,* 766–771.

Feshbach, M., & Friendly, A., Jr. (1992). *Ecocide in the USSR: Health and nature under siege.* New York: Basic Books.

Flynn, C. B. (1981). Local public opinion. In T. H. Moss & D. L. Sills (Eds.), The Three Mile Island nuclear accident: Lessons and implications. *Annals of the New York Academy of Science 365,* 146–158.

Green, B., Lindy, J., Grace, M., Gleser, G. C., Leonard, A. C., Korol, M. et al. (1990). Buffalo Creek survivors in the second decade: Stability of stress symptoms. *American Journal of Orthopsychiatry 60*, 43–54.

Hatch, M. C., Beyea, J., Nieves, J. W., & Susser, M. (1990). Cancer near the Three Mile Island nuclear plant: Radiation emissions. *American Journal of Epidemiology, 132*, 397–412.

Havenaar, J. M., Rumyantzeva, G. M., Vandenbrink, W., Poelijoe, N. W., Vandenbout, J., Vanengeland, H. et al. (1997). Long-term mental health effects of the Chernobyl disaster: An epidemiologic survey in two former Soviet regions. *American Journal of Psychiatry, 154*, 1605–1607.

Havenaar, J. M., & van den Brink, W. (1997). Psychological factors affecting health after toxicological disasters. *Clinical Psychology Review, 17*, 359–374.

Houts, P. S., Cleary, P. D., & Hu, T-W. (1988). *The Three Mile Island crisis: Psychological, social, and economic impacts on the surrounding population.* University Park: Pennsylvania State University Press.

Lifton, R. J. (1967). *Death in life: Survivors of Hiroshima.* New York: Random House.

Litcher, L., Bromet, E. J., Carlson, G., Squires, N., Goldgaber, D., Panina, N. et al. (2000). School and neuropsychological performance of evacuated children in Kiev eleven years after the Chernobyl disaster. *Journal of Child Psychiatry and Psychology, 41*, 219–299.

McFarlane, A., Policansky, S., & Irwin, C. (1987). A longitudinal study of the psychological morbidity in children due to a natural disaster. *Psychological Medicine, 17*, 727–738.

Misao, T., Hattori, K., Shirakawa, M., Suga, M., Ogawa, N., Ohara, Y. et al. (1961). Characteristics in abnormalities observed in atom-bombed survivors. *Journal of Radiation Research, 2*, 85–97.

Nikiforov, Y., Gnepp, D. R., & Fagin, J. A. (1996). Thyroid lesions in children and adolescents after the Chernobyl disaster: Implications for the study of radiation tumorigenesis. *Journal of Clinical Endocrinology and Metabolism, 81*, 9–14.

Phelan, J., Schwartz, J. E., Bromet, E. J., Dew, M. A., Parkinson, D. K., Schulberg, H. C. et al. (1991). Work stress, family stress and depression in professional and managerial employees. *Psychological Medicine, 21*, 999–1012.

Spitzer, R., Endicott, J., & Robins, E. (1978). Research diagnostic criteria: Rationale and reliability. *Archives of General Psychiatry 35*, 773–782.

Stiehm, E. R. (1992). The psychologic fallout from Chernobyl. *American Journal of Diseases of Children, 146*, 761–762.

Tarabrina, N., Lazebnaya, E., Zelenova, M., & Lasko, N. (1996). Chernobyl clean-up workers' perception of radiation threat. *Radiation Protection Dosimetry, 68*, 251–255.

Viinamäki, H., Kumpusalo, E., Myllykangas, M., Salomaa, S., Kumpusalo, L., Kolmakov, S. et al. (1995). The Chernobyl accident and mental wellbeing—a population study. *Acta Psychiatrica Scandinavica, 91*, 396–401.

Whitcomb, R. C., & Sage, M. (1997). Nuclear reactor incidents. In E. K. Noji (Ed.), *The public health consequences of disasters* (pp. 397–418). New York: Oxford University Press.

Yamada, M., Kodama, K., & Wong, F. L. (1991). The long-term psychological sequelae of atomic-bomb survivors in Hiroshima and Nagasaki. In R. Ricks, M. E. Berger, & R. M. O'Hara (Eds.), *The medical basis for radiation preparedness III: The psychological perspective* (pp. 155–163). New York: Elsevier.

Yevelson, I. I., Abdelgani, A., Cwikel, J., & Yevelson, I. S. (1997). Bridging the gap in mental health approaches between East and West: The psychosocial consequences of radiation exposure. *Environmental Health Perspectives, 105(suppl.)* (6), 1551–1556.

5

The Chaotic Aftermath of an Airplane Crash in Amsterdam

A Second Disaster

JORIS YZERMANS and BERTHOLD P. R. GERSONS

INTRODUCTION

At the time of the 1992 Bijlmermeer plane crash, no one would have dreamt that more than 6 years after the event, the entire country would be glued to the television to witness the demise of what could only be characterized as a chaotic aftermath of the disaster. In 1998, the Dutch Parliament decided to organize a Parliamentary inquiry to determine the causes and consequences of the crash and its possible ramifications for public health. An inquiry committee was appointed, exhaustive investigations were launched, and public hearings were broadcast on primetime national television. Half a million viewers followed the 6 weeks of "the Bijlmer Inquiry"—named after the Bijlmermeer district of Amsterdam—where the crash occurred. Front pages were filled with pictures and reports of breathtaking interrogations. The climax came when an air traffic controller testified that he

JORIS YZERMANS • Academic Medical Center/University of Amsterdam, Division Public Health, Department of General Practice. 3500 BN Utrecht, The Netherlands. BERTHOLD P. R. GERSONS • Academic Medical Center/University of Amsterdam/de Meren Department of Psychiatry, 1100 DD Amsterdam, The Netherlands.

Toxic Turmoil: Psychological and Societal Consequences of Ecological Disasters, edited by Johan M. Havenaar, Julie G. Cwikel, and Evelyn J. Bromet. New York, Kluwer Academic/Plenum Publishers, 2002.

had been instructed shortly after the crash to keep information about lethal substances that were possibly on board the cargo airplane "under his hat." Although this statement was later proven to be false, rescue workers had not been warned at the time to take extra precautions. Since that day, the expression "keeping something under your hat" has become part of the everyday household vernacular. It captured the widespread conviction that information was deliberately being withheld.

Disasters are not only characterized by the death and destruction they inflict, but also by their traumatic effects on survivors, eyewitnesses, and rescue workers. Similar traumatic effects have been observed after combat experiences, peacekeeping operations, and other UN missions.

The purpose of this chapter is to reconstruct the events of the Amsterdam airplane crash and to analyze them specifically from the mental and public health perspectives. We will examine the chronology of events and the narratives that accompanied them. Then, we will tentatively offer explanatory models for the uncontrolled aftermath of the crash and will attempt to draw some conclusions and lessons for the future.

FACTS AND CHRONOLOGY

The First Period (1992–1994)

On October 4, 1992, an El Al Boeing 747 cargo jet lost two engines from its right wing without being noticed by the crew. The captain, confronted with his airplane being out of control, decided to return to Schiphol Airport but the plane crashed onto two apartment buildings in Amsterdam's densely populated Bijlmermeer district, also known as "the Bijlmer." At a time when most people were enjoying their evening meal, the tranquillity of the late summer Sunday was transformed into a horrific inferno. Buildings were obliterated and human beings incinerated in the towering sea of flames that arose from the tanks of the jumbo jet. Some 39 residents and 4 crew members lost their lives. An enormous rescue operation got under way to combat the blaze and bring the survivors to safety. The nearby Bijlmer sports hall was taken over to provide initial relief to the survivors.

Remarkably enough, very few of the survivors had suffered immediate physical injuries from the crash. Hundreds of doctors and nurses at the Amsterdam Academic Medical Center (AMC), University of Amsterdam, only a few miles away, were on duty throughout the evening without having to provide services.

This first period was characterized by the issues who did it and what caused it. Journalists asked a lot of questions why a damaged plane was allowed to try to return to Schiphol Airport over a densely populated city and did not, for instance, attempt a forced landing on a nearby lake (the IJsselmeer). When the rubble was cleared at the end of the week, the final count of victims proved to be far lower than had been feared. Initially, estimates of some 1,500 victims were calculated. When the total figure of 43 victims was established after one week, rumors mounted that numerous illegal foreigners, living in the apartment buildings, had presumably died out of view of public knowledge. Likewise, there were rumors about victims who had been totally incinerated. After a few weeks of public debate and wild guessing about the actual number of victims, a general pardon was granted by the Dutch government to all illegal foreigners who could prove they lived in the buildings concerned. This paved the way for illegal aliens to come forward and report the loss of relatives and friends and eventually led to the final estimated death toll. At that time, little attention was given to the third issue, namely what hit us.

As the public debate subsided, relief work and aftercare services were implemented. The bulk of the initial relief work consisted of arranging for shelter for those who had lost their homes and financial support for those who needed it. The Salvation Army, churches, and residents' organizations set up support facilities for the dazed survivors and eyewitnesses of the disaster. The following Sunday, 10,000 people took part in a silent march in the Bijlmermeer, and a memorial ceremony—in the presence of Queen Beatrix and the prime minister—was held in a large hall elsewhere in the city.

The emphasis in the relief work soon shifted toward the psychological aftereffects of the disaster. Based on the state of the art at the time, a campaign was launched in the media and leaflets were distributed in many languages to inform people about post-traumatic stress disorder (PTSD). General practitioners and mental health care professionals were instructed about potential psychological effects. The slogan "A normal reaction to an abnormal event" was coined to prepare people for the impending psychological aftereffects and simultaneously to reassure them that such effects were normal. The implicit expectation was that long-term psychological damage would be limited by this short-term "normalization" of the emotional responses. The Southeast Amsterdam Institute for Community Mental Health Care (RIAGG) promptly set up a direct intervention program for the victims and was also active in providing care to children in local schools. The Amsterdam Municipal Health Service (GG&GD) coordinated the provision of aftercare and deployed professionals to make home visits and to look after victims who were relocated to houses farther away. The AMC took charge of the public education campaign and the training and instruction of professionals. In addition, the Department of Psychiatry AMC initiated research into the effects of the disaster on the victims and eyewitnesses and on the care provided to police officers.

The combined effect of all these efforts was that several hundred adults and children received some form of trauma intervention. The estimated total number of people who had directly experienced the crash, including rescue workers who had come into the area during the early hours after the crash, was somewhere between 1,000 and 1,500. A research convenience sample of 340 of the affected population was assembled six months after the crash. The sample was composed of volunteers who experienced the crash at close range; they were given monetary compensation for participating in the research. It was not possible to create a random sample because of Dutch legislation on individual privacy. Eighteen months after the crash, 136 of the 340 subjects were selected for a follow-up interview, including 73 individuals with 0–5 post-traumatic stress (PTS) symptoms and 63 individuals with 6 or more PTS symptoms (Table 5.1).

Respondents' post-traumatic stress reactions were expressed in two diagnoses: PTSD and partial PTSD. A structured diagnostic interview for PTSD was conducted; this so-called PTSD interview addressed the 17 PTSD-symptoms according to DSM-III-R. The term partial PTSD refers to cases in which respondents had PTS symptoms but did not meet criteria for all three of the required symptom clusters (Carlier & Gersons, 1995).

These findings resulted in several recommendations in 1993, none of which was acted upon at the time. When the report of the inquiry committee was debated in Parliament in June 1999, these recommendations were repeatedly cited (Carlier & Gersons 1997; Carlier, van Uchelen, Lamberts, & Gersons, 1993; Carlier, van Uchelen, Lamberts, & Gersons, 1995; Gersons & Carlier, 1993, 1994; Yzermans et al., 1999):

1. *Information about the aftercare of victims.* It is important to inform victims about all available services (victim and peer support), for example in a leaflet.

2. *Central information point.* It is very important to have a central advise and information point. All possible victims should be made aware of its existence and it should be operational for several years. It should be outreaching and inform victims about all relevant issues. A small newspaper could be distributed regularly to keep victims informed.

3. *Monitoring.* Long-term monitoring of aftercare provision is essential. It is also important to monitor (developments in) health problems, preferably using existing registration systems and databases.

4. *Mental health care provision following disasters.* A large proportion of the survivors had persistent, chronic PTSD. In most cases, treatment had been too brief and too discontinuous to achieve a satisfactory outcome. Moreover, PTSD often does not stand alone in the diagnosis, but occurs in combination with other disorders. It is important for

both the referring general practitioners and for the care providers at the receiving end, to know that is taking care for medical costs for victims of a disaster. Victims do not always find their way to mental health services (see 1 and 2).

5. *Peer support.* Many victims were offered dwellings outside the area, so they could avoid a daily confrontation with the disaster scene. However, many of them missed the ease of bumping into friends and acquaintances in the well-known "ethnic subculture," and years later, many of them moved back to the area.

6. *Financial problems.* An emergency fund has to be established for long-term problems to which people could apply.

Despite the fact that the wide range of opportunities to receive care offered to the public was generally considered to be quite satisfactory, this did not result in a low rate of post-traumatic stress reactions. The percentage of respondents with PTSD remained virtually unchanged across the two waves of assessment, and the needs for psychological help were greater than the care that was actually utilized. Although the large majority of respondents did make use of mental health care at some time, treatments were often terminated prematurely, notably because of financial constraints or perceived ineffectiveness of the treatments.

It is also unclear to what degree the emotional disturbances were partly attributable to a disruption of the social environment. Beyond all the emotional distress brought on by the loss of friends or relatives, for many of the victims the disaster also meant the loss of an entire subculture that was characteristic of the Bijlmermeer. The Bijlmermeer neighborhood consists of 90,000 people originating from 50 different countries, especially Surinam, the Netherlands Antilles, and Ghana. Once removed from this subculture, many victims were thrown into social isolation, at least temporarily, which was exacerbated by the emotional problems. In addition, some victims suffered from other mental disorders that may or may not have been trauma related. Indeed, our data showed that most such respondents had already experienced psychological problems *before* the disaster.

One tenth of our respondents (Carlier, van Uchelen, & Gersons, 1995) saw their claims for compensation of psychological damage denied by Boeing, the aircraft manufacturer. The reasons given were that the respondent had not been at home on the evening of the crash or had "lived outside the disaster area as defined by Boeing" (the so-called danger zone). Also not eligible for compensation were people who had experienced the crash from very nearby (eye- and earwitnesses) but who lived outside the official danger zone. On the whole, little is actually known about the association between the severity of illness in victims and the honoring or denial of damage claims.

Table 5.1 Shifts in Estimated Number of Victims, Study Aims, and Main Health Problems Reported/Investigated Over Time

Period	Estimated number of victims at the time	Type of study	N	Sample characteristics	Main results[1]
Immediately after crash (October 1992)	1,000–1,500 (figures from local authorities)	counting	90,000	39 residents and 4 crew members died	Not applicable
April 1993	1,000–1,500 (not counted since 1992)	Convenience sample among people who experienced the crash at close range (N = 136; a selection of the cohort N = 340)	136	57% men; 43% women; mean age 35 years (SD 12.6)	26% PTSD 44% partial PTSD
April 1994	1,000–1,500 (not counted since 1992)	See April 1993	115	59% men; 41% women; mean age 36 years (SD 11.8)	24% PTSD 32% partial PTSD
June–July 1998	1,000–1,500 (not counted since 1992)	Interviews among 52 GPs in region (Amsterdam SE)	90,000 patients on the list	Not applicable	Some 300 patients presented symptoms possibly related to the crash (psychological and unspecified problems)

| June–July 1998 | 1,000–1,500 (not counted since 1992) | Exploratory telephone survey to assess health effects attributed to the crash among people who phoned open call center | 846 | 66% men; 34% women; mean age 42 years (SD 12) 39% residing in apartments concerned, 12% in neighbourhood and 49% elsewhere | 3,463 symptoms presented (mean 4.1, SD 2.9) Five clusters of symptoms: General unspecified 77% Psychological 42% Respiratory 33% Skin 25% Musculoskeletal 22% |
| March–April 1999 | 6,280 | Registered for large-scale physical examinations | | 42% residents 52% rescue workers 6% Schiphol Airport/KLM | In progress |

¹See text for case definitions and method of assessment.

The *persistence* of the post-traumatic stress reactions has major implications for relief work and aftercare in the wake of future disasters. It was concluded that the persistence of PTSD for as long as 18 months after the disaster may have been related to a variety of adverse circumstances that subsequently arose, as covered in the next section. These could have caused the victims' symptoms to worsen and greatly impeded them in dealing with the trauma effectively (see also Groenjian et al., 1995). Furthermore, the mental health interventions provided to many victims were much too short in duration to achieve any lasting result, did not follow an explicit protocol, and, in many cases, did not prove to be effective even in the short term.

Several lessons were learned from this period: Victims repeatedly need to be provided with information. The trauma interventions themselves should focus on how to cope with symptoms over a much longer period. Mental health care services, in particular, need to prepare themselves for prolonged emotional distress in a large percentage of the victim population. Care professionals should receive more thorough instruction about the appropriate actions to take, the appropriate treatments to give, and the most effective ways of dealing with the symptoms over an extended period.

The Second Period (1995–1999)

The preceding period was dominated by the interactions between post-traumatic symptoms and psychosocial problems in the wake of the airplane disaster. The second period was no longer characterized by determining the causes of the accident or the number of victims, but by growing suspicions about the plane's cargo and the potentially harmful *physical* effects this might have had on victims and rescue workers. The black boxes, containing cockpit voice recorders and data flight recorders, were never found, which is very unusual in an accident on the ground. Rumors started about men in white "space suits"—Mossad agents it was assumed—who, within 30 minutes after the crash, took things from the crash scene and disappeared in a helicopter. The initial information on the cargo (e.g., flowers, computers, and perfume) had been based on an incomplete list. Extensive detective work by journalists revealed that the plane had also been fitted with depleted uranium in its tail, as a counterweight. The next discovery was that the plane had even contained military goods, among them the chemical dimethylmethylphosphonate (DMMP), a component of the nerve gas Sarin. Such reports, coupled with the Dutch and Israeli government's inability to produce the full cargo specifications, greatly stirred the fears of Bijlmermeer residents and rescue workers. Action groups were set up, which launched their own investigation of toxic substances and radioactivity. Some of the worried residents and rescue workers publicly aired their physical complaints, such as skin rashes, respiratory problems, and fatigue, linking these to their presence at the disaster scene. Similar concerns arose among employees of Schiphol Airport who had worked in a hangar where the plane's wreckage had been stored. Tests carried out in the hangar detected slightly elevated levels of ionizing radiation near the wreckage.

A virtually unstoppable, tragic chain of events ensued, in which the public authorities (at least in the perceptions of the general public) responded too slowly and were too uncoordinated, at times even supplying factually incorrect information. Meanwhile, one of the action groups, named Visie (Vision) attempted to collect information on its own. It commissioned a Swedish laboratory to test the blood and feces of the victims and rescue workers for traces of uranium. Suspicions toward the authorities grew when this private investigation revealed traces of depleted uranium in the subjects' feces. Even though the scientific community was quick to point out the shortcoming of the Swedish study (e.g., there was no mention of a control group or other reference data and at least one of the subjects used antacids), the result was that information from the government was no longer trusted.

At this point, it seemed that everybody was making some contribution to the uproar. Specifically individuals attributed their medical problems to the crash; tenacious journalists were determined to leave no stone unturned and often generalized from individual cases; and members of Parliament put the matter back on the political agenda after several years of neglect.

By 1997, so many press reports about physical complaints attributable to the crash had appeared that the national chief health care inspector commissioned the AMC to conduct an investigation into the health problems. The study was headed by a professor from the Department of Psychiatry, who directed the previous study of the psychological consequences in residents and rescue workers (BPRG). The hospital appointed a team of investigators who initially considered performing a comprehensive clinical screening of the victim population. In the discussions that followed, the team concluded that such action should not be taken until it was certain that the cargo had contained toxic substances, since that information was required for any focused physical examination. Another methodological problem was the specific number of victims and rescue workers was unknown.

Therefore, because it was impossible to conduct a targeted epidemiological or toxicological investigation, the research team decided first to conduct an exploratory study focused on describing the number of persons who attributed their health complaints to the disaster and the nature of those complaints.

The following method was used: In the Netherlands, every citizen is required to be on the list of *one* general practitioner who acts as a gatekeeper to specialist care. Therefore, it was reasoned that an increase in morbidity in the stricken area should be apparent in their medical files. General practitioners (GPs) in the Bijlmermeer were interviewed to see whether they had noticed an increase in disaster-related illnesses. In addition, a toll-free call center was opened for 2 months to enable people to report their health symptoms. The Symptom Checklist-90 (SCL-90) was sent to all people who presented their complaints to the call center. Analysis of the data so obtained would help to answer the question of whether a focused physical examination was advisable. As an additional precaution, after obtaining informed consent, the medical files of the people who called the toll-free center and completed the SCL-90 were checked to determine whether the GPs were informed about the health complaints.

The AMC call center was open in June and July 1998. A total of 903 people phoned the line, 846 of whom presented at least one health problem attributed to the disaster (Table 5.1). The nature of the health problems pointed exclusively to PTSD and to medically unexplained physical symptoms. A doctor was visited for the majority of the health problems. According to the medical files, 13% of the health problems were already known to the general practitioner before the crash in 1992. On the other hand, 15% of the health problems originated in the previous 6 months and, in total, 60% originated in what we call "the second period." The results of the SCL-90 showed a lot of distress (2 standard deviations higher than a Dutch reference population on average. The five symptom clusters bore a striking resemblance to the so-called Gulf War syndrome and were classified as "unexplained physical symptoms," suggesting a possible psychological origin.

The AMC concluded that these results gave no grounds to proceed with medical screening of the victims: no specific pattern of symptoms was detected, and 87% of the problems were treated by (AMC-)doctors. Its primary recommendation was that the general practitioners should devote special attention to patients with PTSD. A special protocol-based treatment program (state of the art in 1999) was set up for PTSD. A few weeks later the parliamentary inquiry committee presented their results (Eindrapport Bijlmermeer Enquête, 1999), in which, finally, the complete cargo list was published: no unknown toxic substances were aboard the plane.

Despite this, further intense political pressure induced KLM Arbo Services—the department that monitors working conditions at the airline—to conduct a large-scale physical examination of the affected population. At the time of this writing this is still in progress. It is hoped that this will finally allay the fears of the residents and rescue workers.

DISCUSSION

Clearly the Bijlmermeer plane crash was a unique and instructive experience for the Netherlands in many ways. The uniqueness lay especially in the two distinct periods in the crash's aftermath. The initial disaster relief

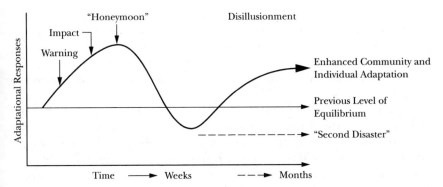

Figure 5.1. Phases of response to a disaster. *Source:* B. Raphael, *When disaster strikes: A Handbook for the Caring Professions.* Boston: Unwin Hyman, 1986, p. 8.

period, focused on the post-traumatic effects, was followed by a second period of deepening mistrust, centering around what was commonly called unexplained physical symptoms (Barsky & Borus, 1999; Havenaar & van den Brink, 1997; Wessely, Nimnuan, & Sharpe, 1999). A virtually unmanageable political crisis resulted, which seriously undermined public confidence in the government.

On the basis of our knowledge of PTSD and disaster psychology, we would like to suggest some possible explanations for the uncontrolled aftereffects of the crash. Several different adaptational phases can be distinguished in the aftermath of a disaster: a warning phase in specific conditions as tornadoes; an impact phase, a "honeymoon" phase (including the so-called cry-out phase), a disillusionment phase, and finally, what we will add, a reintegration phase (Figure 5.1).

The impact phase is the 24–36–hour period of recoil and shock immediately following the disaster, in which the urge to survive is paramount. This is followed by a cry-out phase characterized by a need to talk at length about the experience and give vent to rage and grief. This gives rise to a feeling of intense solidarity among survivors and other people involved in the disaster. For this reason, it is also called the "honeymoon" phase. In the wake of the Bijlmermeer crash, such solidarity could be seen in the silent march and the national memorial ceremony. The disillusionment phase is reached when the nonvictims resume their normal lives. Victims feel cut off from the solidarity and compassion. Bureaucratic structures, which had temporarily geared themselves to respond flexibly to the victims' needs, shut themselves off again and return to the formal procedures in place before the disaster. The difficulty then is whether the authorities and care organizations are still able to provide enough services to minimize the victims' feeling of rejection. We therefore recommend that an advice and information center must be kept open for an extended period, to coordinate the response to the victims' problems. Victims in this phase can easily turn into complainers. The suspicion promptly arises that they are using lawyers and insurance companies to "exploit their victimhood." This has been described as secondary victimization. First they fall victim to the disaster, then they are stigmatized as profiteers.

Figure 5.1 clearly illustrates how a "second disaster" occurred after the Bijlmermeer crash. A process of collective secondary victimization was set in motion, and the authorities and care services lost control of it. It was this second disaster that ultimately led to the parliamentary inquiry. By that time, restoring public confidence and achieving "enhanced community adaptation" had become virtually impossible tasks for the government.

It is also important to assess the course of events in light of what is now known about the etiology of PTSD. Characteristic of PTSD is a perceived loss of control. The accustomed sense of security has vanished. The victim fears being struck by a new calamity. PTSD, which probably plagued many of the victims to a greater or lesser extent, is characterized by symptoms such as reexperiencing, hypervigilance, and poor concentration. The last two symptoms are curious, because victims are sharply alert to danger but have trouble focusing on more trivial matters. This all leads to sleep disturbances and intense fatigue. Presumably such complaints are perpetuated by feelings of rage about what has happened and by feelings of grief—not only at the loss of loved ones, but at the destruction of a life perspective and fundamental sense of security. Another common symptom is the emotional volatility of both the victims and many of the people affected by the disaster's aftermath. In short, emotions prevail over reason. The parliamentary inquiry was a clear reflection of such a phenomenon. Even the parliamentarians themselves came under the spell of emotions. They took on the rage of the victims, and somebody had to be blamed. Both authors testified under oath, one to explain the state of the art of diagnosing and treating PTSD, the other to explain the preliminary results of the AMC exploratory study. They, and the AMC staff with them, were also the center of criticism by victims, action groups, lawyers, and colleagues in the scientific community. They were put under considerable political pressure to conduct medical screening of the victims who they did not judge to be desirable from a scientific or clinical point of view.

The aftermath of the Bijlmermeer crash also teaches us a third lesson. Beyond the post-traumatic complaints that arise from the acute stress of a disaster, a number of studies have also shown that *chronic* stress can arise out of a persistent fear of bodily harm from exposure to noxious stimuli such as radiation or poisons (Carlier & Gersons, 1995; Havenaar & van den Brink, 1997). The chronic anxiety is then maintained by nagging suspicion and the spread of physical symptoms. Although the Gulf War produced a minimum of fatal casualties for U.S. forces, many soldiers returned home with "unexplained physical complaints" quite similar to those reported to the AMC call center by the Bijlmermeer victims. In British veterans the threat of SCUD missiles containing poison gas was found to be a risk factor for unexplained symptoms (Unwin et al., 1999).

Persons who are exposed to traumatic events, report (nonspecific) psychological and general physical symptoms that stem from a comparable, restricted symptom repertoire. Similar symptoms are reported following different types of traumatic events, civil and military, among victims and rescue workers. In our opinion, the common factor across these incidents is an ineffective and/or disconnected response by authorities that leads to chronic stress-related health problems.

Persons suffering from medically unexplained symptoms confront the health care services with a difficult problem. Patients demand a physical explanation for their illness. Although the doctors tell them time and again that they do not have any "real" disease, the information seldom reassures them and their symptoms usually persist. They must have a disease, and if the doctors can't find it, the suspicions continue to gnaw. The victims fear they are being "psychologised." Despite the frequent use of the words "trauma" and "stress" in the public debate, the mental health care sector stood conspicuously on the sidelines during the aftermath of the Bijlmermeer crash. To make matters worse, prominent spokespeople for the victims reacted angrily at any attempt to give psychological explanations for their physical complaints. To say that their physical ailments were "in their heads" was similar to not taking them seriously. The inquiry committee implicitly acknowledged that psychological factors were behind the health complaints, but shied from actually stating so. Rarely has such an abrupt line been drawn between body and mind in a public debate.

A special role was fulfilled by the media. There was a tendency to produce more fears than facts, suggesting that people were exposed, resulting in major health effects. On television, 7 years after the crash, even in 30-second items, images of the inferno were shown (many persons told the interviewers of the call center this to be untenable). Individual cases were generalized, and "new" diseases and syndromes were discovered and attributed to the disaster. A few individuals (members of action groups, lawyers, and members of Parliament) were asked to comment on nearly everything, often unprepared. In some cases, when the news turned out to be false, no rectifications were published.

In every respect, the events that followed the Bijlmermeer plane crash culminated in a second disaster. Patterns of acute and chronic stress brought forth an amalgam of psychological and physical complaints. The parliamentary inquiry on the disaster functioned as a mirror, reflecting the unresolved emotions left behind by the disaster and all the uncertainties that arose in its aftermath. The phenomenon of loss of control was observable not only in the victims themselves. It manifested itself in public institutions, health care organizations, media, national and local authorities, the health ministry, and the Parliament. Stopping a downward spiral like this one costs many times the amount of money and effort that would be required for early interventions to restore the disaster victims' sense of control. Besides taking the belated steps that are still needed today to overcome the lingering consequences of the Bijlmer crash, we should avoid unnecessary mistakes in future. For caregivers and for the authorities it does not hurt to be alert. For patients suffering from PTSD, on the contrary, it hurts to be alert. On a societal level the aftermath of the Bijlmermeer crash may be interpreted as a lack of balance between hypervigilance (on the part of victims and their advocates, including the media) and denial and repression, later also followed by hypervigilance and outcry in other sections of society.

In May 2000 the Netherlands was visited by another disaster: In the city of Enschede, a depot of fireworks exploded sweeping away a neighborhood in the center of the city, killing 22 persons and wounding another 1,000 people. In the aftercare of this disaster, authorities try to put in practice the lessons learned from the Bijlmermeer crash, in which the recommendations delineated earlier in the chapter played an important role.

REFERENCES

Barsky, A. J., & Borus, J. F. (1999). Functional somatic syndromes. *Annals of Internal Medicine; 130*, 910–921.

Carlier, I. V. E., & Gersons, B. P. R. (1995). Partial posttraumatic stress disorder (PTSD): The issue of psychological scars and the occurrence of PTSD symptoms. *Journal of Nervous and Mental Disease, 183*, 107–109.

Carlier, I. V. E., & Gersons, B. P. R. (1997). Stress reactions in disaster victims following the Bijlmermeer plane crash. *Journal of Traumatic Stress, 10*, 329–335.

Carlier, I. V. E., Lamberts, R. D., van Uchelen, A. J., & Gersons, B. P. R. (1998). Disaster-related post-traumatic stress in police officers: A field study of the impact of debriefing. *Stress Medicine, 14*, 143–148.

Carlier, I. V. E., van Uchelen, J. J., Lamberts, R. D., & Gersons, B. P. R. (1993). *De Bijlmervliegramp. Een onderzoek naar de psychische gevolgen bij getroffenen en hun commentaar op de geboden nazorg*. Internal report, Academic Medical Centre, University of Amsterdam, Department of Psychiatry.

Carlier, I. V. E., van Uchelen, A. J., & Gersons, B. P. R. (1995). *De Bijlmermeer-vliegramp; een vervolgonderzoek naar de lange termijn psychische gevolgen en de nazorg bij getroffenen*. Academic Medical Center, University of Amsterdam, Department of Psychiatry.

Carlier, I. V. E., van Uchelen, J. J., Lamberts, R. D., & Gersons, B. P. R. (1995). *Het langetermijn effect van debriefen. Een vervolgonderzoek bij de Amsterdamse politie naar aanleiding van de Bijlmerramp*. Internal report, Academic Medical Center, University of Amsterdam, Psychiatry Division, Psychotrauma Group.

Eindrapport Bijlmermeer Enquête. (1999). *Een beladen vlucht.* The Hague: Sdu.

Gersons, B. P. R., & Carlier, I. V. E. (1993). Plane crash crisis intervention: A preliminary report from the Bijlmermeer, Amsterdam. *Journal of Crisis Intervention and Suicide Prevention, 14,* 109–116.

Gersons, B. P. R., & Carlier, I. V. E. (1994). Treatment of work related trauma in police officers: Posttraumatic stress disorder and post-traumatic decline. In M. B. Williams & J. F. Sommer, *Handbook of post-traumatic therapy* (pp. 325–333). Westport, CT: Greenwood.

Goenjian, A. K., Pynoos, R. S., Steinberg, A. M., Najarian, L. M., Asarnow, J. R., Karayan, I. et al. (1995). Psychiatric comorbidity in children after the 1988 earthquake in Armenia. *Journal of the American Academy of Child Psychiatry, 34,* 1174–1183.

Havenaar, J., & van den Brink, W. (1997). Psychological factors affecting health after toxicological disasters. *Clinical Psychology Review, 17,* 359–374.

Raphael, B. (1986). *When disaster strikes: A handbook for the caring professions.* Boston: Unwin Hyman.

Unwin, C., Blatchley, N., Coker, W., Ferry, S., Hotopf, M., Hull, L. et al. (1999). Health of UK servicemen who served in Persian Gulf War. *Lancet, 353,* 169–178.

Wessely, S., Nimnuan, C., & Sharpe, M. (1999). Functional somatic syndromes: One or many? *Lancet, 354,* 936–939.

Yzermans, C. J., van der Zee, J., Oosterhek, M., Spreeuwenberg, P., Kerssens, J., Donker, G. et al. (1999). *Gezondheidsklachten en de vliegramp Bijlmermeer: een inventariserend onderzoek naar aard en omvang van, volgens mensen en/of huisartsen aan de ramp gerelateerde klachten.* Amsterdam: AMC/Utrecht:Nivel.

6

The Gulf War and Its Aftermath

SIMON WESSELY

Last year marked the 10th anniversary of Operation Desert Storm, the start of the Persian Gulf War. The facts are clear. Iraq occupied Kuwait on August 2, 1990. Shortly after, Coalition Forces, led by the United States, began a military deployment known as Operation Desert Shield. On January 17, 1991, an active air campaign began against Iraq, Operation Desert Storm, and on February 24 a ground war began, lasting only four days. For the Coalition it was a military success. Iraqi forces were beaten in the field and expelled from Kuwait. The main contributor to the Coalition was the United States, with 697,000 personnel. Substantial contributions also came from the United Kingdom (53,000), Saudi Arabia, Egypt, Oman, France, Syria, Kuwait, Pakistan, Canada, Bahrain, Morocco, and Qatar. Twenty-five other countries also contributed smaller numbers.

Not only was the campaign a military success, it was also a medical success. It is only during the modern era that deaths from battle have exceeded deaths from disease for most armies. Traditionally, fighting in hostile environments such as the desert has been associated with morbidity and mortality, often substantial, from causes not related to enemy action such as heat stroke, dehydration, and infectious disease. Yet during the Gulf campaign

SIMON WESSELY • On behalf of the King's College Gulf War Illness Research Unit: Anthony David, Kate Davies, Lydia Farrin, Matthew Hotopf, Lisa Hull, Khalida Ismail, Edgar Jones, Ian Palmer, Steven Reid, Catherine Unwin. Guy's King's and St. Thomas' School of Medicine, London, SE5 8AF, United Kingdom.

Toxic Turmoil: Psychological and Societal Consequences of Ecological Disasters, edited by Johan M. Havenaar, Julie G. Cwikel, and Evelyn J. Bromet. New York, Kluwer Academic/Plenum Publishers, 2002.

there is no evidence of any deaths from those sources among American or British personnel (Hyams, Hanson, Wignall, Escamilla, & Oldfield, 1995). Hence, the military medical authorities must have ended the campaign relieved not to have had to deal with large-scale casualties and delighted with the success of their preventive measures.

GULF WAR SYNDROME

Now more than ten years later those achievements, both military and medical, have become tarnished. Military success was not reflected by political change—Saddam Hussein remains firmly in charge of Iraq. Few will remember the genuine medical achievements of the campaign, and instead most people when asked about the Gulf War and health, will answer "ah yes, that's where Gulf War syndrome began."

It was shortly after the cessation of hostilities that reports started to emerge from the United States of clusters of unusual illnesses occurring among Gulf War veterans. Claims were made that previously fit veterans had developed unusual diseases, illnesses, and symptoms. Reports emerged also of children with birth defects being born to Gulf War veterans.

These reports were invariably anecdotal and impressionistic. Details remain obscure—when many of these clusters were formally investigated there was no objective evidence of any new illness, or alternatively it could not be shown that these represented anything more than normally occurring conditions. Meanwhile, formal epidemiological research was at last commissioned (vide infra), but by the time these studies had started to report, Gulf War syndrome had captured the public imagination.

Long before the machinery of scientific research had rolled into action, Gulf War syndrome had been the focus of a remarkable barrage of publicity and media attention. We have found it impossible to document the number and range of this coverage, but there can be no doubt that the Gulf War syndrome became a media cause célèbre on both sides of the Atlantic.

In this chapter we put forward a tentative explanation of Gulf War–related illnesses. We will argue for the importance of three related factors. The first factor we propose are the events of the Gulf War itself. We argue that the initial trigger for Gulf-related illnesses were the peculiar hazards of modern warfare and the methods used to protect troops from such hazards. We give particular prominence to the threat of chemical and biological warfare and the methods used to reduce that threat.

The second factor relates to events after the conflict and the interaction among the media, government, and military, which served to foster a climate of suspicion and rumor. The third factor we propose links the particular hazards of modern warfare to Western contemporary societal attitudes on environmental risks and concerns. Many of the hazards encountered during the Gulf campaign had resonances with a common, and often passionate, societal agenda, which gave the narratives of the Gulf veterans a particular resonance and link to wider civilian concerns

THE EVIDENCE SO FAR

The Results of the Case Studies

The first coordinated response to the problem was to invite any veteran with health problems to come forward for detailed medical evaluation. This began in the United States and was then repeated in the United Kingdom with the establishment of the Medical Assessment Programme (MAP).

There have now been several analyses of those attending these programs, which now amount to over 2,000 in the United Kingdom and more than 40 times that number in the United States. The results have not suggested any unusual pattern of illness—instead the largest diagnostic category has been medically unexplained symptoms and syndromes (Coker, Bhatt, Blatchley, & Graham, 1999; Joseph, 1997; Roy, Koslowe, Kroenke, & Magruder, 1998).

Such evaluations can only give limited information because of their nonrandom selection. However, one would expect that if service in the Gulf was associated with either disease new to medical science (as with the first appearance of AIDS at the beginning of the 1980s), or a dramatic elevation of a recognized but hitherto rare condition, then this would have been detected. Neither has happened.

The Results of the Studies II: Epidemiology

The most comprehensive analyses have been made of the mortality of both the U.S. and UK Gulf cohorts. The results show that, contrary to media reports, there has been no increase in mortality in either cohort (Kang & Bullman, 1996; MacFarlane, Thomas, & Cherry, 2000), other than an increase in accidental death (U.S. and UK) or suicide (U.S. only) as observed in the aftermath of other conflicts (Boyle, Decoufle, & O'Brien, 1989).

The first epidemiological study of Gulf-related illness was a questionnaire-based study of a random sample of Gulf veterans and appropriate military controls from the state of Iowa (Iowa Persian Gulf Study Group, 1997). This showed increased rates of symptom reporting in the Gulf cohort. Symptom-defined conditions ranging from chronic fatigue syndrome, depression, post-traumatic stress disorder, and others were all elevated.

In our UK study we compared a random sample of 4,246 UK Gulf War veterans, drawn from all three armed services branches, including both serving and nonserving, with similar numbers of nondeployed personnel ("ERA"), but also with an active duty control group—namely members of the UK armed forces who had served in the difficult and dangerous environment of Bosnia from the start of the UN peacekeeping mission (1992–1997; Unwin et al., 1999).

The results were striking. UK Gulf veterans were between two and three times more likely to report each and every one of the 50 symptoms that were inquired about. Whatever the symptom, the rate was at least twice as high in the Gulf cohort than either the nondeployed cohort or the Bosnia cohort. Self-rated health was substantially decreased in the Gulf cohort, but physical functioning was only very slightly decreased and still above expected nonmilitary norms. Hence, the Gulf veterans experienced more symptoms, endorsed more conditions, felt worse, but were still physically functioning better as a group than either the nondeployed cohort or those deployed to an unpleasant and stressful Bosnia (Unwin et al., 1999).

Other epidemiologically based samples from Hawaii and Pennsylvania (Stretch et al., 1995), Boston (Proctor et al., 1998), active service USAF personnel (Fukuda et al., 1998), naval construction units (Sea Bees) (Gray, Kaiser, Hawksworth, Hall, & Barrett-Connor, 1999), and the large U.S. Veterans Administration study (Kang, Mahan, & Murphy, 2000) all show essentially the same findings.

Significantly, all these studies, including our own, are limited by the use of self-report measures. Self-reported symptoms are not, of course, a good guide to findings on clinical examination (McCauley, Joos, Lasarev, Storzbach, & Bourdette, 1999). High rates of reported symptoms do not necessarily reflect high rates of physical disorder. Indeed, if that were the case it would contradict a considerable body of literature on the nature of somatic symptoms in the community. These symptoms are exceedingly common and often persistent. Yet fewer than 1 in 5 are found to have a discrete physical explanation (Kroenke & Mangelsdorff, 1989), suggesting that simple assumptions linking symptom with disease are frequently misleading (Mayou, Bass, & Sharpe, 1995).

Is There a Gulf War Syndrome?

The term Gulf War syndrome (GWS) has acquired remarkable media and popular salience, but is there such a thing? A syndrome implies a unique constellation of signs and/or symptoms. For there to be a Gulf War syndrome then, not only must there be evidence of such a unique constellation, but it must also be found in the context of the Gulf conflict and not elsewhere (Wegman, Woods, & Bailar, 1998).

Robert Haley, a Dallas-based epidemiologist, was the first to argue in favor of a unique Gulf War syndrome (Haley, Kurt, & Hom, 1997), using factor analysis. However, his data came from a single naval reserve construction battalion, already known to have high rates of illness, which had a 41% response rate and a sample size of 249. Haley also did not have a control group, military or nonmilitary. As numerous commentators have pointed out, this makes it difficult to establish whether the proposed new syndrome is indeed linked to Gulf service or not (Landrigan, 1997).

Since then studies that use population-based subjects and appropriate controls have generally not found evidence of a Gulf War syndrome. For example, in our study we did indeed find evidence to support a particular factor structure to symptoms in the Gulf cohort, but this was no different from the factor structure in the Bosnia or ERA controls. The Gulf group had more symptoms experienced at greater intensity, but there was no difference in the way these symptoms could be organized (Ismail et al., 1999). Three controlled U.S. studies draw similar conclusions (Doebbeling et al., 2000; Fukuda et al., 1998; Knoke, Smith, Gray, Kaiser, & Hawksworth, 2000).

The balance of evidence is currently against there being a distinct Gulf War syndrome. In many ways, it is a side issue that has attracted more interest and polemic than it deserves. The key question is whether service in the Gulf War affected health, and this is established beyond reasonable doubt. Whether this amounts to a unique syndrome, identifiable only by complex statistical techniques, seems to be a secondary issue.

The argument among academics is nevertheless academic, since irrespective of the emerging professional consensus, Gulf War syndrome is established as a popular, media, and social reality. Investigating how and why this concept developed is important, but the answers will not come from epidemiology, let alone the laboratory, but rather from the social sciences.

Further Studies

So far we have considered the position solely from a U.S./UK perspective. But many countries participated in the Coalition Forces, and we are now starting to hear from them as well. The first non– U.S. country to publish a detailed examination of its Gulf veterans was Canada (Anonymous, 1998). The results were remarkably consistent with what had already been reported from the United States and would be reported from the United Kingdom.

Each country's experience has also given examples of natural variations and experiments, which will in time, prove informative. For example, Canada sent three vessels to the Gulf—two used pyridostigmine prophylaxis and one did not. Yet rates of illness were identical among the three ships (Anonymous, 1998). Likewise, Danish Gulf veterans also have elevated rates of symptomatic ill-health (Ishoy et al., 1999), yet nearly all were only involved

in peacekeeping duties after the end of hostilities and neither used pyridostigmine prophylaxis nor received vaccinations against biological agents.
   The largest enigma remains the French. French authorities have consistently denied that any health problems have emerged in their Gulf forces.
Likewise, although one or two articles have appeared in the French press
about Gulf War syndrome in other countries, there have been no media
reports of similar stories in France. If this is indeed the case (and as we write
this appears to be changing [Anonymous, 2000]), then this would be vital
epidemiological evidence, since the pattern of forces protection used by
the French differed from that of both the Americans and the British. One
must, however, be cautious about the lack of evidence. First, no systematic
study has even been undertaken, and one should recall official denials of
any problem in this country prior to the publication of systematic studies.
Second, the cultural pattern of illnesses in the Francophone world differs
from that in the English-speaking and Scandinavian world (Payer, 1988).
Illness entities such as chronic fatigue syndrome are rarely acknowledged
or recognized as legitimate (Bamforth, 1997; Cathebras, 1994).

Summary

   The conclusion of these studies is that something about Gulf service has
affected the symptomatic health of large numbers of those who took part
in the campaign from most of the Coalition countries. At the same time, no
evidence has emerged to date of neither distinct biomedical abnormalities
nor premature mortality.
   Is it that some veterans have been significantly affected while the rest
have not? It seems not. There are certainly small numbers of veterans, often
with a high media profile, who have developed substantial disability. But on
a population basis we need to note the larger numbers of veterans who have
experienced small changes in their health. One useful analogy is to imagine
that it is as if the entire population of Gulf veterans has experienced a small
increase in blood pressure. For some this will have had serious effects, but
the main influence is the relative modest increase in symptoms that has
affected the majority, rather than the severe deterioration in function that
has affected a minority.

THE EXPLANATIONS

   We do not know, and probably never will know, the precise explanation
for the increase in ill-health seen in members of the armed forces of several
Coalition countries who took part in the Gulf War. It is almost certain there

is no single explanation. Instead, we propose three different explanatory models, each of them a different approach and conceptualization of the problem.

The First View: Gulf War Illness Is the Result of Hazards Encountered during the Gulf War

The most popular explanation for the Gulf health effect among the media, and, we suspect, the general public, is that the cause of Gulf War syndrome lies in the particular hazards of that conflict. Most attention has been given to the measures taken to protect the combatants from the threat of chemical and biological warfare (CBW). These included immunizations against biological weapons such as plague and anthrax, and pyridostigmine tablets to protect against exposure to anticholinesterase–based nerve agents such as Sarin. Other hazards included exposure to depleted uranium or to the smoke from the oil fires ignited by the retreating Iraqi forces.

Evidence is conflicting. A small group of U.S. Gulf veterans were definitely exposed to depleted uranium in the form of shrapnel fragments and are being intensively monitored. Some subtle changes have been seen in neuropsychological and neuroendocrine function (McDiarmid et al., 2000). No evidence relevant to the vast majority of those deployed has been presented to date.

Smoke from the burning oil wells received much publicity at the end of the land war, and perhaps for that reason was closely monitored on the spot. A series of environmental monitoring studies concluded that in general most toxins were below accepted lower limits, but there was an increase in the level of fine particulates, although even that was not unusual for a desert region (U.S. Army Environmental Hygiene Agency, 1994). A recent paper reported that levels of polycyclic aromatic hydrocarbon biomarkers, which would be expected to be elevated, were actually lower in Gulf veterans exposed to the oil fires than controls who had remained in Germany (Poirier et al., 1999).

Pyridostigmine bromide (PB), a reversible inhibitor of acetyl cholinesterase, was used as a prophylaxis against exposure to nerve gas. Although side effects were frequently reported during its use in the Gulf campaign, these were short-lived. No acute toxicity was observed (Keeler, Hurst, & Dunn, 1991). This is important, since long-term organophosphorus toxicity, which is certainly a hazard, has only been clearly documented in the aftermath of acute toxicity (Fulco, Liverman, & Sox, 2000). The Canadian experience (vide supra) also argues against a prominent role for PB. PB has been used in civilian practice for the treatment of myasthenia gravis for many years, and in higher doses than used by the armed forces, without apparent adverse effect. It has even been used as a treatment for the fatigue associated with postpolio syndrome (Trojan & Cashman, 1995). The extensive cumulative experience with PB in civilian neurological practice argues against an important role for PB per se in Gulf-related illnesss (Ablers & Berent, 2000; Anonynmous, 1997a, 1997b).

Thus the evidence does not support an important role for PB administration, but with two caveats. An elegant mouse experiment has suggested that PB, which normally does not penetrate the blood brain barrier, may do so under stressful conditions (Friedman et al., 1996), but this was not confirmed in guinea pigs (Grauer, Alkalia, Kapon, Cohen, & Ravey, 2000). Second, hazard may have resulted from interactions with other agents. A study of chickens confirmed the safety of pyridostigmine, permethrin, and DEET (the latter two being a pesticide and insect repellent respectively) individually, but reported neurotoxicity when given in combination, albeit in high dosage (Abou-Donia, Wilmarth, Jensen, Oehme, & Kurt, 1996), while rats given similar combinations have slower locomotion rates (Hoy, Cornell, Karlix, Tebbett, & van Haaren, 2000).

Perhaps host variation may explain differences in individual susceptibility. Haley, Billecke, and la Du (1999) have claimed that polymorphisms in the enzyme detoxification pathways for organophosphate compounds are related to symptoms, which is theoretically plausible (Furlong, 2000) but has not been confirmed (Mackness, Durrington, & Mackness, 2000).

The role of pesticides, and in particular organophosphate pesticides, has also been much discussed. Large quantities of pesticides in various forms were used by all the combatants to reduce the risk of infectious disease. In general, providing these were used appropriately and by trained personnel, little hazard should have followed (Anonynmous, 1997a, 1997b). But whether this actually happened in practice is unclear. There have now been numerous expert committee reports on both sides of the Atlantic, but most particularly in the United Kingdom. In general the conclusions are that there is no disputing the acute toxic effects of organophosphates on the human nervous system, but there remains considerable uncertainty and controversy about the effects of low-level chronic exposure (Anonynmous 1997b; Committee on Toxicity of Chemicals in Food, 1999; Joint Working Party, 1998; U.S. General Accounting Office, 1997). Information mismanagement has played a part in making this a controversial issue.

In the United States, but not in the United Kingdom, there was much attention given to the possibility that troops had been exposed to low levels of the nerve agent Sarin following the probable accidental destruction of an Iraqi arms dump at Khamisiyah. Little evidence has been found that those possibly exposed to the plume thought to have resulted from the incident had any difference in postwar illness (Gray, Smith et al., 1999). A recent animal study failed to show any adverse effects from low-dose Sarin (Pearce,

Crofts, Muggleton, Ridout, & Scott, 1999). There is no reliable evidence to suggest deliberate use of CBW weapons during the conflict.

Some of the most suggestive evidence comes from studies of the possible effects of the vaccination program used to protect the armed forces against the threat from biological weapons, although this may partly reflect the fact that quantifying exposure to vaccines, although difficult, is not impossible, unlike some of the other postulated hazards.

The U.S. program involved immunization against anthrax and botulism, while the United Kingdom chose to protect its armed forces against plague and anthrax, with the additional use of pertussis vaccine as adjuvant to speed up the response to anthrax (Ministry of Defence, 2000). We found a relationship between receiving both multiple vaccinations in general and those against CBW agents in particular and the persistence of symptoms, despite controlling for obvious confounders. The finding that multiple vaccinations in other contexts, including deployment to Bosnia, was not associated with any increased experience of symptoms, suggesting some interaction between multiple vaccination and active service deployment to the Gulf (Hotopf et al., 2000; Unwin et al., 1999).

There are also some general objections to the argument that Gulf-related illness is due to the particular biological hazards of the Gulf War (Anonynmous, 1997b). Some studies have found that certain symptom patterns are related to certain self-reported exposures (Haley & Kurt, 1997; Wolfe et al., 1998), but others have not (Gray, Kaiser et al., 1999; Iowa Persian Gulf Study Group, 1997; Kroenke, Koslowe, & Roy, 1998; Unwin, et al., 1999). The time latency between the war and onset of symptoms is also unusual if symptoms were related to war exposure (Kroenke et al., 1998).

In summary then there is some evidence to suggest that some of the new hazards to which the armed forces were exposed during the Gulf War may be associated with unexpected side effects, and perhaps later ill-health. Some claims need replication, and others remain implausible. Position 1 has partial support.

The Second View: Gulf War Is a Modern Manifestation of Postconflict Ill-Health

Our first argument, that the cause of the Gulf health effect lies in the unique nature of modern warfare, would be substantially weakened if it could be shown that similar clinical syndromes have arisen after other conflicts that did not involve the particular hazards of the Gulf War.

That similar syndromes have indeed been found after other conflicts has been most clearly argued by Craig Hyams in a seminal paper (Hyams, Wignall, & Roswell, 1996). Interpretable medical records and accounts really only commence from the middle of the 19th century, but from then onward the literature does contain clinical descriptions of ex-servicemen (and it is always men) with conditions that do show considerable similarities to the Gulf narratives. These conditions have received many different labels—Soldier's Heart, later termed Effort syndrome, which owes its provenance to the Crimean and U.S. Civil Wars. Shell shock and neurasthenia dominate the writings of the First World War, while Agent Orange syndrome and post-traumatic stress disorder emerge after Vietnam.

Hyams's argument rests entirely on a reading of secondary sources, but we have begun the task of assembling primary sources as well. Already we have located clinical case histories from the Crimean War and Indian Mutiny (Jones & Wessely, 1999), which begin the theme of chronic, unexplained symptoms, and are assembling more detailed analyses of medical records from the Boer War, and the First and Second World Wars.

The second position, therefore, states that sending young men to war invariably results in some casualties that cannot be explained on a solely physical injury basis, and that the symptoms experienced are similar to those experienced by Gulf War veterans.

The implication is that this reflects the psychological cost of warfare on the combatants. Yet the Gulf War was not a particularly "stressful" conflict in the traditional sense. The active ground war lasted only a few days. Casualties among the Coalition Forces were exceptionally light. It would be historically wrong to extrapolate from the prolonged privation, fear, and danger of, for example, the Western Front or the Italian campaign of the Second World War, to the Gulf War.

But it would be equally wrong to claim that Gulf veterans were not exposed to stress or fear of any sort. Most particularly, the real threat posed by CBW cannot be underestimated (Betts, 1998; Stokes & Banderet, 1997). Such weapons "engender fear out of all proportion to their threat" (O'Brien & Payne, 1993)—they are as much, if not more, weapons of psychological as physical warfare (Holloway, Norwood, Fullerton, Engel, & Ursano, 1997). Even in training up to 20% of those who took part in exercises using simulated exposure to irritant gases showed moderate to severe psychological anxiety (Fullerton & Ursano, 1990).

There was no doubt that Iraq possessed such weapons and had used them extensively during the Iran-Iraq War and against Kurdish civilians. It was anticipated that they would be used in the forthcoming campaign. Counter-measures were untested and probably insufficient. Effective measures, such as wearing the full nuclear-biological-chemical (NBC) suits were uncomfortable and induced a state of partial sensory deprivation. Surveys during Desert Shield of U.S. forces confirmed that the threat of CBW was the most commonly expressed fear of the coming conflict. The ground war may have only taken a few days, but the deployment itself lasted many months. During Desert Storm there were several thousand documented chemical alarm alerts. Subsequently, the consensus of opinion is that none were true positives, and that Iraq did not use its CBW arsenal. But at the time each alert had to be assumed to be genuine. Thus even if traditional military stressors were not a prominent feature of the active campaign, a well-founded and realistic anxiety about the threat of dreaded weapons could still be important. Believing oneself to be exposed to such weapons has been frequently found to be associated with the development of symptoms (Nisenbaum, Barrett, Reyes, & Reeves, 2000; Unwin et al., 1999), sometimes very strongly (Haley et al., 1997; Proctor et al., 1998).

The Third View: Gulf War Syndrome Can Be Found in People Who Have Never Been to the Gulf or Served in the Armed Forces

Our first argument was that either some hazard of Gulf War service alone (our first view) or war service in general (our second view) is linked to subsequent ill-health. But could the features of Gulf War illness actually have nothing to do with warfare at all?

This seems a surprising proposition. However, patients with multiple unexplained symptoms, all of them reported in the narratives of Gulf veterans, are also encountered in civilian medical practice and literature. In the popular literature first-person accounts and patient-oriented literature (in the media and on the Internet) exist with considerable similarities to those of some Gulf veterans. One finds such material under diverse headings such as "ME," total allergy syndrome, electrical hypersensitivity, dental amalgam disease, silicon breast implant disease, hypoglycaemia, chronic Lyme disease, sick building syndrome, and many more.

Turning to the professional literature, studies are now reporting that the rates of various symptom-defined conditions originally described in the civilian population are also elevated in the Gulf cohorts. Chief among these are chronic fatigue syndrome (CFS; Kipen, Hallman, & Natelson, 1999) and multiple chemical sensitivity (MCS; Black et al., 2000). These syndromes, which also include fibromyalgia, irritable bowel syndrome (IBS), and others, overlap not only with each other (Wessely, Nimnuan, & Sharpe, 1999), but also with Gulf War illnesses.

That symptom-based conditions overlap with Gulf War illness is not surprising, given that all the epidemiological studies confirm that Gulf veterans experience an increase reporting of each and everyone of the symptoms that make up the case definitions of all these syndromes found in civilian practice. This does not mean, however, that either CFS/IBS/MCS and the others are all the same, or that Gulf War illness is the same either. It does mean that they all overlap, that discrete boundaries cannot be drawn between them (or if they can, we currently have no idea where these boundaries are). It also means that any explanation of Gulf War illness must explain how similar conditions can be found either in nondeployed military personnel or in civilians as well.

ATTRIBUTIONS AND EXPLANATIONS

The Military: From Effort Syndrome to Gulf War Syndrome

It is a truism to state that people, whether civilians or soldiers, need to explain their distress. Indeed, an intriguing body of research confirms that in the clinical setting patients prefer a firm, albeit inaccurate, label for their symptoms as opposed to an honest expression of uncertainty (Thomas, 1978). We have already discussed the various labels given in the past to postconflict syndromes and suggested that there is considerable overlap between the different names given at different times. But where did those labels come from, and can one read any significance into the choice of label?

We believe so. Some of the labels applied to unexplained illnesses in the armed services clearly are related to the particular nature of the recent conflict. Hence Soldier's Heart arose because of the contemporary concern that the straps securing the heavy back packs worn by the Unionist soldiers in the U.S. Civil War were compressing the muscles, arteries, and nerves in the region of the heart. The epidemic of "rheumatic" conditions that we have documented after the Boer War was a response to the presumed health dangers of sleeping out in wet conditions on the High Veldt. Shell shock took its name from the presumed effects of concussion caused by the passage of the shell, let alone its actual detonation. Again, one must remember that the exploding shell remains the predominant image of the First World War and epitomized both then and now the particular trauma and anxiety of that conflict—for the first time the main cause of death was the unseen enemy.

Another popular term was neurasthenia. As originally described in civilian life, neurasthenia was a condition affecting successful people, usually males, and was a response to the stresses and strains of contemporary life. Overwork, exhaustion, long hours, the new demands of capitalism, and so on were the kinds of explanations that dominated the early (but not late) literature—it was an illness of successful men, "captains of industry." Hence, when it emerged that army captains on the Western front were developing similar unexplained conditions associated with extreme exhaustion, it was not difficult to translate the civilian neurasthenia concept into the military context. Sir Frederick Mott (1919), one of the most influential medical figures of the period, wrote that "neurasthenia . . . was more likely to be acquired in officers of a sound mental constitution than men of the ranks, because in the former the prolonged stress of responsibility which, in the officer worn out by the prolonged stress of war and want of sleep, causes anxiety less he should fail in his critical duties."

After Vietnam came two new syndromes, one ostensibly psychological, the other somatic. Post-traumatic stress disorder (PTSD) was socially created to deal with the guilt and trauma of an unpopular, lost campaign (Young, 1995). The other, Agent Orange syndrome (Hall, 1989), can be seen as the forerunner of Gulf War syndrome.

So the labels given to previous postconflict syndromes can be seen to derive from both the specifics of that particular campaign, but also the general health beliefs of the time. We have already listed the main health concerns of the Gulf campaign—depleted uranium, vaccinations, pollution, chemical warfare, and so on. How do these map onto wider civilian, health concerns?

The Civilian Perspective

People who feel ill need an explanation for their malaise. Sometimes doctors can provide such an explanation, often they cannot (Kroenke & Mangelsdorff, 1989). And in those circumstances, when Medical experts fail to provide clear answers, people most often turn to their environment to provide those explanations. The choice they make is culturally determined, since it must depend on contemporary and accepted views of health and disease.

In a previous time ill-health and misfortune were commonly interpreted in terms of demonic possession, spirits, and satanic influence. Such explanations have now lost their cultural resonance in the developed world. To a large extent these have been replaced by explanations based on environmental hazards and threats.

It is evident that the range and scope of symptoms, illnesses, and conditions blamed on the environment have increased over the course of the past decade or so. There are many social, historical, and cultural reasons why this should be—reflecting increasing global concern about the effects of chemicals, radiation, and infectious diseases, and the collective memories of recent health disasters. The generation that fought the Gulf War was born in a world already sensitized by *Silent Spring* and the thalidomide tragedy, and had come to maturity in a background of the AIDS epidemic, mad cow disease, and numerous well-publicized environmental tragedies, such as Chernobyl, Seveso, and Bhopal. It is a moot point indeed if our environment really is more threatening than it was—the food, water, and air of any given postindustrial revolution city of the 19th century does not bear comparison with their modern counterparts (Dalrymple, 1998; Shorter, 1997)—but we are certainly more aware of these dangers than our predecessors.

It is the role of environmental attribution that provides a link between the otherwise varied new illnesses and health hazards that figure so prominently in the media, such as dental amalgam disease, electromagnetic radiation, ME, organophosphate toxicity, candida, sick building syndrome, multiple chemical sensitivity, and so on. Although the postulated pathophysiological mechanisms are many and varied, all are associated with the presence of multiple unexplained symptoms, and all are in one way or another blamed on some unwelcome external environmental hazard, such as chemicals, pollution, viruses, radiation, and so on. Alternatively, it is an internal toxic substance introduced from outside, such as silicon breast implants or dental amalgam. Thus in civilian life we argue that what unites these disparate conditions is not only the clinical evidence of multiple unexplained symptomatology, but also the cognitive schema linking them with ideas of environmental hazard and toxicity.

One result of this heightened environmental awareness has been a gradual transformation of popular models of illness and disease. In place of the demons and spirits comes the belief that we as a society are oppressed by mystery gases, viruses, and toxins, all of which are invisible, and some of which are as elusive as the demons of old. One can see this in the changing pattern of attributions given by patients with unexplained symptoms (Stewart, 1990). Guy's Poisons Unit, for example, reported that it is only in the past two decades that they have started to see patients with multiple symptoms attributed to environmental poisoning (Hutchesson & Volans, 1989).

Many scientists now profess themselves baffled by the public anxieties expressed over the possible adverse effects of pesticides, not to mention genetically modified foods and cell phones (Burke, 1999), but these make sense when seen in light of the previous paragraph. At the turn of the Past century science and technology held great hopes for the future—the introduction of chemicals into food was to be welcomed as it promised greater, and not lesser, food safety, and chemical was not the term of abuse it has now become. But those days have passed. Science is certainly not a force for evil, nor have we become a nation of Luddites, but both science and technology are clearly seen in more ambiguous terms than previously.

Few can deny the heightened anxiety by the public and mass media over the safety of the environment and the suspicions about the food we eat, the water we drink, and the air we breathe. As Barsky points out, "the world seems generally filled with peril, jammed with other health hazards in addition to disease.... nothing in our environment can be trusted, no matter how comfortable or familiar" (1988b, p. 63).

Likewise, few can doubt the growing strength of the environmental movement. We are far more aware of the risks of our environment than ever before. Activism to combat environmental pollution and toxic waste has been described as a new social movement (Matterson-Allen & Brown, 1990). There is even an epidemic of the word risk in the scientific, and most particularly epidemiological, journals (Skolbekken, 1995).

There is a complex relationship between environmental concerns and symptoms. There is no doubt that being exposed to environmental hazard, such as chemicals, leads to increased fears and concerns (Bowler, Mergler, Huel, & Cone, 1994). This increase occurs whether the exposure is real or perceived. These concerns in turn lead to increased symptom reporting, perhaps via activation of the stress response. The strength of a subject's opinions on environmental matters was associated with symptom reporting in those exposed to a hazardous waste site but also in those who were not (Lipscomb, Satin, & Neutra, 1992; Roht et al., 1985). Those who described themselves as "very worried" about local environmental conditions were 10 times more likely to complain of headaches than those not so concerned (Shusterman, Lipscomb, Neutra, & Satin, 1991). Finally, people who experience more symptoms, for whatever reason, may have an increased level of concern about their environment as they look for explanations for their ill-health. The consequence is a vicious circle linking exposure (whether real or perceived), beliefs, and symptoms.

It is therefore possible that as the general level of concern increases, so might the overall burden of symptoms—perhaps one explanation for the oft-observed "paradox of health"—that we live longer, healthier lives than at any time in human history, but experience more symptoms and feel worse (Barsky, 1988a).

Reproductive Fears

At the same time as concerns over health surfaced, so did concerns about reproductive health. Numerous emotional media stories emerged of veterans fathering children with severe birth defects. It was impossible not to be moved by these individual tragedies, and impossible not to understand and sympathize why the parents of children so afflicted should search for explanations and generally find these in the father's military service. These concerns remain prominent—a common response we have encountered among the veterans who have completed our qualitative survey is the intention to delay having children until these issues are resolved. Fortunately, there is no evidence of any increased risk at present (Cowan, Gray, & DeFraites, 1997). But the longer families delay fertility, the greater the chance that such a risk will develop.

Reproductive concerns are one area in which there is a lack of historical continuity. These concerns are largely absent from the voluminous records and narratives of the First World War. The first example we can find is an isolated report that Australian veterans returning from the Pacific war expressed these fears, blamed on the malaria prophylaxis they had taken, but concerns about hazard to the next generation is not a common Second World War–belief either. It first surfaces as a major issue in veteran's health during the Vietnam era, as part of the Agent Orange controversy. We suspect that it was the cumulative and widespread knowledge of the medical effects of radiation post–Hiroshima and the thalidomide tragedy that are the triggers for this change. Now such concerns seem to be an integral part of most environmental accidents and exposures. Following the Chernobyl radiation disaster there was a decrease in the birthrate across Western Europe and an increase in induced abortions (Bertollini, Di Lallo, Mastrolacovo, & Perucci, 1990; Knudson, 1991). The International Atomic Energy Agency estimated that somewhere between 100,000 and 200,000 pregnancies were medically aborted in Western Europe for this reason (Ketchem, 1987). There was also a major increase in therapeutic abortions after the Seveso incident (Pocchiari, Silano, & Zampieri, 1979). Spontaneous abortions and delayed pregnancy became an issue in the Balkans during aerial bombing of chemical plants (Fineman, 1999).

The Soldier Becomes a Civilian Again

The situation of the soldier returning from war, especially if accompanied by rapid separation from service, is a complex one. Upon enlistment individuals enter military society and become part of a group where their loss of autonomy is offset by a feeling of belonging and a clearly defined role within the organization. Deployment to war is a unique experience of shared adversity, when the reality of military service cannot be avoided and where individual concerns are shared and managed by group membership.

Following combat everything changes. Readjustment to routine soldering occurs and the process of assimilation and accommodation of the experience of war continues. Some may experience guilt or shame at acts of commission or omission. Pride and a feeling of achievement may be felt by some, while others may become angry and accusatory at those who they see as letting them down in time of threat. The search for meaning may continue for years.

Leaving the service may be desired for many reasons. These include the simple end of their engagement; but also both being unable to equal the combat experience or desiring never to have to repeat it. Once "separated," modern servicemen and -women will return to a risk aversive society where individual rights, not duties or obligations, count—the obverse of military society. A realistic knowledge of military experience by civilian society has become less with the end of national conflicts or national service—fewer and fewer civilians will have any contact with the military. Contemporary understanding of military service is more likely to be driven by Hollywood's depictions than personal experience. Films that portray the veteran as victim are common, a situation abhorrent to most servicemen and -women. A few, however, will construe their experience in this way, encouraged by the media.

Military and veteran culture also reflects the general changing relationship between individual and society. One sign of this is the loss of Crown indemnity by the Ministry of Defence and the subsequent avalanche of litigation against the military authorities. However, it is simplistic, and probably erroneous, to assume that the rise in symptoms among Gulf veterans is related to the rise in litigation, as some skeptics have suggested. Instead, it is more likely that litigation arises as a consequence, rather than a cause, of these concerns. Furthermore, there is little difference in the health complaints and concerns of U.S. versus UK veterans (Kang et al., 2000), but whereas UK veterans can, and are, litigating against the military, their U.S. counterparts are by statute barred from any similar activity.

We do not subscribe to simplistic notions of war, stress, and posttraumatic stress, but neither do we see war as having no psychological or social significance. We suggest that nearly everyone is changed by exposure to combat, either for better or worse. In the words of one Second World War veteran "everything since (war) has just been a footnote."

The Gulf War and Modernity

Turning to the hazards of the Gulf War, we can also see that these have particular resonance to general societal issues and concerns. There is, for example, a powerful antivaccination lobby that receives frequent media coverage, as exemplified by the controversy over whooping cough vaccination, and more lately the measles-mumps-rubella vaccination (Jefferson, 2000).

All commentators agree that the Gulf War was the most high-tech military conflict to date, which might be expected to reduce traditional military stressors of more direct, low-tech combat. However, the introduction of new technologies is not without risks of its own—the introduction of new technologies into civilian industries is often accompanied by a rise in nonspecific complaints and is also blamed by many for particular syndromes such as repetitive strain injury (RSI; Smith & Carayon, 1996). Scandinavian researchers have coined the term "techno stress" to describe this phenomenon (Arnetz & Wiholm, 1997; Berg, Arnetz, Liden, Eneroth, & Kallner, 1992).

One reason why natural disasters seems to have a lesser association with long-term subjective health effects than technological/chemical disasters may relate to the differing time courses of the threats. Technological threats or disasters give rise not only too more health-related fears, there is also genuine uncertainty about the long-term risks from such exposures. Hence, it is difficult for experts to confirm or deny such concerns, particularly related to possible outcomes that occur endemically in affected communities anyway, such as cancer, miscarriage, or reproductive abnormalities. The lack of certainty of long-term health risks, such as seen in the Three Mile Island episode (Prince-Embury & Rooney, 1988), can be applied to many of the nontraditional military hazards of the Gulf campaign, providing a further link between civilian and military health (Bowler & Schwarzer, 1991).

Distrust, Conspiracy, and Confidence

The importance of public confidence and political (mis)judgment in shaping health concerns may be illustrated by one U.S./UK comparison. In the United States there has been considerable concern and outcry over the role of the probably accidental discharge of Sarin gas at the Khamisiyah arms dump, but this has not been a major issue in the United Kingdom. What has been a major issue there is the role of exposure to organophosphate pesticides. One reason may be that both issues were accompanied by misinformation. In Great Britain it was originally denied that any organophosphate pesticides had been used—a clear misjudgment. This was corrected, but the result was to focus attention on this particular risk and fuel the cries of "coverup." Something rather similar transpired regarding Khamisiyah in the United States.

Indeed, one can go further and say that the initial actions of the UK authorities could hardly have been worse in terms of maintaining the confidence and trust of the armed forces and the populace. First, records that now would give crucial information, such as vaccination records, were destroyed. We do not generally subscribe to the conspiracy theorists, and instead see this as a low-level decision to get rid of unnecessary paperwork that was no longer of interest. Armies fight wars, not plan epidemiological surveys. But it handed a weapon to every Internet conspiracy buff, who have flocked to the Gulf issues in droves.

Second, when concerns first began to surface in the United Kingdom, there was an attitude, expressed in Parliament that this was a "storm in a teacup." There were also coded hints that rotten apples could be found in every basket, those complaining really should be able to "pull themselves together," and that this would not happen to troops that were properly lead and trained. This was not expressed in so many words, but the meaning was clear. This is not a new view—similar sentiments were expressed to and by the Shell Shock Commission of 1922, but the modern change in the balance between the duties and rights of individuals and media scrutiny, on a previously unknown scale, means such views are now less acceptable. Finally, there was a delay in commissioning research that might allay concerns.

The result of all these events was a serious and understandable lack of trust of governmental and military authorities. This was partly a response to the specific errors related to Gulf War illness, and partly a result of other known misjudgments or denials usually from the Cold War era, including such events as involuntary experiments carried out on some service personnel during that period. Given that risk communication and management are critically dependent upon a trust between the community that feels exposed and those responsible for managing that risk (Slovic, 1999), we believe these misjudgments were integral to the further development and shaping of Gulf War syndrome after the conflict.

If the complaints of Gulf War syndrome are indeed related to general popular views on health and disease, then one would expect to find some evidence of social and media transmission. There is some, albeit scanty, evidence to provide some support (Chalder et al., 2001).

This is not to say that the media are responsible for Gulf War syndrome. Public concern and media coverage go hand-in-hand—the Gulf War syndrome was a "good story" precisely because it touched on so many contemporary issues of general public concern. Public concerns and media coverage are consistent with each other, even if neither necessarily reflects an "objective" appraisal or reality (Funkhouser, 1973). It is, however, true that the news media are more likely to report negative, trust destroying stories than ones that enhance trust (Slovic, 1999).

CONCLUSIONS

Questions Remaining

Many important research questions remain unanswered. Some will be addressed in the next few years. Key epidemiological studies, most particularly those conducted by the U.S. Veterans Administration and by Manchester University in the United Kingdom, will begin to report. The experience of other countries will start to become clearer. Numerous clinical and animal studies will also report, and we anticipate a flood of reports on neuropsychological, neurological, immunological, and other investigations of Gulf veterans. If these are based on well-defined and preferably epidemiologically based samples, the interpretation of these results will be far easier.

Having·said this, we must also face reality. At the time of writing we have passed the 10th anniversary of the Gulf conflict. The possibilities of further direct etiological research diminish with each year. The chances of finding new evidence on exposures during the conflict becomes increasingly unlikely.

The Lessons

It might be argued that each military deployment is unique in its historical and military context, and so it is. But the story of Gulf War syndrome can only make sense when seen in the wider context. Sadly we suspect that it is not a "one off." The origins of Gulf War syndrome can be traced to factors outside the 1991 conflict, and these same factors continue to operate today, perhaps even heightened by the Gulf experience, both in reality and mythology. Will the future hold more "Gulf War syndromes"? We suspect so.

Already newspaper reports have appeared concerning, for example, the "horrendous range of symptoms" now experienced by Canadian UN peacekeepers in Croatia (Gilmour, 1999) and Dutch peacekeepers in Cambodia (De Vries, Soetekouw, Bleijenberg, & van der Meer, 2000; Soetekouw et al., 1999). Similar reports have emerged in the German and Belgian press concerning their soldiers in Kosovo. Concerns include exposure to depleted uranium munitions, contaminated sandbags (Kondro, 1999), or to pollutants released from the destruction of factories during the NATO bombing campaign against Serbia. And as I write this chapter, the newspapers across Europe are once again leading on stories of the possible health effects of depleted uranium munitions.

There has likewise been an epidemic of papers in the medical journals concerning preparations to deal with a chemical or biological terrorism incident—all of which have been concerned with the acute emergency response. We have argued elsewhere that the insidious but perhaps ultimately more damaging long-term effects have been ignored (Hyams, Murphy, & Wessely, in press).

The current uncertainty over the chronic health effects of low-level exposure to chemical and nuclear materials will continue and will further increase public anxiety. Because health officials cannot provide blanket assurances that harm will not result from acute, nonsymptom producing exposure, distrust of medical experts and government officials can result (Prince-Embury & Rooney, 1988). The potential effects of low-level chemical and radiation exposure is a long-standing controversy (Birchard, 1999). It is unlikely that these complex scientific and political issues will be resolved in the near future. Nor is it likely that research studies conducted after well-publicized disasters will convincingly answer basic scientific questions because of the difficulties of eliminating research biases in highly charged circumstances (David & Wessely, 1995; Neutra, 1985; Roht et al., 1985). As a result, numerous unconfirmed and controversial hypotheses about the effects of low-level exposures will flourish, just as they did after the Gulf campaign.

Gulf War Syndrome: The Postmodern Illness

In a provocative article Muir Gray (1999) describes the features of what he calls "postmodern medicine"—a distrust of science, a readiness to resort to litigation, a greater attention to risk, and better access to information (of whatever quality). He also points out, as indeed have many commentators, how consumer and patient values have already replaced paternalistic and professional values, and where doctors used to lead, they now follow. The monolithic role of the doctor has been challenged by "lay experts," whose ability to influence public debate and policy increases just as that of the doctor or scientist diminishes—the "lay expert" may be the survivor of a disaster or the sufferer from a disease (Bury, 1998). The Gulf War veteran may fulfill both roles.

We suggest that Gulf War syndrome is therefore a paradigmatic postmodern illness. It is perhaps the first major health condition that was constructed almost entirely without the assistance of medicine in any shape or form. This is postmodern. Previous syndromes in the military have arisen for many reasons—"shell shock" was not invented by Myers in his seminal 1915 paper, but without his contribution it is improbable that the term would have gained widespread acceptance. In modern civilian practice the success of chronic fatigue syndrome depended in part on the rise in patient consumerism and the reaction against medical paternalism, but key triggers were the paper describing the original Royal Free epidemic that gave rise to the term "myalgic encephalomyelitis" in the United Kingdom, or the NIH papers on "chronic Epstein Barr" virus infection in the United States (Wessely, Hotopf, & Sharpe, 1998). Without them CFS would have taken a different course, if it had emerged at all. Sick building syndrome, like Gulf War syndrome, arose out of confusion, but a key part in its success was the persistent and vocal activities of a handful of doctors and scientists who, in the words of one commentator, "unequivocally diagnosed as a pathologic state something that had not been scientifically demonstrated" (Bardana, 1997, p. 290).

Yet for Gulf War syndrome, as far as we can tell, the shape of the syndrome had been determined in the popular and political imaginations long before scientists or doctors had anything to say on the matter. Gulf War syndrome, we suggest, developed without the assistance of science or medicine. Certainly populist and occasionally maverick scientists have emerged into the limelight of Gulf War syndrome and have played roles in subsequent events; but Gulf War syndrome may be the first truly postmodern illness, in that it developed from the congruence of veterans' narratives, veterans' disquiet and distrust, and a powerful media agenda. Medical professionals and scientists generally have reacted to events and not shaped them.

We end with our own speculations. We propose that the story began with the experiences of veterans' reporting symptoms. These may have been triggered as an unexpected reaction to measures taken to protect the armed forces against modern warfare, reinforced by the social and psychological pressures and changes that war brings to all it touches. These narratives were taken up by a powerful media and shaped into a particular syndrome, under the influence of popular views of health, disease, and illness. Further impetus came from the actions, or inactions, of government, and only recently by the activities of doctors and scientists. How the story will end remains to be seen.

ACKNOWLEDGMENT. A shortened version of this chapter was published in the January–February issue of the *Journal of the Royal College of Physicians*.

REFERENCES

Ablers, J., & Berent, S. (2000). Controversies in neurotoxicology. *Neurologic Clinics, 18*, 741–763.

Abou-Donia, M., Wilmarth, K., Jensen, K., Oehme, F., & Kurt, T. (1996). Neurotoxicity resulting from coexposure to pyridostigmine bromide, DEET, and permethrin: implications of Gulf War chemical exposures. *Journal Toxicol and Environmental Health, 48*, 35–56.

Anonymous. (1997a). *Gulf war illnesses: Dealing with the uncertainities*. London: Parliamentary Office of Science and Technology.

Anonymous. (1997b). *Presidential advisory committee on Gulf War veterans' illnesses: Final report*. Washington, DC: U.S. Government Printing Office.

Anonymous. (1998). *Health study of canadian forces personnel involved in the 1991 conflict in the Persian Gulf*. Ottawa: Goss Gilroy.

Anonymous. (2000, May 29). French army wary of first Gulf War syndrome charge. Reuters.

Arnetz, B., & Wiholm, C. (1997). Technological stress: Psychophysiological symptoms in modern offices. *Journal of Psychosomatic Research, 43*, 35–42.

Bamforth, I. (1997). Life as an omnipraticien in France. *British Medical Journal Classified*, 2–3.

Bardana, E. (1997). Sick building syndrome—a wolf in sheeps' clothing. *Annals of Allergy Asthma and Immunology, 79*, 283–293.

Barsky, A. (1988a). The paradox of health. *New England Journal of Medicine, 318*, 414–418.

Barsky, A. (1988b). *Worried sick: Our troubled quest for wellness.* Toronto: Little, Brown.

Berg, M., Arnetz, B., Liden, S., Eneroth, P., & Kallner, A. (1992). Techo-Stress: A Psychophysiology Study of Employees with VDU-Associated Skin Complaints. *Journal of Occupational Medicine, 34,* 698–700.

Bertollini, R., Di Lallo, D., Mastrolacovo, P., & Perucci, C. (1990). Reduction in births in Italy after the Chernobyl accident. *Scandinavian Journal of Work and Environmental Health, 16,* 96–101.

Betts, R. (1998). The new threat of mass destruction. *Foreign Affairs, 77,* 26–41.

Birchard, K. (1999). Experts still arguing over radiation doses. *Lancet, 354,* 400.

Black, D., Doebbeling, B., Voelker, M., Clarke, W., Woolson, R., Barrett, D. et al. (2000). Multiple chemical sensitivity syndrome: Symptom prevalence and risk factors in a military population. *Archives of Internal Medicine, 160,* 1169–1176.

Bowler, R., Mergler, D., Huel, G., & Cone, J. (1994). Psychological psychosocial and psychophysiological sequelae to a community affected by a railroad disaster. *Journal of Traumatic Stress, 7,* 601–624.

Bowler, R., & Schwarzer, R. (1991). Environmental anxiety: Assessing emotional distress and concerns after toxin exposure. *Anxiety Research, 4,* 167–180.

Boyle, C., Decoufle, P., & O'Brien, T. (1989). Long term health consequences of military service in Vietnam. *Epidemiologic Reviews, 11,* 1–27.

Burke, D. (1999). The recent excitement over genetically modified food. In P. Bennett & K. Calman (Eds.), *Risk communication and public health* (pp. 140–151). Oxford: Oxford Medical Publications.

Bury, M. (1998). Postmodernity and health. In G. Scambler & P. Higgs (Eds.), *Modernity and health* (pp. 1–28). London: Routledge.

Cathebras, P. (1994). Neurasthenia, spasmophilia and chronic fatigue syndromes in France. *Transcultural Psychiatric Research Review, 31,* 259–270.

Chalder, T., Hotopf, M., Hull, L., Ismail, K., Unwin, C., David, A. et al. (2001). Who believes they have Gulf War syndrome? *British Medical Journal, 323,* 473–476.

Coker, W., Bhatt, B., Blatchley, N., & Graham, J. (1999). Clinical findings for the first 1000 Gulf war veterans in the Ministry of Defence's medical assessment programme. *British Medical Journal, 318,* 290–294.

Committee on Toxicity of Chemicals in Food. (1999). *Organophosphates.* Retrieved from http://www.doh.gov.uk/cot/op.htm

Cowan, D., Gray, G., & DeFraites, R. (1997). Birth defects among children of Persian Gulf War veterans. *New England Journal of Medicine, 337,* 1175–1176.

Dalrymple, T. (1998). *Mass listeria: The meaning of health scares.* London: Andre Deutsch.

David, A., & Wessely, S. (1995). The legend of Camelford: Medical consequences of a water pollution accident. *Journal of Psychosomatic Research, 39,* 1–10.

De Vries, M., Soetekouw, P. M., Bleijenberg, G., & van der Meer, J. (2000). Fatigue in Cambodia veterans. *Quarterly Journal of Medicine, 93,* 283–289.

Doebbeling, B., Clarke, W., Watson, D., Torner, J., Woolson, R., Voelker, M. et al. (2000). Is there a Persian Gulf War syndrome? Evidence from a large population-based survey of veterans and nondeployed controls. *American Journal of Medicine, 108,* 695–704.

Fineman, M. (1999, July 6). Yugoslav city battling toxic enemies. *Los Angeles Times.*

Friedman, A., Kaufer, D., Shemer, J., Hendler, I., Soreq, H., & Tur-Kaspa, I. (1996). Pyridostigmine brain penetration under stress enhances neuronal excitability and induces early immediate transcriptional response. *Nature Medicine, 2,* 1382–1385.

Fukuda, K., Nisenbaum, R., Stewart, G., Thompson, W., Robin, L., Washko, R. et al. (1998). Chronic multisymptom illness affecting air force veterans of the Gulf War. *Journal of the American Medical Association, 280,* 981–988.

Fulco, C., Liverman, C., & Sox, H. (Eds.). (2000). *Gulf war and health: Volume 1. Depleted Uranium, Sarin, Pyridostigmine Bromide, Vaccines.* Washington DC: Institute of Medicine.

Fullerton, C., & Ursano, R. (1990). Behavioral and psychological responses to chemical and biological warfare *Military Medicine, 155,* 54–59.

Funkhouser, G. (1973). The issues of the sixties: An exploratory study in the dynamics of public opinion. *Public Opinion Quarterly, 37,* 62–75.

Furlong, C. (2000). PON1 status and neurologic symptom complexes in gulf war veterans. *Genome Research,* 153–155.

Gilmour, B. (1999, September 9). Hazardous duty. *Edmonton Journal.*

Grauer, E., Alkalia, D., Kapon, J., Cohen, G., & Ravey, L. (2000). Stress does not enable pyridostigmine bromide to inhibit brain cholinesterase after parenteral administration. *Toxicology and Applied Pharmacology, 164,* 301–304.

Gray, G., Smith, T., Knoke, J., & Heller, J. (1999). The postwar hospitalization experience of Gulf War veterans possibly exposed to chemical munitions destruction at Khamisiyah, Iraq. *American Journal of Epidemiology, 150,* 532–540.

Gray, G. C., Kaiser, K. S., Hawksworth, A. W., Hall, F. W., & Barrett-Connor, E. (1999). Increased postwar symptoms and psychological morbidity among US navy Gulf War veterans. *American Journal of Tropical Medicine and Hygiene, 60,* 758–766.

Gray, J. (1999). Postmodern medicine. *Lancet, 354,* 1550–1553.

Haley, R., Billecke, S., & la Du, B. (1999). Association of low PON1 type Q (type A) arylesterase activity with neurologic symptom complexes in Gulf War veterans. *Toxicology and Applied Pharmacology, 157,* 227–233.

Haley, R., & Kurt, T. (1997). Self-reported exposure to neurotoxic chemical combinations in the Gulf War: A cross-sectional epidemiologic survey. *Journal of the American Medical Association, 277*(3), 231–237.

Haley, R., Kurt, T., & Hom, J. (1997). Is there a Gulf War syndrome? Searching for syndromes by factor analysis of symptoms. *Journal of the American Medical Association, 277,* 215–222.

Hall, W. (1989). The logic of a controversy: The case of Agent Orange in Australia. *Social Science and Medicine, 29,* 537–544.

Holloway, H., Norwood, A., Fullerton, C., Engel, C., & Ursano, R. (1997). The threat of biological weapons: Prophylaxis and mitigation of psychological and social consequences. *Journal of the American Medical Association, 278,* 425–427.

Hotopf, M., David, A., Hull, L., Ismail, K., Unwin, C., & Wessely, S. (2000). The role of vaccinations as risk factors for ill-health in veterans of the Persian Gulf War. *British Medical Journal, 320,* 1363–1367.

Hoy, J., Cornell, J., Karlix, J., Tebbett, I., & van Haaren, F. (2000). Repeated coadministrations of pyridostigmine bromide, DEET, and permethrin alter locomotor behavior of rats. *Veterinary and Human Toxicology, 42,* 72–76.

Hutchesson, E., & Volans, G. (1989). Unsubstantiated complaints of being poisoned: Psychopathology of patients referred to the National Poisons unit. *British Journal of Psychiatry, 154,* 34–40.

Hyams, K., Hanson, K., Wignall, F., Escamilla, J., & Oldfield, E. (1995). The impact of infectious diseases on the health of US troops deployed to the Persian Gulf during Operations Desert Shield and Desert Storm. *Clinical Infectious Diseases, 20,* 1497–1504.

Hyams, K., Murphy, F., & Wessely, S. (in press). Combatting terrorism: Recommendations for dealing with the long term health consequences of a chemical, biological or nuclear attack. *Journal of Health Politics, Policy and the Law.*

Hyams, K., Wignall, F., & Roswell, R. (1996). War syndromes and their evaluation: From the US Civil War to the Persian Gulf War. *Annals of Internal Medicine, 125,* 398–405.

Iowa Persian Gulf Study Group. (1997). Self-reported illness and health status among Persian Gulf War veterans: A population-based study. *Journal of the American Medical Association, 277,* 238–245.

Ishoy, T., Suadicani, P., Guldager, B., Appleyard, M., Hein, H., & Gyntelberg, F. (1999). State of health after deployment in the Persian Gulf: The Danish Gulf War study. *Danish Medical Bulletin, 46,* 416–419.

Ismail, K., Everitt, B., Blatchley, N., Hull, L., Unwin, C., David, A. et al. (1999). Is there a Gulf War syndrome? *Lancet, 353,* 179–182.

Jefferson, T. (2000). Real or perceived adverse effects of vaccines and the media—A tale of our times. *Journal of Epidemiology and Community Health, 54,* 402–403.

Joint Working Party of the Royal College of Physicians and Psychiatrists. (1998). *Organophosphate sheep dip: Clinical aspects of long-term low-dose exposure.* Salisbury, Wiltshire: Royal College of Physicians.

Jones, E., & Wessely, S. (1999). Chronic fatigue syndrome after the Crimean War and the Indian Mutiny. *British Medical Journal, 319,* 1545–1547.

Joseph, S. (1997). A comprehensive clinical evaluation of 20,000 Persian Gulf War veterans. *Military Medicine, 162,* 149–156.

Kang, H., & Bullman, T. (1996). Mortality among U.S. Veterans of the Persian Gulf War. *New England Journal of Medicine, 335,* 1498–1504.

Kang, H. K., Mahan, C. M., & Murphy, F. M. (2000). Illnesses Among United States veterans of the Gulf War: A population-based survey of 30,000 veterans. *Journal of Occupational and Environmental Medicine, 42,* 491–501.

Keeler, J., Hurst, C., & Dunn, M. (1991). Pyridostigmine used as a nerve agent pretreatment under wartime conditions. *Journal of the American Medical Association, 266,* 693–695.

Ketchem, L. (1987). Lessons of Chernobyl: SNM members dry to decontaminate world threatened by fallout. *Journal of Nuclear Medicine, 6,* 933–942.

Kipen, H. M., Hallman, W., & Natelson, B. H. (1999). Prevalence of chronic fatigue and chemical sensitivities in Gulf registry veterans. *Archives of Environmental Health, 54,* 313.

Knoke, J., Smith, T. C., Gray, G, Kaiser, K. S., & Hawksworth, A. W. (2000). Factor analysis of self reported symptoms: Does it identify a Gulf War syndrome? *American Journal of Epidemiology, 152,* 379–388.

Knudson, L. (1991). Legally induced abortions in Denmark after Chernobyl. *Biomedicine and Pharmacotherapy, 45,* 229–232.

Kondro, W. (1999). Soldiers claim ill health after contact with contaminated soil in Croatia. *Lancet, 354,* 494.

Kroenke, K., Koslowe, P., & Roy, M. (1998). Symptoms in 18.495 Persian Gulf War Veterans. *Journal of Occupational and Environmental Medicine, 40,* 520–528.

Kroenke, K., & Mangelsdorff, A. (1989). Common symptoms in ambulatory care: Incidence, evaluation, therapy and outcome. *American Journal of Medicine, 86,* 262–266.

Landrigan, P. (1997). Illness in Gulf War veterans: Causes and consequences. *JAMA, 277*(3), 259–261.

Lipscomb, J. A., Satin, K. P., & Neutra, R. R. (1992). Reported symptom prevalence rates from comparison populations in community-based environmental studies. *Archives of Environmental Health, 47,* 263–269.

McCauley, L., Joos, S., Lasarev, M., Storzbach, D., & Bourdette, D. (1999). Gulf War unexplained illnesses: Persistence and unexplained nature of self-reported symptoms. *Environmental Research, 81,* 215–223.

McDiarmid, M., Keogh, J., Hooper, F., McPhaul, K., Squibb, K., Kane, R. et al. (2000). Health effects of depleted uranium on exposed gulf war veterans. *Environmental Research, 82,* 168–180.

MacFarlane, G., Thomas, E., & Cherry, N. (2000). Mortality amongst United Kingdom Gulf War veterans. *Lancet, 356*, 17–21.

Mackness, B., Durrington, P., & Mackness, M. (2000). Low paraoxonase in Persian Gulf War veterans self reporting Gulf War syndrome. *Biochemical and Biophysical Research Communications, 276*, 729–733.

Matterson-Allen, S., & Brown, P. (1990). Public reaction to toxic waste contamination: Analysis of a social movement. *International Journal of Health Services, 20*, 484–500.

Mayou, R., Bass, C., & Sharpe, M. (1995). Overview of epidemiology, classification and aetiology. In R. Mayou, C. Bass, & M. Sharpe (Eds.), *Treatment of functional somatic symptoms* (pp. 42–65). Oxford: Oxford University Press.

Ministry of Defence. (2000). *British chemical warfare defence during the Gulf conflict (1990–1991)*. Retrieved from www.mod.uk/policy/gulfwar/index.htm

Mott, F. (1919). *War neuroses and shell shock*. London: Hodder & Stoughton.

Neutra, R. (1985). Epidemiology for and with a distrustful community. *Environmental Health Perspectives, 62*, 393–397.

Nisenbaum, R., Barrett, D. H., Reyes, M., & Reeves, W. C. (2000). Deployment stressors and a chronic multisymptom illness among Gulf War veterans. *Journal of Nervous and Mental Diseases, 188*, 259–266.

O'Brien, L., & Payne, R. G. (1993). Prevention and management of panic in personnel facing a chemical threat—lessons from the Gulf. *Journal of Royal Army Medical Corps, 139*, 41–45.

Payer, L. (1988). *Medicine and culture: Varieties of treatment in the United States, England, West Germany and France*. New York: Henry Holt.

Pearce, P., Crofts, H., Muggleton, N., Ridout, D., & Scott, E. (1999). The effects of acutely administered low dose sarin on cognitive behaviour and the electrocephalogram in the common marmoset. *Journal of Psychopharmacology, 13*, 128–135.

Pocchiari, F., Silano, V., & Zampieri, A. (1979). Human health efftcs from accidental release of tetrachlorordibenzo-p-dioxin (TCDD) at Seveso, Italy. *Annals of the New York Academy of Sciences, 320*, 311–320.

Poirier, M., Weston, A., Schoket, B., Shamkhani, H., Pan, C. F., McDiarmid, M. et al. (1999). Polycyclic aromatic hydrocarbon biomarkers of internal exposure in US army soldiers serving in Kuwait in 1991. *Polycyclic Aromatric Compunds, 17*, 197–208.

Prince-Embury, S., & Rooney, J. (1988). Psychological symptoms of residents in the aftermath of the Three-Mile Island nuclear accident in the aftermath of technological disaster. *Journal of Social Psychology, 128*, 779–790.

Proctor, S., Heeren, T., White, R., Wolfe , J., Borgos, M., Davis, J. et al. (1998). Health status of Persian Gulf War veterans: Self-reported symptoms, environmental exposures, and the effect of stress. *International Journal of Epidemiology, 27*, 1000–1010.

Roht, L., Vernon, S., Weir, F., Pier, S., Sullivan, P., & Reed, L. (1985). Community exposure to hazardous waste disposal sites: Assessing reporting bias. *American Journal of Epidemiology, 122*, 418–433.

Roy, M., Koslowe, P., Kroenke, K., & Magruder, C. (1998). Signs. symptoms and ill-defined conditions in Persian Gulf War veterans: Findings from the comprehensive clinical evaluation program. *Psychosomatic Medicine, 60*, 663–668.

Shorter, E. (1997). Multiple chemical sensitivity: Pseudodisease in historical perspective. *Scandinavian Journal of Work and Environmental Health, 23* (Suppl. 3), 35–42.

Shusterman, D., Lipscomb, J., Neutra, R., & Satin, K. (1991). Symptom prevalence and odor-worry interaction near hazardous waste sites. *Environ Health Perspect, 94*, 25–30.

Skolbekken, J. (1995). The risk epidemic in medical journals. *Social Science and Medicine, 40*, 291–305.

Slovic, P. (1999). Trust, emotion, sex, politics, and science: Surveying the risk assessment battlefield. *Risk Analysis, 19*, 689–702.

Smith, M., & Carayon, P. (1996). Work organization, stress and cumulative trauma disorders. In S. Moon & S. Sauter (Eds.), *Beyond biomechanics: Psychosocial aspects of musculoskeletal disorders in office work* (pp. 23–44). London: Taylor & Francis.

Soetekouw, P., De Vries, M., Preijers, F., Van Crevel, R., Bleijenberg, G., & van der Meer, J. (1999). Persistent symptoms in former UNTAC soliders are not associated with shifted cytokine balance. *European Journal of Clinical Investigation, 29*, 960–963.

Stewart, D. (1990). The changing faces of somatization. *Psychosomatics, 31*, 153–158.

Stokes, J., & Banderet, L. (1997). Psychological aspects of chemical defense and warfare. *Military Psychology, 9*, 395–415.

Stretch, R., Bliese, P., Marlowe, D., Wright, K., Knudson, K., & Hoover, C. (1995). Physical health symptomatology of Gulf War-era service personnel from the states of Pennsylvania and Hawaii. *Miltiary Medicine, 160*, 131–136.

Thomas, K. (1978). The consultation and the therapeutic illusion. *British Medical Journal, 1*, 1327–1328.

Trojan, D., & Cashman, N. (1995). An open trial of pyridostigmine in post poliomyelitis syndrome. *Canadian Journal of Neurological Sciences, 22*, 223–227.

Unwin, C., Blatchley, N., Coker, W., Ferry, S., Hotopf, M., Hull, L. et al. (1999). The health of United Kingdom servicemen who served in the Persian Gulf War. *Lancet, 353*, 169–178.

U.S. Army Environmental Hygiene Agency. (1994). *Biological surveillance initiative. Appendix F of final report Kuwait oil fire health risk assessment, 5 May–3 December 1991* (39-26-L192-91). Aberdeen Proving Ground, MD: Author.

U.S. General Accounting Office. (1997). *Gulf War illnesses: Improved monitoring of clinical progress and reexamination of research emphasis are needed* (GAO/NSIAD-97-163). Washington, DC: Author.

Wegman, D., Woods, N., & Bailar, J. (1998). Invited commentary: How would we know a Gulf War syndrome if we saw one? *American Journal of Epidemiology, 146*, 704–711.

Wessely, S., Hotopf, M., & Sharpe, M. (1998). *Chronic fatigue and its syndromes.* Oxford: Oxford University Press.

Wessely, S., Nimnuan, C., & Sharpe, M. (1999). Functional somatic syndromes: One or many? *Lancet, 354*, 936–939.

Wolfe, J., Proctor, S., Duncan Davis, J., Borgos, M., & Friedman, M. (1998). Health symptoms reported by Persian Gulf War veterans two years after return. *American Journal of Industrial Medicine, 33*, 104–113.

Young, A. (1995). *The harmony of illusions: Inventing post-traumatic stress disorder.* Princeton, NJ: Princeton University Press.

7

Bhopal Gas Leak Disaster
Impact on Health and Mental Health

R. SRINIVASA MURTHY

INTRODUCTION

Bhopal's gas leak disaster is the worst recorded industrial disaster in human history. On the night between December 2–3, 1984, methyl isocyanate leaked at the Union Carbide India Limited (UCIL) factory at Bhopal, in central India, spreading into the surrounding environment. This leak of an "extremely hazardous chemical" covered the city of Bhopal in a cloud of poisonous gas over the span of a few hours, killing more than 2,000 people.

The Bhopal disaster is important from a mental health perspective for a number of reasons: (1) It is one of the largest man-made disasters in a developing country. (2) The adverse health effects of the disaster were due to a combination of the substances inhaled and the psychological effects of living through a disaster experience. (3) No formal mental health infrastructure was available to provide postdisaster mental health care. (4) A number of innovative approaches were developed to provide mental health care, which may be especially suitable for use in other developing countries. (5) This disaster was the subject of intensive prospective health research for

R. SRINIVASA MURTHY • Department of Psychiatry, National Institute of Mental Health and Neurosciences, Bangalore 560029, India.

Toxic Turmoil: Psychological and Societal Consequences of Ecological Disasters, edited by Johan M. Havenaar, Julie G. Cwikel, and Evelyn J. Bromet. New York, Kluwer Academic/Plenum Publishers, 2002.

the first 5 years. This research included mental health aspects of the disaster on the population.

The aims of this chapter are to describe the disaster, the physical health effects, the mental health effects, the interventions undertaken, and to identify issues for future research and interventions in this area, especially those relevant to developing countries.

THE DISASTER

The Union Carbide factory at Bhopal was part of India's response to the severe food shortages in the 1960s. A green revolution involving major changes in agricultural practices was one of the methods adopted to increase agricultural productivity. As part of this effort, chemical fertilizers and pesticides came to be common and used extensively.

In 1969, Union Carbide set up the UCIL pesticide plant at Bhopal, the capital of the state of Madhya Pradesh. Bhopal is located in the central part of India. In 1984, the population of Bhopal was about 700,000. The city was chosen by Union Carbide because of its central location in the country, good railway services connecting the city to rest of India, and the availability of a large natural lake to provide adequate water supply. The chemical plant was located only about 2 kilometres from the railway station and not far from the residential neighborhoods.

Until 1979, the factory was importing methyl isocyanate (MIC) from the parent company. After 1979, MIC was manufactured at the Bhopal factory. MIC is one of the many intermediates used in the production of the powerful pesticide Sevin. MIC is a dangerous chemical. It is lighter than water and very hygroscopic (quick to absorb moisture). It is also twice as heavy as air and as a result in a open environment, it remains close to the ground. At the time, the factory employed about 800 workers. Ironically, the Indian government had extended the plant's license for 7 years in 1983 (one year prior to the disaster), after a promise that the plant would secure from its parent company the technology to handle "emergency situations like toxic gas release, sometimes accompanied with fire, endangering the safety of the community" (Jayaraman, 1984, p. 581). There are reports that 4 months before the tragedy, the U.S. multinational had decided to dismantle its Bhopal installations and relocate them in Brazil and Indonesia (Lapierre & Moro, 2001).

In the early morning hours of December 3, 1984, about 40 tons of MIC from tank number 610 leaked into the atmosphere. The gas spread and covered about a 7 kilometer radius of the plant and affected about 200,000 people. More than 2,000 people died on the night of the disaster. The disaster was the result of a combination of factors. The direct cause is thought to be the entry of water into the tank or the spontaneous polymerization (in the absence of inhibitors) of the liquid of MIC, which had been in storage for over a month, a period longer than normal (Jayaraman, 1984, 1985, 1987). In addition to this, the gauges measuring the temperature and pressures were not functioning properly; the refrigeration unit for keeping the tank of MIC cool had been shut off for some time; the gas scrubber had been shut off for maintenance; and the flare tower that could have burned off the escaping MIC was not functioning (MacKenzie, 1985; Tachakra, 1987). Thus, the disaster was the result of a combination of factors including negligence and poor operational procedures.

Though the estimated number of persons who died immediately was around 2,000, in the years following the leak, more than 10,000 persons are estimated to have died from the exposure. In addition, 200,000 persons who were exposed to the gas leak and survived have a wide variety of health problems and disabilities (Jayaraman, 1984).

During the past 18 years, the Bhopal disaster continues to be an important public health and legal issue. The major milestones in the legal responsibility were the passing of the Bhopal Gas Relief Act in 1985 and the settlement by the government of India and the company for a onetime compensation payment of $470 million. However, the legal battles for the rights and relief to the survivors continue and are the source of much public debate (Menon, 1999). In 2000, developments in India reflect the public's concern about the legal liability of the company: "Union carbide shields former chairman Warren Anderson" (2000) and "Bhopal gas leak survivors launch cyber protest" (2000). Questions about the damage to the population, legal liability of the company, and the continuing needs of the affected population continue to be active public issues in India.

IMPACT ON HEALTH

Physiological effects were immediately apparent primarily in the eyes, lungs, and the gastrointestinal systems. Individual doctors, researchers from India and abroad, as well as the Indian official medical research organization, namely the Indian Council of Medical Research (ICMR), New Delhi, have been systematically recording the health effects. The reported health effects of the toxic chemical inhalation are summarized in the following section.

Specific Health Effects Related to the Exposure

Immediately after the gas leak, eyes were most commonly affected. The acute conjunctivitis came to be known as the Bhopal eye (Anderson, Muir, & Mehra, 1984). Subsequently, there were reports of persistent watery eyes among survivors 2 years after exposure (Andersson, Muir, Ajwani, Mahashabde, Salmon, Vaidyanathan, 1986; Maskati, 1986). There were also reports of chronic lesions such as chronic conjunctivitis, refractive changes, deficiency of tear secretion, and persistent ocular opacities (Raizada & Dwivedi, 1987).

Acute respiratory complaints immediately following the gas exposure were observed in the form of coughing, dyspnea, pulmonary oedema, with evidence of chronic damage to the lungs. These are seen as fibrosing bron-chiolitis obliterans. Several exposed subjects were found to have a sub-clinical alveolitis characterized by accumulation and possibly activation of macrophages in the lower respiratory tract. Radiological studies demon-strated evidence of lung fibrosis. There was a direct relationship between the changes in the lungs and the degree of exposure to the chemical toxin (Bhargava, Verma, Saini, Misra, Tiwari, Vijayan, Jain, 1987; Kamat, Patel, Kol-hatkar, Dave, & Mahashur, 1987; Rastogi, Gupta, Husain, Kumar, Chandra, Ray, 1988; Vijayan, Pandey, Sankaran, Mehrotra, Darbari, Mi, 1989; Vijayan & Sankaran, 1996; Vijayan, Sankaran, Sharma, & Misra, 1995; Weil, 1987). In a study conducted 10 years after the disaster among 454 randomly selected subjects, respiratory symptoms and reduced lung function were significantly more common among those exposed to the gas compared to a nonexposed comparison group. The greater the exposure to the gas, the more likely com-promised lung function was observed. In addition, lung function was lower among those complaining of symptoms (Beckett, 1998; Cullinan, Acquilla, & Dhara, 1997).

The general health impact among the affected population has been reported at various time points following the disaster. The ICMR set up the Bhopal Gas Research Centre to study the health effects of the disaster. This center began longitudinal health monitoring at the time of the dis-aster, which continued for a 5-year period. Dissatisfied with the closure of the ICMR studies after 5 years, independent research groups have carried out studies and continue to follow up on the health status of the exposed population.

A number of investigators have reported on the higher physical morbidity in the affected population as compared with unexposed groups (Andersson, Muir, Mehra, & Salmon, 1988; Gupta, Rastogi, Chandra, Mathur, Mathur, Mahendra, Pangley, Kumar, Kumar, Seth, 1988; Laxmipuram & Srivatsa, 1987; Naik, Acharya, Bhulerao, Kowli, Nazareth, Mahashur, Shah, Potnis, Mehta, 1986; Misra, Nag, Nath, Khan, Gupta, Ray, 1988). Studies reported on the health status of the population after 1 year (Misra, 1986; Sainani, Joshi, Mehta, & Abraham, 1985) and after 10 years (Cullinan, Acquilla, & Dhara, 1996). They all reported a higher morbidity in the affected population and a dose-response of adverse effects in relation to the exposure.

A high incidence of spontaneous abortions (24.2%) among pregnant women exposed to the toxic gas was reported in comparison to the control population. The perinatal and neonatal mortalities were significantly higher in the affected area (6.9% and 6.1% respectively) as compared to the control area (5% and 4.5%) (Bajaj, Misra, Rajalakshmi, & Madan, 1993; Bhandari, Syal, Kambo, Nair, Beohar, Saxena, Dabke, Agarwal, Saxena, 1990). Fetal loss was also abnormally high (26.3%) as compared to the control area (7.8%) (Kapoor, 1991).

Higher incidence rates of cancer of the lungs, oropharynx, and oral cavity (Dikshit & Kanhere, 1999), chromosomal variations including Robertsonian translocations (Goswami, Chandorkar, Bhattacharya, Vaidyanath, Parmar, Sengupta, Patidar, Sengupta, Goswami, Sharma, 1990), and immunological changes have been reported (Saxena, Singh, Nagle, Gupta, Ray, Srivastav, Tewari, Singh, 1988).

IMPACT ON MENTAL HEALTH

The Bhopal disaster was the first disaster in India to be studied systematically for its mental health effects. Information about the mental health effects is available from a number of sources, including studies as part of general health surveys as well as specific mental health studies. The direct involvement of the psychiatrists/neurologists in the field did not occur until about 8 weeks after the disaster. By coincidence the Fourth Advisory Committee on Mental Health of ICMR was scheduled to meet on December 12–14, 1984. The experts in the meeting recognized the need of the affected population as follows:

> The recent developments at Bhopal involving the exposure of "normal" human beings to substances toxic to all the exposed and fatal to many, raises a number of mental health needs. The service needs and research can be viewed both in the short-term and long-term perspectives. The acute needs are the understanding and provision of care for confusional states, reactive psychoses, anxiety-depression reactions and grief reactions. Long term needs arise from the following areas, namely, (i) psychological reactions to the acute and chronic disabilities, (ii) psychological problems of the exposed subjects, currently not affected, to the uncertainties of the future, (iii) effects of broken social units on children and adults, and (iv) psychological problems related to rehabilitation. (Srinivasa Murthy, Isaac, Chandrasekar, & Bhide,1987, p. 1)

However, in spite of this early recognition of the need for mental health interventions there was a delay of 6–8 weeks before mental health professionals were involved. An important reason for this was the lack of mental health professionals in the state of Madhya Pradesh and the city of Bhopal. At that point of time none of the five medical colleges had a psychiatrist on their faculties.

Andersson and Muir (1988) conducted the first community survey within 2 weeks of the disaster. The survey was carried out in eight exposed areas and two nonexposed clusters of households. There was a 2-month follow-up. The focus of the survey was eye and lung problems. As part of this study authors noted that the pupillary reflex was normal. Based on this, they concluded, "the fact that this reflex was normal in all groups can not be taken as evidence that neurotoxicity did not occur" (p. 470). Misra et al. (1988) reported on 33 adult patients treated during the acute phase at the Medical College Hospital. They found that symptoms of severe cough and dyspnea were followed by fainting in 55% of the patients. The duration of unconsciousness ranged from 30 minutes to 3 days. At the 3-month follow-up of this group of patients, depression and irritability were commonly reported symptoms.

Gupta et al. (1988) systematically studied 687 affected persons from various age groups in the general population and from different affected areas at two months after the disaster and another 592 persons after a 4-month period. These studies included behavioral studies and a control population. The behavioral studies were carried out with 350 adults. An extensive neuropsychological test battery examined various aspects of personality and cognitive function. The behavioral tests showed that memory, mainly visual perceptual and attention/response speed along with attention/vigilance were severely affected in the gas-exposed population. Further statistically significant differences were observed between the controls and the exposed groups on all the parameters tested. The gas-exposed groups, especially the females, had poor scores in the auditory memory tests. The exposed male group showed significantly lower visual memory scores as compared to controls and females. The Visual memory was more affected than auditory memory. Perceptual motor speed was significantly lower in the gas-exposed group. All these changes were associated with subjective complaints of lack of concentration and poor attention. In the manual dexterity tests there were no differences across the groups.

The Eysenck Personality Inventory (EPI) questionnaire results showed that 79.6% had poor scores on general lability items as measured by the EPI, whereas 88.6% with poor scores also had a tendency to general fatigue with somatic complaints on the EPI. Only 4.5% had neurotic tendencies as measured by EPI. As a group, women were more affected than men, and this difference was statistically significant.

Cullinan et al. (1996) carried out an epidemiological study of a representative gas-exposed population in January 1994, 9 years after the disaster. They studied 474 subjects and a control group. Of this sample, 76 participated in detailed neurological testing, which included vestibular and peripheral sensory function and tests for short-term memory. In this study a high proportion of subjects reported a wide variety of neuropsychiatric symptoms like abnormal smell, abnormal taste, faintness, headache, difficulty staying awake, and abnormal balance. Headache was reported by 80% of the subjects as compared to 50% in the control population. Neurological examination showed that a high proportion was judged to have clinical evidence of central, peripheral, or vestibular neurological disease. The mean short-term memory scores were lowest among the heavily exposed group (1.0 vs. 3.0). There was some evidence of impaired extrapyramidal functions. There was also an abnormal vertical drawing test among the exposed.

In this group, the psychological symptoms reported were fatigue (88%), anxiety (65%), and difficulty in concentration (64%). Difficulty in decision making was reported in 80% as compared to 35% in the control population. Irritability was reported by 33% compared with none in the control group. There was a consistent dose-response gradient across the separate exposure groups for all symptoms except depression. Approximately 25% reported symptoms of depression.

The initial assessment of mental health was carried out in the first week of February 1985 (about 8 weeks after the disaster) by R. Srinivasa Murthy of the National Institute of Mental Health and Neuro Sciences, Bangalore, and B. B. Sethi of K. G. Medical College, Lucknow. They visited Bhopal and interacted with the general population, including the patients attending the health facilities and the medical personnel, to understand the magnitude and nature of the mental health problems in the affected population. Their observations were based on clinical and unstructured interviews with a nonrepresentative sample that took place over the course of a week. Based on their findings, they estimated the magnitude of mental health needs of the population at 50% of those in the community and of about 20% of those attending medical facilities (Srinivasa Murthy, 1990).

Immediately following these observations, during February–April 1985, the K. G. Medical College team carried out systematic studies. Ten general medical clinics in the disaster-affected area were chosen in the first stage. A team, consisting of a psychiatrist, a clinical psychologist, and a social worker, visited one clinic a day, by rotation in a randomized fashion, on three occasions and screened all the newly registered adult patients with the help of a self-report questionnaire (SRQ). Subjects identified as probable psychiatric patients were then evaluated in detail by the psychiatrist with the help of a standardized psychiatric interview, the Present State Examination (PSE) (Wing, Cooper, & Sartorius, 1975). Clinical diagnoses were based on the International Classification of Diseases (9th revision) (ICD-9) (WHO, 1975).

During a period of 3 months (February–May 1985), 259 of the 855 patients screened at the 10 clinics were identified as having a potential mental disorder on the basis of their SRQ scores. Of these identified persons, 44 could not be evaluated and 215 were assessed using the PSE. The confirmed number of psychiatric patients was 193, yielding a prevalence rate of 22.6%. Most of the patients were females (73.6%) under 45 years of age (79%). The main diagnostic categories were anxiety neurosis (25%), depressive neurosis

(37%), adjustment reaction with prolonged depression (20%), and adjustment reaction with predominant disturbance of emotions (16%). Cases of psychosis were rare, and they were not related to the disaster (Sethi, Sharma, Trivedi, & Singh, 1987).

During the same period, in the third month of the postdisaster period, neurological studies were carried out (Bharucha & Bharucha, 1987). This was a survey of the gas-affected patients admitted to the various hospitals in Bhopal. A total of 129 adults and 47 children were studied for neurological problems. Evidence of involvement of the central nervous system was present in three patients in the form of stroke, encephalopathy, and cerebellar ataxia. The peripheral nervous system was affected in six patients. Vertigo and hearing loss occurred in four patients. Many patients reported transitory symptoms like loss of consciousness (50%), muscle weakness, tremors, vertigo, ataxia, and easy fatigability. Most of these symptoms diminished after varying periods of time. Of the 47 gas-affected children, loss of consciousness at some time occurred in half the patients. Fits occurred during the course of the illness in three children. Mental regression was observed in one child who had commenced speaking in sentences but stopped talking after the disaster. There were no abnormalities in the neurological examination in all the children. An important observation by the doctors who had examined the children during the early phase of illness was generalized hypotonia and weakness. Two children were noted to be "floppy" with weakness of limb movements and had difficulty in getting up from the ground. Of the three patients who had central nervous system involvement, the patient with stroke died. His autopsy showed intense congestion and petechial hemorrhages of the gray and white matter with frank hemorrhage in the circle of Willis area, perhaps indicating the sustained microvascular damage by the circulating MIC.

Subsequently, from June 1985, the Lucknow team with funding from ICMR and a New Delhi team conducted a detailed longitudinal epidemiological study in the general population to assess the mental health impact of the accident, along with the community level epidemiological study for other health effects. This study included recording the complaints of subjects and recording illnesses and deaths in 100,000 people in the different areas, selected randomly from the population census lists of Bhopal. A fresh census of the total population was undertaken prior to the study. The sampling frame was drawn up in such a manner that populations variously exposed to the disaster were included along with a control group located far from the gas-exposed area, but from within Bhopal itself.

The methodology used for screening the households was an interview with the head of the household for the presence of symptoms from a standardized checklist. Those found to have symptoms were then seen by a qualified psychiatrist who administered a detailed mental status examination instrument (PSE-9th version) and arrived at the ICD-9th version diagnosis. Each year a new set of families were sampled and studied in addition to the follow-up of the patients diagnosed in the previous years.

The first-year survey included 4,098 adults from 1,201 households. Most of the sample consisted of females (71%); 83% were in the age group 16–45 years. A total of 387 patients were diagnosed to be suffering from mental disorders, giving a prevalence rate of 94/1,000 population. Ninety-four percent of the patients received a diagnosis of neurosis (neurotic depression, 51%; anxiety state, 41%; hysteria, 2%) and had a temporal correlation with the disaster. For the next 3 years, the team repeated the annual surveys and follow-up of the initial patients identified by the community survey. Detailed case vignettes and descriptive accounts of the patients from the Bhopal disaster were prepared.

These general population psychiatric epidemiological studies showed that the gas-exposed population had significantly higher prevalence rates for psychiatric disorders in comparison to the general population. The dose-response relationship of higher rates of psychiatric morbidity with severity of exposure to the poisonous gas was maintained throughout the 5 years of the survey period. At the end of the 5-year period only a small number were fully recovered and large numbers continued to experience symptoms along with significant disability in functioning.

MENTAL HEALTH INTERVENTIONS

One of the challenges faced by the team of psychiatrists was the provision of psychiatric services to the affected population. There was no psychiatric help available in the city for a total population of 700,000 and affected population of about 200,000. A number of measures were taken to meet this challenge. First, Srinivasa Murthy and Sethi worked to prepare clinical vignettes of patients to sensitize the medical professionals and the administrators. The majority of the administrators and medical professionals considered the complaints, especially the psychiatric symptoms, imaginary and compensation related. This misconception was corrected by demonstrating the real nature of the symptoms and the universality of the adverse effects of the accident on the mental health of the affected population. Second, starting from February 1985, teams of psychiatrists, clinical psychologists, and psychiatric social workers from Lucknow were located in the city for periods of 2–4 weeks to provide psychiatric care to the affected population. This was a short-term measure (Sethi et al., 1987). The third response was to train the general medical officers working with the affected population with the essential skills for mental health care. This was indeed very challenging but was a rapid way of increasing the mental health care in the city. In view of its importance and since this was the first time it had been done in India, and possibly in other developing countries, it is described in detail.

Soon after the disaster, additional physicians were moved to the city and located in the different gas-affected areas to provide general medical care to the population. In April 1985, about 50 medical officers were providing health care services to the affected populations, most of them with no prior training in mental health. In their initial medical training there were no teachers of psychiatry in the state medical colleges.

This lack of training was reflected in their difficulty to understand the emotional needs of the disaster-affected population. The basic orientation of these doctors was highly medical/biological. In the pretraining interviews, most of them expressed the view that distribution of monetary compensation would solve the physical complaints of a large number of their patients. Some expressed the view that the free rations (food grains and other essentials) provided by the state was the reason for the complaints of weaknesses and inability to work reported by many patients. The doctors believed that the "lethargy" of their patients would disappear not by medical treatment or by the use of drugs but by "stopping the free rations and distribution of compensation money."

The training was designed to enhance the sensitivity of the medical officers to the emotional needs of individuals and to provide the skills to recognize, diagnose, treat, and refer (when required) the mental health problems (Srinivasa Murthy & Isaac, 1987). The period of initial training was 6 working days. It was decided that the training should be as practical as possible and should be imparted to groups not exceeding 20 persons. The methodology of training took into account principles of "adult learning," that is, an open learning environment in which participants were free to share their needs and experiences, with greater emphasis on interactive learning. The predominantly lecture approach was changed to the use of case studies and group discussions facilitated by audio-visual, audiotaped material of the affected population with maximum student involvement.

The actual training was carried out in two series by the two consultant psychiatrists. A manual was prepared on the basis of experience in training primary care physicians at the National Institute of Mental Health and Neurosciences (NIMHANS) in Bangalore (Isaac, Chandrasekar, & Srinivasa Murthy, 1984). Additional sections on emotional reactions to sudden severe stress, emotional reactions of children to stress, and emotional reactions to physical problems were written and incorporated into the manual, which was used in its draft form for the training. A revised manual incorporating the experience of the training and the needs of the medical officers was prepared subsequently and distributed to all the doctors working with the gas-affected population (Srinivasa Murthy, Isaac, Chandrashekar, & Bhide, 1987). For the purpose of the evaluation of the existing pretraining psychiatric knowledge, a video presentation of 10 cases was utilized. These included video interviews of the gas-affected population and standard interviews with those having different psychiatric problems.

Each morning the two faculty members visited the different health facilities and worked with the medical officers to help them learn the interview techniques and counseling methods. This "live" experience was considered very useful by the medical officers. Post-training evaluation was carried out by a simple questionnaire. A total of 38 medical officers took part in the training.

The main objectives for the first session were to facilitate faculty-participant interaction. The trainee doctors were asked to share their expectations from the program. The pretraining responses of all the doctors were obtained on a structured response sheet. Subsequently, a detailed introduction to the training program was given highlighting the mental health problems among the gas-affected community and the possibilities for feasible interventions. In the introduction, the work carried out by a team of psychiatrists in Bangalore on the victims of the Venus Circus Fire tragedy in 1981 was also discussed (Narayana, 1986).

The aim of the second session was to give the doctors an understanding of normal and illness behaviors. The biological (brain anatomy, physiology, and chemistry), psychological, and the social basis and dimensions of normal human behavior were discussed. In light of this, symptoms presented by psychiatric patients were discussed. Patients with different symptoms and presentations were shown using videos. Types, features, and causes of mental illnesses were outlined.

During the third session, approaches to patients with emotional disturbances, history taking, and the mental examination were taught. Audiotaped and videotaped interviews facilitated this part. Following a short 20–minute video on psychosis, the topic was discussed at length. The topic of neurosis with special emphasis on anxiety, depression, and grief reactions was discussed in detail.

The fourth session was critical as the trainee doctors discussed their experiences in their daily clinical work. The training during the first three days provided the basic background required to understand the psychological nature of many of the complaints of the patients. During this session, various clinical presentations of the gas-affected patients were discussed. All the audio and video material used pertained to the patients seen in the various clinics in Bhopal. Since emotional reactions of people to disasters, irrespective of the nature of the disaster, have a similar pattern the world over, some of the classic documents on psychological sequeae of disaster were also reviewed and discussed. Many children were brought for consultation for various kinds of complaints and therefore some time was given to the discussion of the emotional reactions of children to sudden severe stress. Many interviews with children both on audiotape and videotape were presented. The assessment of persons with varying degrees of physical disability due to proven gas-related physical illnesses (such as fibrosis of the lungs) posed a problem for many doctors. Emotional responses to physical disability and chronic physical illnesses were also covered. The availability of patients (on video) from the local clinics for discussion greatly enhanced the interest and involvement of the participants. The emotional dimension to the complaints of patients was completely new to most of the participant doctors.

By the fifth day of training, most of the participants were able to recognize the psychological needs of a large number of patients attending their clinics. The participants were able to elicit, in many patients, various psychiatric symptoms. At this stage of training, the approaches to management of such patients were presented. This session emphasized the importance of psychological management. After the initial introduction by the faculty, the session began with role-play exercises where interviewing of patients was simulated. The basic principles of psychological management, the importance of appropriate interview techniques to establish a satisfactory doctor-patient relationship, and the methods of providing reassurance, use of suggestion, and psychological support were demonstrated. Audio recordings of psychotherapy by the faculty with some of the local patients were used to illustrate the techniques.

During the last session, pharmacological management and other approaches and referral guidelines were covered. A good part of the time was occupied by discussion on "the implementation of the mental health care program" among the affected population in Bhopal. The last 30 minutes was devoted to obtaining post-training responses from the participants.

Some of the comments of the participants in the post-training evaluation supported the usefulness of the training. Most of them felt that with the training, they would be much more capable of treating psychiatric illness and other patients having medical problems as well. Some doctors expressed that earlier they used to give the patients only symptomatic treatment, but after the training they were able to think and diagnose the condition in terms of a psychological approach. Some doctors mentioned that prior to the training, they were not aware of any psychiatric problems and were of the opinion that the patients were malingering and giving vague symptoms to evoke a sympathetic response and get more medicines. All the doctors who took part in the training agreed that there was need for privacy during interviews, support from psychiatrists for difficult cases, and a regular supply of psychotropic drugs.

There are a number of unresolved issues of the Bhopal disaster. The Bhopal disaster continues to provoke public debate and the people continue to demand relief and rehabilitation. Three social issues are of importance. First, there is an international-level debate about the right to know. (Jasanoff, 1988). The Bhopal disaster jolted activist groups around the world into renewing their demands for right-to-know legislation granting broader access to information about hazardous technologies (Bader, 1987; Bhopal Working Group, 1987; Levenstein & Ozonoff, 1987; Walker, 1987). Second, there is a need for continued study of the health effect of the exposure on the population. This need has been voiced by a number of researchers and human rights activists. However, except for limited efforts, large-scale systematic studies are not forthcoming. Long–term monitoring of the affected community should be done for at least the next 50 years. Formal studies of ocular, respiratory, reproductive, immunologic, genetic, and psychological health must be continued to elucidate the extent and severity of long-term effects (Delvin, 1996; Dhara, 1992a, 1992b; Dhara, Acquilla, & Cullinan, 2001; Dhara & Dhara, 1995; Dhara & Kriebel, 1993a, 1993b; *Lancet*, 2000; Srinivasa Murthy, 2001). Third, appropriate medical services to the affected population are still needed. It is now 18 years after the disaster and thousands of men, women, and children are still suffering from respiratory illnesses, precocious blindness, cancers, and so many other related ailments for which they receive no treatment (Harshmander, 2001; Lapierre & Moro, 2001). The efforts to date have set up specialized centers (Percival, 2001) without a clear link to community services. It has been repeatedly emphasized that a health care–pyramid approach needs to be adopted to deal with health problems resulting from the gas leak. Community-level health units should be developed to serve only a maximum of 5,000 people. Local hospitals with specialized departments may be used to provide secondary care. A specialized medical center should be established, dedicated to treatment and research of the more serious problems arising from the gas leak. There is clearly an urgent need to develop standard protocols of treatment for the unique problems of the gas-affected population (International Medical Commission on Bhopal, 1994; Srinivasa Murthy, 2001).

LESSONS FROM THE BHOPAL DISASTER

One of the big challenges for a mental health professional working in a developing country is the low priority given to mental health. This is mainly because it is thought of as a marginal problem affecting only a small proportion of people who lack voice. However, the recognition of mental health of disaster-affected populations switches the value of mental health from a deviant model to a normalcy model. The recognition that each and every person has a potential risk for mental health problems, following severe stress, makes attention to mental health important to everyone on the individual as well as community levels. For example, in India in the state of Madhya Pradesh, with a population of over 60 million, there were less than a handful of psychiatrists at the time of the disaster. Following the disaster, there was greater awareness of mental health. There has been a significant improvement in the mental health infrastructure; most of it created as a consequence of the disaster. Currently all the medical colleges have psychiatrists on their staff.

This innovative approach utilized to study the mental health effects of disasters by using existing health personnel to provide mental health care, initiated at Bhopal, has become the accepted pattern in the country to meet the mental health needs of the subsequent disaster-affected populations (Acharya, 2000; Ali & Jaswal, 2000; Gandevia, 2000; Joseph, 2000; Juvva & Rajendran, 2000; Pande, Phadke, Dalal, & Agashe, 2000; Pande, Phadke, Dalal, Gadkari et al. 2000; Patel, 2000; Parasuraman & Unnikrishnan, 2000; Sharma, Chaudhury, Kavathekar & Saxena, 1996).

A good example of this innovation reaching its full potential was the Orissa cyclonic disaster in October 1999 and the Gujarat earthquake in January 2001. A supercyclone hit the Orissa coast on October 29, 1999. The wind force was of more than 250 kilometers per hour. The sea waves were 20–30 feet high. This disaster affected over 15 million people living in 12 districts. The estimated number of people who lost their lives was about 10,000. Another aspect of this disaster was the extensive damage to the trees, animals, and houses. As a result of the cyclone there were millions without a roof over their heads. In addition most of the schools in the affected area were totally destroyed, disrupting the school system. Mental health initiatives started soon after the disaster, unlike the 2-month hiatus following the Bhopal disaster. A series of studies were carried out following the disaster. The first one was within 4 weeks of the disaster covering 1,000 persons from a total population of 10,000. This study showed that 65% have identifiable mental health problems and 25% have severe mental health problems. In addition, the staff of the local medical college reported an increase in the number of people presenting with psychiatric problems as compared to a normal period. In addition, there were a wide variety of disorders ranging from anxiety states to severe psychosis. The subject matter of symptoms and the time of occurrence of the illness indicate an association with the disaster. The number of mental health resources available in the whole state of Orissa was extremely small. For a population of over 30 million, there were only

31 psychiatrists and an insignificant number of clinical psychologists and psychiatric social workers. A very positive outcome of this disaster was the very recognition given to psychosocial problems and psychiatric problems in the affected population.

A specific program to meet the needs of the population was initiated with the following components. At the level of all the affected population a simple information booklet has been prepared describing how they can take care of their own health by measures that are within their reach. (Srikala et al., 2000) A more detailed booklet was prepared for all categories of community-level workers to provide support, first aid, and referral or severe cases and stimulation of community support systems (Kishorekumar et al., 2000). A program was established for training the primary care doctors so that they can provide mental health care as part of primary health care. A manual was prepared for teachers to provide mental health care to affected children and especially to help them understand the disaster as well as the mechanisms they can use to recover. All of these efforts were carried out both by voluntary organizations as well as the government as part of the total relief work. A system of monitoring and evaluation was planned for all of these activities.

It is important to recognize the mental health needs and interventions as part of the other needs of the disaster population. The integration has significant advantages in terms of utilizing the available resources, providing psychiatric care without stigma, as well as harmonizing the physical, social, and psychological services. This requires training of all personnel who are working with disaster populations in mental health care.

The mental health professionals have the challenge of simplifying the information as well as the intervention skills suitable to the affected population, community-level helpers, schoolteachers, primary care health workers, primary care doctors, and other developmental personnel. These programs have to be short, focused, and practical rather than theoretical. In addition, they have to be routed in the local cultural ethos of the affected population. As noted above, nonprofessionals particularly from the local area should provide the bulk of initial counseling, rather than moving volunteers from different parts of the country to the disaster area. In this approach the professionals will have to accept a partnership with laypeople so that there is no conflict between professionals and nonprofessionals. The training should be located in the field area, should include a lot of practical work, and the professionals should be able to demonstrate the interventions in the actual community situation.

Mental health professionals have a very important role in evaluating interventions. Currently most of the interventions are based on face validity. Short-term and long-term evaluations have not been done beyond evaluation of the training programs. Such evaluations should not only look at clinical symptoms but at the quality of life of the affected population. There is also need for developing simple tools for evaluation that can be used by nonprofessionals.

There is a need to study various aspects of the psychiatric problems in disaster–affected populations. Recent reviews of literature in this area have identified variables like family support, kinship help, and subsequent events in the affected populations as being important for the long-term outcome (Bromet and Dew, 1995). The cross-cultural aspect of disaster is only recently recognized as being important (Patel, 2000). WHO (1992) identified the following areas for research in this field especially relevant to developing countries.

1. Much of the research on the psychosocial effects of disasters has been carried out among western populations. It is therefore imperative to carry out extensive research with populations from developing countries, those that are most affected by natural and man-made disasters, both large and smallscale; this research will allow the study of cross-cultural variations in frequency, symptomatology, temporal patterns and outcome of psychological disorders, and will clarify the moderating effect of culture on these disorders. This research, to be practically and ethically feasible, needs to follow strict guidelines, and should adopt a rigorous research methodology. To achieve this, every effort should be made to obtain reliable pre-disaster baseline health data (preferably from various sources); to have a control group; to have high follow up response rates; to use a longitudinal design, and to find valid screening instruments to be employed as a first step in mass screening programs in the acute post-disaster phase.

2. Although there is agreement that social support and intense kin relationships are highly supportive and facilitate post-disaster recovery among victims, little empirical evidence is available in this regard. Therefore, the specific role of these variables in modifying the overall frequency, severity and course of psychological disorders needs to be further explored, as do the importance of personal vulnerability and prior psychopathology in their occurrence. Specific groups, particularly dependent on social support (such as children, the elderly, and the physically ill) should be carefully investigated.

3. Investigations into physiological determinants and correlates of psychological and psychiatric disorders, especially PTSD, so far mainly laboratory-based, should be strengthened and should be mainly clinically based. It would therefore be useful to find reliable, valid and feasible physiological measures of stress to be used as diagnostic tools. For practical reasons, this research is more feasible with individual victims of a single trauma or in more limited accidents or disasters occurring in developed countries.

4. The diagnostic specificity of the symptoms of PTSD also needs to be further explored, as does the natural history of this disorder.

5. An important area of research is comorbidity, especially among persons suffering from PTSD: for instance, substance abuse, frequently associated with PTSD, has been interpreted as a long-term attempt to numb oneself against intrusive images and nightmares, thus representing a secondary response to primary PTSD symptoms.

6. The experience of facing a trauma as an individual, versus the effect of trauma when experienced with others needs to be investigated.

7. Finally, treatment of the main psychological and psychiatric posttraumatic disorders is an important area for research. The main psychotherapeutic and pharmacological treatment methods deserve detailed consideration and need to be adequately tested and verified for cross-cultural applicability as well as for general effectiveness. (p. 22)

CONCLUSIONS

Ecological disasters are a challenge everywhere for both the affected populations as well as health care professionals. However, they represent special challenges and opportunities in developing countries. The Bhopal disaster is a turning point in understanding the mental health aspects of disasters. The research has shown the high physical and mental morbidity in the general population and the continuing need for longitudinal health studies. Using a public health approach in priority setting, identification of interventions, training of existing personnel, and utilizing existing community resources, the needs of the population can be addressed. Such situations offer mental health professionals both challenges and opportunities for innovation.

REFERENCES

Acharya, N. (2000). Double victims of Latur eartquake. *Indian Journal of Social Work, 61,* 558–564.

Ali, N., & Jaswal, S. (2000). Political unrest and mental health in Srinagar. *Indian Journal of Social Work, 61,* 598–618.

Andersson, N., Kerr Muir, M., Ajwani, M. K., Mahashabde, S., Salmon, A., & Vaidyanathan, K. (1986). Persistent eye watering among Bhopal survivors, *Lancet 2,* 1152.

Andersson, N., Muir, M. K., & Mehra, V. (1984). Bhopal eye. *Lancet 2,* 1481.

Andersson, N., Muir, M. K., Muir, M., Mehra, V., & Salmon, A. (1988). Exposure and response to methyl isocyanate: Results of a community based survey in Bhopal. *British Journal of Industrial Medicine, 45,* 469–475.

Bader, M. (1987). The Bhopal working group report. *American Journal of Public Health, 77,* 878–879.

Bajaj, J. S., Misra, A., Rajalakshmi, M., & Madan, R. R. (1993). Environmental release of chemicals and reproductive ecology. *Environmental Health Perspective* (Suppl. 2), 125–130.

Beckett, W. S. (1998). Persistent respiratory effects in survivors of the Bhopal disaster. *Thorax,* *53* (Suppl. 2), S43–46.

Bhandari, N. R., Syal, A. K., Kambo, I., Nair, A., Beohar, V., Sexena, N. C., Dabke, A. T., Agarwal, S. S., & Saxena, B. N. (1990). Pregnancy outcome in women exposed to toxic gas at Bhopal. *Indian Journal of Medical Research, 92,* 28–33.

Bhargava, D. K., Verma, A., Saini, G., Misra, N. P., Tewari, V. C., Vijayan, V. K., & Jain, J. K. (1987). Early observations on lung function studies on symptomatic gas exposed population of Bhopal. *Indian Journal of Medical Research, 86* (Suppl.), 1–10 .

Bharucha, E. P., & Bharucha, N. E. (1987). Neurological manifestations among those exposed to toxic gas at Bhopal. *Indian Journal of Medical Research, 86* (Suppl.), 59–62.

Bhopal gas leak survivors launch cyber protest. (2000). Retrieved on August 16, 2000, from Indya.com

Bhopal Working Group. (1987). The public health implications of the Bhopal disaster: Report to the program development board, American Public Health Association. *American Journal of Public Health, 77,* 230–236.

Bromet, E., & Dew, M. A. (1995). Review of psychiatric epidemiological research on disasters. *Epidemiologic Reviews, 17,* 113–119.

Cullinan, P., Acquilla, S. D., & Dhara, V. R. (1996). Long term morbidity in survivors of the 1984 Bhopal gas leak. *National Medical Journal of India, 9,* 5–10.

Cullinan, P., Acquilla, S., & Dhara, V. R. (1997). Respiratory morbidity 10 years after the Union Carbide gas leak at Bhopal: A cross sectional survey. The International Medical Commission on Bhopal. *British Medical Journal, 314,* 338–342.

Delvin, N. (1996). Call to alleviate long-term effects of Bhopal gas disaster. *Lancet, 348,* 1652.

Dhara, R. (1992a). Health effects of the Bhopal gas leak: A review. *Epidemiologia e prevenzione, 52,* 22–31.

Dhara, R. (1992b). On the bioavailability of methyl isocyanate in the Bhopal gas leak. *Archives of Environmental Health, 47,* 385–386.

Dhara, R., Acquilla, S., & Cullinan, P. (2001). Has the world forgotten Bhopal? Letter to the Editor. *Lancet, 357,* 809–810.

Dhara, R., & Dhara, V. R. (1995) Bhopal—A case study of international disaster. *International Journal of Occupational Enviornmental Medicine, 1,* 58–69.

Dhara, R. V., & Kriebel, D. (1993a). An exposure-response method for assessing the long-term health effects of the Bhopal gas disaster. *Disasters, 17,* 281–290.

Dhara, R. V., & Kriebel, D. (1993b). The Bhopal gas disaster: It is not too late for sound epidemiology. *Archives of Environmental Health, 48,* 436–437.

Dikshit, R. P., & Kanhere, S. (1999). Cancer patterns of lung, oropharynx and oral cavity cancer relation to gas exposure at Bhopal. *Cancer Causes Control, 10,* 627–636.

Gandevia, K. (2000). Psychosocial health of a village ravaged by an earthquake. *Indian Journal of Social Work, 61,* 652–663.

Goswami, H. K., Chandorkar, M., Bhattacharya, K., Vaidyanath, G., Parmar, D., Sengupta, S., Patidar, S. L., Sengupta, L. K., Goswami, R., & Sharma, P. N. (1990). Searya for chromosomal variations among gas-exposed persons in Bhopal. *Human Genetics,* 84: 172–176.

Gupta, B. N., Rastogi, S. K., Chandra, H., Mathur, A. K., Mathur, N., Mahendra, P. N., Pangley, B. S., Kumar, S., Kumar, P., & Seth, R. K. (1988). Effect of exposure to toxic gas on the population of bhopal: Part I—Epidemiological, clinical, radiological and behavioral studies. *Indian Journal of Experimental Biology, 26,* 149–160.

Harshmander, (2001). *Unheard voices.* New Delhi: Penguin.

International Medical Commission on Bhopal. (1994). Press release, January 24. New Delhi, India.

Isaac, M. K., Chandrasekar, C. R., & Srinivasa Murthy, R. (1984). *Manual of mental health care for primary care doctors.* Bangalore: National Institute of Mental Health and Neurosciences.

Jasanoff, S. (1988). The Bhopal disaster and the right to know. *Social Science and Medicine, 27,* 1113–1123.

Jayaraman, K. S. (1984). Pesticide plant leak wreaks disaster in India. *Nature, 312,* 581.

Jayaraman, K. S. (1985). Bhopal disaster: Technical inquiry underway. *Nature, 313,* 89.

Jayaraman, K. S. (1987). Bhopal aftermath re-assessed. *Nature, 329,* 752.

Joseph, H. (2000). Salokha: A response to communal riots, a social disaster. *Indian Journal of Social Work, 61,* 664–674.

Juvva, S., & Rajendran, P. (2000). Disaster and mental health: A current perspective. *Indian Journal of Social Work, 61,* 521–526.

Kamat, S. R., Patel, M. H., Kolhatkar, V. P., Dave, A. A., & Mahashur, A. A. (1987). Sequential respiratory changes in those exposed to the gas leak at Bhopal. *Indian Journal of Medical Research, 86* (Suppl.), 20–38.

Kapoor, R. (1991). Fetal loss and contraceptive acceptance among the Bhopal victims. *Social Biology, 38,* 242–248.

Kishorekumar, K. V., Chandrashekar, C. R., Chowdhury, P., Parthasarathy, R., Girimaji, S., Sekar, K. et al. (2000). *Supercyclone: Psychosocial care for community level helpers. Information manual 2.* Bangalore: Books for Change.

Lancet. (2000). Has the world forgotten Bhopal? Editorial. *Lancet, 356,* 1863.

Lapierre, D., & Moro, J. (2001). *It was five past midnight in Bhopal.* Delhi: Full Circle.

Laxmipuram, P., & Srivatsa, L. P. (1987). Bhopal—What is their suffering? *Journal de Toxicalogie Clinique et Experimentale, 7,* 323–329.

Levenstein, C., & Ozonoff, D. (1987). Levenstein and ozonoff respond. *American Journal of Public Health, 77,* 879.

MacKenzie, D. (1985). Design failings that caused Bhopal disaster. *New Scientist, 28,* 3–4.

Maskati, O. B. (1986). Ophthalmic survey of Bhopal victims 104 days after the tragedy. *Journal of Postgraduate Medicine, 32,* 199–202.

Menon, M. N. R. (1999, September 2). Law according to injustice. *The Telegraph,* Kolkata, P. 7.

Misra, N. P. (1986). Bhopal tragedy—A year later. *Journal of the Association of Physicians of India, 34,* 307.

Misra, N. P., Nag, D., Nath, P., Khan, W. A., Gupta, B. N., & Ray, P. K. (1988). A clinical study of toxic gas poisoning in Bhopal, India. *Indian Journal of Experimental Biology 26,* 201–204.

Naik S. R., Acharya V. N., Bhalerao R. A., Kowli S. S., Nazarath H., Mahas A. A., Mahashur, A. A., Shah, S., Potnis, A. V., & Mehta, A. C. (1986). Medical survey of methyl isocynate gas affected population Bhopal. Part II. Pulmonary effects in Bhopal victims as seen weeks after M.I.C. exposure. *Journal of Postgraduate Medicine, 32,* 185–191.

Narayana, H. S. (1986). Grief reaction among bereaved relatives following a fire disater in circus. *NIMHANS Journal, 5,* 13–22.

Pande, N. R., Phadke, S. S., Dalal, M. S., & Agashe, M. M. (2000). Mental health care in Marathwada earthquake disaster-1: Organisation of services. *Indian Journal of Social Work, 61,* 640–651.

Pande, N. R., Phadke, S. S., Dalal, M. S., Gadkari, P. J., Nagapurkar, U. S., & Agashe, M. M. (2000). Mental health care in Marathwada earthquake disaster-2: Short-term outreach counselling. *Indian Journal of Social Work, 61,* 640–651.

Parasuraman, S., & Unnikrishnan, P. V. (2000). *India Disasters report: Towards a policy initiative.* New Delhi: Oxford University Press.

Patel, V. (2000). Culture and mental health consequences of trauma. *Indian Journal of Social Work, 61,* 619–630.

Percival, R. (2001). Has the world forgotten Bhopal? Letter to the Editor *Lancet, 357,* 810.

Raizada, J. K., & Dwivedi, P. C. (1987). Chronic ocular lesions in Bhopal gas tragedy. *Indian Journal of Ophthalmology, 35,* 453–454.

Rastogi, S. K., Gupta, B. N., Husain, T., Kumar, A., Chandra, S., & Ray, P. K. (1988). Effect of exposure to toxic gas on the population of Bhopal: II Respiratory impairment. *Indian Journal of Experimental Biology, 26,* 161–164

Sainani, G. S., Joshi, V. R., Mehta, P. J., & Abraham, P. (1985). Bhopal tragedy—A year later. *Journal of Association of Physicians of India, 33,* 755–756.

Saxena, A. K., Singh, K. P., Nagle, S. L., Gupta, B. N., Ray, P. K., Srivastav, R. K., Tewari, S. P., & Singh, R. (1988). Effect of exposure to toxic gas on the population of Bhopal: IV—Immunological and chromosomal studies. *Indian Journal of Experimental Biology, 26,* 173–176.

Sethi, B. B., Sharma, M., Trivedi, J. K., & Singh, H. (1987). Psychiatric morbidity in patients attending clinics in gas affected areas in Bhopal. *Indian Journal of Medical Research, 86* (Suppl.), 45–50.

Sharma, P., Chaudhury, G., Kavathekar, S. A. & Saxena S. (1996). Preliminary report of psychiatric disorders in survivors of a severe earthquake. *American Journal of Psychiatry, 153,* 556–558.

Srikala, B., Chandrashekar, C. R., Kishore Kumar, K. V., Chowdhury, P., Parthasarathy, R., Girimaji, S. et al. (2000). *Supercyclone: Psychosocial care for individuals. Information manual 1.* Bangalore: Books for Change.

Srinivasa Murthy, R. (1990). Bhopal. *International Journal of Mental Health, 19,* 30–35

Srinivasa Murthy, R. (2000). Disaster and mental health: Responses of mental health professionals. *Indian Journal of Social Work, 61,* 675–692.

Srinivasa Murthy, R. (2001). Has the world forgotten Bhopal? Letter to the Editor. *Lancet, 357,* 810.

Srinivasa Murthy, R., & Isaac, M. K. (1987). Mental health needs of Bhopal disaster victims and training of medical officers in mental health aspects. *Indian Journal of Medical Research, 86* (Suppl.), 51–58.

Srinivasa Murthy, R., Isaac, M. K., Chandrashekar, C. R., & Bhide, A. S. (1987). *Manual of mental health for medical officers—Bhopal disaster.* New Delhi: ICMR.

Tachakra, S. S. (1987). The Bhopal disaster. *Journal of Royal Society of Health, 107*(1), 1–2.

Union Carbide shields pharma Chairman Anderson. (2000, May 28). *Asian Age,* p. 8.

Vijayan, V. K., Pandey, V. P., Sankaran, K., Mehrotra, Y., Darbari, B. S., & Mi, N. P. (1989) Bronchoalveolar lavage study in victims of toxic gas leak at Bhopal. *Indian Journal of Medical Research, 90,* 407–414.

Vijayan, V. K., & Sankaran, K. (1996). Relationship between lung inflammation, changes in lung function and severity of exposure in victims of the Bhopal tragedy. *European Respiratory Medicine, 9,* 1977–1982.

Vijayan, V. K., Sankaran, K., Sharma, S. K., & Misra, N. P. (1995). Chronic lung inflammation in victims of toxic gas leak at Bhopal *Respiratory Medicine, 89,* 105–111.

Walker, B. (1987). Spectre of the Bhopal disaster. *American Journal of Public Health, 77,* 878.

Weil, H. (1987). Disaster at Bhopal: The accident, early findings and respiratory health outlook in those injured. *Bulletin European Physiopathologie Respiratoire, 23,* 587–590.

Wing, J. K., Cooper, J. E., & Sartorius, N. (1975). Measurement and classification of psychiatric symptoms. Cambridge: Cambridge University Press.

World Health Organization. (1975). *International statistical classification of diseases* (9th edition). Geneva: Author.

World Health Organization. (1992). Psychosocial consequences of disasters prevention and management. WHO/MNH/PSF/91.3.

8

Psychological and Physical Health Effects of the 1995 Sarin Attack in the Tokyo Subway System

NOZOMU ASUKAI and KAZUHIKO MAEKAWA

INTRODUCTION

In June 1994, a terrorist group released Sarin gas in the residential area of Matsumoto in central Japan, killing 7 people and affecting about 600 residents and rescue personnel (Morita, Yanagisawa, & Nakajima, 1995). In March 1995, another Sarin attack occurred in the Tokyo subway system (Okumura, Takasu, & Ishimatsu, 1996). Both cases had deleterious effects on Japanese society. The perpetrator of the Matsumoto case was not identified until the Aum Shinrikyo cult leader, Shoko Asahara, and members of his entourage were arrested just after the Tokyo subway case and their clandestine Sarin factory was discovered on the premises of their rural cult compound. Japan's courts are now trying both cases and the national media are giving them extensive coverage almost on a daily basis.

Lethal nerve gas agents, such as Tabun, Sarin, Soman, and VX, are organophosphate anti-cholinesterases. German scientists synthesized Tabun

NOZOMU ASUKAI • Department of Stress Disorders Research, Tokyo Institute of Psychiatry, Tokyo, Japan. KAZUHIKO MAEKAWA • Department of Traumatology and Critical Care Medicine, University of Tokyo Faculty of Medicine, Tokyo, Japan.

Toxic Turmoil: Psychological and Societal Consequences of Ecological Disasters, edited by Johan M. Havenaar, Julie G. Cwikel, and Evelyn J. Bromet. New York, Kluwer Academic/Plenum Publishers, 2002.

and Sarin in the late 1930s, and Soman in 1944. VX was synthesized by a British scientist in 1952 and forwarded to the United States for production. The use of nerve agents by the German military in combat never occurred during the Second World War. The first documented use of lethal nerve gas agents on a battlefield was when Iraq used Sarin against the Kurdish people in 1988. Aside from military use, lethal nerve gas agents had never been used on a civilian population in any civilized country not at war (Holstege, Kirk, & Sidell, 1997).

The magnitude of the devastation caused by this "chemical warfare" in the middle of a metropolis in peacetime was quite unprecedented. As such, they have commanded a great deal of media attention in the past decade. Also, for disaster psychiatry and psychology, the possibility of a terrorist attack with the nerve agent is now becoming a great concern and various issues in psychiatric aspects are being examined (DiGiovanni, 1999).

In this chapter we will describe our experiences and findings in the wake of the Sarin attack on the Tokyo subway system to help mental health professionals to prepare against disaster caused by the nerve agent.

OVERVIEW OF THE EVENT

The Sarin Attack on the Subway Trains

On March 20, 1995, Sarin nerve gas was released simultaneously on five trains on three lines of the Tokyo subway system during a Monday morning rush hour. These three lines serve the major governmental and financial districts of Tokyo. Aum Shinrikyo cult members carried sealed plastic packs of Sarin liquid onto the trains, then pierced the packs to spread Sarin on the floor, resulting in poisonous fumes filling the closed subway cars.

Central Tokyo was thrown into chaos when subway commuters started collapsing and staggering out of the trains as the Sarin gas permeated the cars shortly after 8:00 A.M. The first emergency call was received from the Tsukiji subway station at 8:09 at the Command and Control Center of the Tokyo Fire Department. Later, the Control Center received a series of emergency calls from other subway stations in other areas. Hospitals and rescue workers in central Tokyo were initially alerted by the Control Center to the possibility of mass casualties due to what was thought to be some kind of explosion. The Tokyo Metropolitan Police Department announced at a press conference at 11:00 A.M. that all indications pointed to Sarin nerve gas as having been used in the attack.

Passengers suffered from a darkened visual field, coughing and respiratory distress, rhinorrea, headache, and nausea. The subway lines were shut down and passengers were evacuated from the stations. The most severely poisoned victims collapsed on station platforms and fell into a comatose state accompanied with convulsions and foaming from the mouth. Many passengers witnessed the agony experienced by these severely poisoned victims.

In total, approximately 5,500 people visited 280 medical facilities during that day and in the days that followed. Of them, 1,046 people were admitted to 98 hospitals. The total number of poisoned victims, as summed up in official police record, came to 3,795. They included subway passengers, subway workers, firefighters, and police officers. Twelve people died of the Sarin poisoning; 10 of them within 48 hours. All the fatalities were caused by cardio-pulmonary arrest at the scene of the attack. According to the reported data on age and gender distributions of 740 hospitalized patients in 62 hospitals, 65% were males and 35% were females. The male patients were mostly in their 20s to 50s while 60% of the female patients were in their 20s (Maekawa, 1997). The age and gender distributions of the hospitalized patients probably represent those of subway commuters during weekday morning rush hour.

Secondary Contamination

One of the egregious effects of nerve agents is the secondary contamination. As an emergency response to mass exposure, it is said that decontamination should occur near the site of exposure to limit the spread of toxic agents. Decontamination of poisoned victims serves to terminate toxin exposure and the secondary contamination of rescue staff. Staffers should wear air-supplied respirators until the patient is decontaminated (Holstege et al., 1997). In the Tokyo Sarin case, however, it took 3 hours before the toxic substance was identified as Sarin, and, as mentioned above, firefighters and police officers were initially alerted by the Control Center to the possibility of mass casualties due to what was thought to be some kind of explosion. Therefore, emergency workers rushed on site without appropriate protection gear, resulting in the secondary contamination. In this way, many emergency staffers, firefighters, police officers, and hospital staffers were exposed to the secondary contamination.

Apart from disaster workers, passengers who volunteered for rescuing severely poisoned victims also became severely contaminated, and some of those volunteers lost consciousness in their attempt to rescue others.

ACUTE EFFECTS

Acute Symptoms of Poisoning

Nerve agents bring out their effects as anti-cholinesterases. With few exceptions, the poisonings in the Tokyo Sarin attack were due to vapor inhalation. In mild vapor inhalation of the nerve gas, miosis, conjuctival injection, dim vision, rhinorrea, wheezing, and respiratory distress are observed as acute symptoms. In moderate inhalation, in addition to these, more pronounced dyspnea, increasing bronchorrhea and salivation, and generalized muscular weakness appear. In severe inhalation, victims fall into coma, convulsions, paralysis, and/or apnea (Sidell, 1991).

In the Tokyo subway case, vital signs were generally unremarkable in the majority of patients and no more than 20 patients were admitted and treated at intensive care units. The physical symptoms observed on admission among the 740 hospitalized patients, as mentioned above, were found in at least 10% of patients, in order of decreasing frequency: miosis; 90%; headache; 52%; nausea; 35%; dyspnea; 30%; blurred vision; 30%; opthalmoplegia; 29%; narrowed vision; 29%; heavy headedness; 20%; nasal discharge; 20%; fever; 19%; muscle weakness; 17%; conjunctival discharge; 15%; lacrimation; 13%; and vomiting; 10% (Maekawa, 1997). A darkened visual field due to miosis is the most pervasive symptom among poisoned victims. The decrease of serum cholinesterase activity is a marker for nerve gas poisoning. In 53% of the hospitalized patients, the serum cholinesterase activities were lower than the reference activity, and in 16% of the patients, the activities were severely decreased (Maekawa, 1997).

The National Police Agency and the National Research Institute of Police Science (1999, 2001) conducted surveys 3 and 5 years after the event using self-rating questionnaires about somatic and psychological symptoms experienced by victims (one third of them were hospitalized patients). Although the response rates were relatively low, those surveys were the most extensive studies for the victims. On the other hand, St. Luke's International Hospital, located just two blocks from the Tsukiji subway station in Tokyo, treated the largest number of cases (640 patients including 110 hospitalized patients) in the event. Among 610 patients whose addresses were identified, 475 patients responded to self-rating questionnaires for follow-up study one month after the event (St. Luke's International Hospital, 1995). According to the reports by the National Police Agency and St. Luke's International Hospital, the proportion of somatic complaints observed in the acute stage is by and large the same with those reported by Maekawa.

Responses of Victims in the Early Stage

Perplexing Silence. Most of the victims were office workers who were commuting from the outskirts to the central area of Tokyo. The first thing that came to their minds was that the event was hindering them from getting to their offices on time. They had to find an alternative way to reach their offices and look for a public phone to inform their office that they were running late. People rushed outside the stations. However, extensive panic did not occur. A firefighter whom the first author interviewed described the scene: "When we got to the site, we ran into some passengers coming up the stairs with handkerchiefs over their noses and mouths and others were sitting on the ground. Something had happened but people remained silent around the site. I have never experienced such a scene; just victims' coughing heard in the perplexing silence." The same scene was observed in hospitals where victims were transported or had managed to get there by themselves. Victims waited patiently to be treated. This perplexing silence among the victims might be a sign of pervasive psychic numbness.

Interestingly, this response by the victims might contrast with the extreme fear reactions observed following the first SCUD missile attack on Israel during the Gulf War. According to the report by Shalev and Solomon (1996), more people died as a result of fear than from actual exposure to the missiles: 7 from suffocation due to faulty use of gas masks and 4 due to heart attack. Forty people suffered physical injuries while rushing to safety shelters after hearing the warning siren, and 230 patients were admitted after needlessly injecting themselves with atropine (the nerve gas antidote that was distributed to all residents of Israel before the outbreak of the war). Furthermore, 544 patients were admitted to hospital emergency wards with symptoms of acute psychological distress. This fact suggests that warnings and anticipation of attack in a case like this may exacerbate reactions rather than help people behave with composure.

Survivor's Guilt. Some survivors felt guilty for not helping the severely poisoned victims. A woman described her feelings. "I saw a woman crying and falling down on the platform. I hurried out of the station because I felt something bad had happened. I learned later that a woman had died at that station and it seemed to have been the woman I saw. She might have survived if I had helped her. I should have helped her. I used to believe I was a good person, but after the event I cannot feel that way about myself. I may have inadvertently seen the evil in me. I cannot trust myself any more. A police officer who questioned me tried to soothe me by saying that I would have been severely poisoned if I had helped her. I know what he said is true. But I cannot help thinking I should have done something." Her guilty feeling seemed to cause her lingering flashbacks and fear for approaching the subway station where she had been victimized.

Public Reactions. Soon after the event, the cult leader, Shoko Asahara and his entourage were arrested. However, some of his followers were still at large and people were scared of another possible attack. In fact, malevolent gas spraying was reported soon afterward. Trash boxes were removed or sealed in almost every station or public space for quite a while to avoid placement of bombs or toxic substances in them.

Acute Traumatic Stress Responses. The majority of hospitalized patients were discharged within a few days. During their hospitalization, sleep disturbances, nightmares, and anxiety were sometimes reported among the patients as psychologically mediated acute stress responses. However, this conclusion is somewhat controversial. Nerve agent poisoning can produce a variety of neurogenic signs and symptoms because of the widespread presence of such receptors. As neuropsychiatric symptoms, headache, vertigo, anxiety, insomnia, depression, excessive dreaming, and emotional lability have all been reported following exposure to anti-cholinesterases, for example, the organophosphate pesticide or insecticide (Namba et al., 1971; Sidell, 1974). Therefore, psychological symptoms such as sleep disturbance, nightmares, anxiety, and emotional lability in the acute stage of serious Sarin poisoning should be regarded chiefly as toxic neuropsychiatric symptoms rather than as traumatic stress symptoms (Asukai, 1998).

To differentiate neuropsychiatric symptoms from traumatic stress symptoms suffered by victims of the nerve agents, clinicians are required to at least have a basic knowledge about organic psychiatric symptoms caused by the acute organophosphate intoxication.

The National Police Agency and the National Research Institute of Police Science (1999) and St. Luke's International Hospital (1995) reported the proportion of traumatic stress symptoms in the acute stage experienced by the victims. Fears when taking the subway, flashbacks of the event, and sleep disturbance were the three most frequent symptoms observed around 20–30% of the victims.

On the other hand, Asukai, Miyake, and Sawano (1996) studied 45 hospitalized patients with acute Sarin poisoning in a metropolitan hospital one month after the event, using the post-traumatic symptom scale (Weisaeth, 1989). Although the proportion of acute stress responses among patients had decreased in the first month, we determined the proportion one month after the event as follows: fears when approaching the subway; 20%; depressed feelings; 18%; difficulty with sleep; 16%; physical tension; 13%; frequent swings in mood; 9%; and irritability; 7%. Also in our study samples, fear when approaching the subway was the main symptom.

The Incidence of Post-Traumatic Stress Disorder

Although poisoned patients with post-traumatic stress disorder (PTSD) symptoms were reported anecdotally, there is little empirical research that has studied the incidence of PTSD after the Tokyo Sarin attack. Kadokura et al. (2000) conducted a study 6 months after the event using self-report measures for 408 subjects: 65 were hospitalized and 343 were treated only in outpatient clinics. Proportions of the subjects who ever fulfilled DSM-IV PTSD symptom criteria for at least 1 in 6 months after the event were 10.8% of hospitalized patients and 7.3% of outpatients. On the other hand, among 120 patients who visited St. Luke's International Hospital for the screening checkup 2 years after the event, 24 (20%) patients were referred for psychiatric interview. Among them, 12 (10%) were identified in clinical diagnoses as a probable case of current PTSD or subthreshold PTSD, and the others were identified as recovered cases from PTSD symptoms, although their diagnostic method was not precisely described (St. Luke's Hospital, 1997). In our study using the impact of event scale (IES) (Horowitz, Wilner, & Alvarez, 1979), we found that 26% of 35 inpatients indicated 20 or above on the IES total score and were identified as high-risk PTSD cases at 6 months after the event (Asukai et al., 1996). Therefore, we suggest that around 20 to 25% among at least moderately poisoned victims suffered from PTSD or subthreshold PTSD as a clinical concern after the Sarin attack.

Limitations of Early Intervention

DiGiovanni (1999) pointed out that psychiatrists have an important role in the management of a chemical or biological terrorist incident. Their role includes immediate treatment of individual patients and groups of patients who are experiencing the psychological impact of a mass disaster, organizing and managing the delivery of mental health care by others to the community, and assisting local medical facilities and community leaders in the control of widespread anxiety, fear, and perhaps even panic.

In our study mentioned above, we offered psychiatric intervention for the high-risk subjects who indicated 20 or above on the IES total score at the 1-month follow-up and psychiatrists interviewed them once or twice. After psychological intervention, they said they felt relieved. However, contrary to our expectation, their IES score did not improved at the 6-month follow-up carried out by mail. This suggests the difficulty of establishing a mental health care regimen for such disasters. In other types of disasters, victims are inhabitants of local communities or people at the same workplace who are more or less psychologically connected to one another. On the other hand, in a large-scale traffic disaster in an urban area, victims are often accidental sojourners whose psychological connection with one another is diminished when they set out on their separate ways after acute treatment is terminated. Therefore, although a single psychological intervention on site or in a follow-up shortly after the event can take place, it is not feasible to set up a long-term community-based care program. We believe that a new long-term care program should be created for future dispersed victims.

Case Vignette

The case is a 26-year-old male firefighter 5 years into his professional career. He had neither a history of psychiatric illness nor substance abuse and was well adjusted to his job before he contracted Sarin poisoning. He was a fire engine crewmember and also a reserve ambulance staffer. Receiving an emergency call after the Tokyo Sarin attack, he started rescue work at a subway station. His team evacuated several seriously poisoned passengers, including a nearly dead male and a comatose female victim. During rescue operations, he experienced dim vision. Later, he witnessed two ambulance staffers doing cardio-pulmonary resusitation (CRP) for the nearly dead victim, who had collapsed to the ground and lost consciousness due to secondary contamination. He rode in the ambulance to his reserve duty assignment and there with another staffer continued to do CPR. The ambulance left the scene with the two severely poisoned victims. Several minutes later, another staffer was immobilized due to toxic poisoning, crying "I am done for." He alone kept doing CPR for a short while. Then he felt severe nausea and muscle weakness. His consciousness began to cloud. He felt for sure he was going to die. Shortly afterward, the ambulance arrived at an emergency hospital where he was hospitalized together with the other victims. The nearly dead victim died and the comatose female victim has yet to recover consciousness.

His exposure to the traumatic stress was extremely serious. He first witnessed two comatose victims, one of them near death. Then, he witnessed two colleagues who had collapsed and lost consciousness. After that, in the ambulance, he witnessed other colleagues who had serious symptoms. Finally, he felt serious symptoms of poisoning and he thought his death was at hand. His traumatic stress symptoms after this event seemed to epitomize those of severely affected victims of the Tokyo subway Sarin attack.

After one week's hospitalization, his acute toxic symptoms ameliorated. However, he suffered from serious PTSD symptoms for one year. He was having nightmares a few times each week during the first three months. It took one year for the nightmares and sleep disturbances to subside. In his nightmares, he recalled, "I was chased by a big black ball in deep darkness. I heard a captain crying, 'Run away!', and I kept running and running then woke up suddenly." And, "I was talking with colleagues at the fire station. Suddenly, one colleague got his head cut off and the head fell on the floor but kept on talking away." After he returned to duty, whenever he heard an emergency call about suspected gas poisoning, he would freeze up and violently tremble with fear. He never wanted to go near the station where he had been traumatized. Also, he determinedly avoided talking about the event. He also never had any idea of seeking psychological treatment. He felt reluctant to be treated as a helpless victim. He still remains apprehensive about going near that subway station 3 years after the event.

We identified 4 PTSD cases out of 27 poisoned firefighters with structured clinical interviews. In addition to this case, 2 emergency workers collapsed and lost consciousness with severe poisoning, and another moderately poisoned case also suffered from PTSD. All of them complained of nightmares at least several months after the event beyond the acute stage of Sarin poisoning, and these nightmares can be considered as post-traumatic stress symptoms.

LONG-TERM EFFECTS

Apprehension to Unknown Health Effects

Apprehension about long-term health effects of Sarin poisoning is still pervasive among survivors of the Tokyo metro Sarin attack and a substantial number of the survivors have experienced physical complaints as well as post-traumatic stress symptoms. Furthermore, in toxic contamination, the poisoned victim tends to be stigmatized as a contaminated person. In stigmatization, victims are contaminated not only physically but also spiritually; this should be widely recognized among victims of toxic contamination disasters and have an effect on their trauma-related psychopathology. Young males and females also seriously worried about the risk of genetic danger from their Sarin poisoning. One young male who got married after the event confessed to the first author that he was not really relieved until his wife gave birth to a healthy baby.

Sarin and other nerve gas agents belong to the chemical compounds of organophosphates. Organophosphate agents are widely used as pesticides around the world. Acute intoxication with organophosphate pesticides remains a problem for quite a few accidental poisoning in industrialized as well as developing counties. One of the well-known complications of organophosphate poisoning is a delayed peripheral neuropathy. In addition, epidemiological studies suggest that exposure to organophosphate pesticides can induce other chronic effects on the central and peripheral nervous system. While clinical neurological examinations studied epidemiologically have given negative results in the previously poisoned subjects, well-designed studies have shown chronic subclinical effects on the central and peripheral nervous system among the poisoned subjects by organophosphates. Those effects are several cognitive deficits, such as memory, abstraction, sustained attention and speed of information processing on the central nervous system, and decreased vibrotactile sensation and nerve conduction velocity on the peripheral nervous system (Streenland, 1996).

Lingering Somatic Complaints among Poison Victims

In general, clinical examinations have yielded negative results for long-term effects on physical health after the Sarin poisoning except for some complications among severe cases. Although complaints of visual difficulty, general fatigue or tiredness, and headaches were observed in a substantial proportion of patients, the majority of these complaintants recovered within several months after the event. However, some of these complaints were lingering over a long-term period.

The National Police Agency and the National Research Institute for Police Science (1999, 2001) conducted follow-up studies 3 and 5 years after the event. According to those studies, the somatic complaints that did not seem to decrease substantially in the time course from the acute stage to 3 and 5 years after the event were eye strain (51%–34%–43%), weakened eye sight (38%–26%–37%), and easily fatigued (22%–20%–28%). The follow-up study of St. Luke's International Hospital (1997) 2 years after the event showed almost the same proportions of these lingering symptoms: 40%, eye strain; 26%, easily fatigued. However, except a few anecdotal cases, no pertinent objective signs of these lingering subjective complaints were reported in clinical examinations. Ophthalmologic examinations thoroughly done for poisoned and nonpoisoned subjects also showed no positive findings in poisoned subjects (Yamaguchi & Yasuda, 2001).

Possibility of Subclinical Long-Term Health Effects

Consistent to previous findings after organophosphate pesticides poisoning, a few case-control studies have shown asymptomatical effects of the acute Sarin poisoning. Those are the prolonged P300 and visual evoked potential latencies in the patients (Murata et al., 1997) and lowered score of digit symbol test in the neurobehavioral examination (Yokoyama et al., 1998). These studies posited that a chronic effect on psychomotor performance is caused directly by acute Sarin poisoning and concluded acute exposure to Sarin may have neurotoxic actions in addition to the inhibitory action on brain cholinesterase, such as acute exposure to organophosphate pesticide poisoning.

To clarify the chronic effects of Sarin on nervous system, another cross-sectional epidemiological study was conducted 3 years after the event in poisoned versus nonpoisoned male firefighters and police officers (Nishiwaki et al., 2001). In their study, the number of subjects exposed to Sarin was 56 in total: 27 firefighters and 29 police officers, and the number of matched controls without exposure was 52 in total: 29 firefighters and 23 police officers. The result showed that the poisoned group performed less well in the backward digit span test than the nonpoisoned group in a dose-effect manner even after controlling for possible confounding factors. Furthermore, this finding was independent of post-traumatic stress symptoms. On the other hand, none of the stabilometry and vibration perception threshold parameters had any relation to the exposure. The result suggested the chronic decline of memory function after the exposure to Sarin, although the mechanism of memory disturbance due to Sarin remains unclear.

These findings may suggest the long-term neuropsychiatric effect caused by acute Sarin poisoning. However, whether the effect is truly caused by the direct neurotoxicity of Sarin should be determined based on a body of sound evidence in future studies (Nishiwaki et al., 2001).

Long-Term Psychological Effects among Poisoned Victims

According to the report by National Police Agency and the National Research Institute for Police Science (2001), as psychological complaints, 18% of the survivors still suffered from flashbacks; 16%, fear of the subway; 15%, intense distress at exposure to reminders; and 14%, avoidance of thinking about the event.

In another study, Asukai et al. (2002) studied post-traumatic stress symptoms of survivors using the Japanese-language version of the impact of event scale-revised (IES-R) 5 years after the event. Among 658 subjects who responded, including a substantial number of litigant victims, 367 were male with a mean age of 48.5 and 291 were female with a mean age of 35.7. The IES-R can be a useful self-rating diagnostic instrument particularly for survivors with PTSD symptoms as a clinical concern (PTSD + partial PTSD) using 24/25 cut-off in total score. The percentage of subjects at risk scoring 25 or above in the IES-R total score among male and female poisoned victims were 24.6% and 35.8% respectively. Mean values of the total IES-R score were 16.3 in male subjects and 21.8 in female subjects. Female subjects showed significantly higher scores in the IES-R than male subjects. Although the sampling bias due to the litigant population should be considered for this study, these proportions of high-score subjects might indicate that the magnitude of the psychological impact had not yet waned even 5 years after the event.

CONCLUSIONS

A terrorist attack with a nerve agent, such as Sarin, in an urban area brings forth an unfamiliar disaster with particular aspects. One aspect is the risk of secondary contamination that may cause a serious dilemma for people who intend to help affected victims. Another is the apprehension of the unknown effects of the nerve agent's poisoning on survivor's long-term physical health or genes.

Although empirical findings of well-designed research are few, we may suggest that around 20 to 25% among at least moderately poisoned victims suffered from PTSD or subthreshold PTSD as a clinical concern in the wake of the Sarin attack on the Tokyo subway system. Flashbacks and fears when taking the subway or approaching the station where the victimization occurred are chief complaints as post-traumatic stress responses in the long-term as well as in the early stages among survivors. Some of them show lingering phobic reactions to subway lines or stations where they were exposed.

The main physical symptoms in acute Sarin poisoning, such as eye complaints or being easily fatigued, tended to linger as subjective complaints even 5 years after the event among a substantial proportion of poisoned victims. However, clinical examinations found no pertinent objective signs to these lingering subjective complaints. The apprehension for unknown health effects due to Sarin poisoning seems to exacerbate these subjective physical complaints. In addition, the strong memory of acute symptoms seems to be easily revived when they feel minor eye discomfort or general fatigue in their everyday lives.

A few studies suggest the long-term neuropsychiatric effect caused by acute Sarin poisoning. However, this remains to be proven in future studies. Although the delivery of mental health care to control widespread anxiety and fear should be required after a disaster due to the nerve agent attack, our experience from the Tokyo Sarin attack suggests the difficulty of establishing a mental health care regimen for such disasters. When the large-scale attack occurs on people like transient passengers in an urban area, it is not feasible to set up a long-term community-based care program, although a single psychological intervention on site or in a follow-up shortly after the event can take place.

A strategy of the long-term care program for dispersed survivors remains to be developed. In general, it is vital for the relief program to provide poisoned victims with accurate health information and a sound physical checkup system as well as supportive counseling including psychoeducation for post-traumatic stress symptoms.

REFERENCES

Asukai, N. (1998). *Health effects following the Sarin attack in the Tokyo subway system.* Paper presented in the 14th meeting of the International Society for Traumatic Stress Studies. Washington DC.

Asukai, N., Kato, H., Kawamura, N., Kim, Y., Yamamoto, K., Kishimoto, J. et al. (2002). Reliability and validity of the Japanese-language version of the Impact of Event Scale-Revised (IES-R-J): Four studies on different traumatic events. *Journal of Nervous and Mental Disease, 190*, 175–182.

Asukai, N., Miyake, Y., & Sawano, M. (1996). Psychological seaquelae among survivors of Tokyo metro Sarin attack (in Japanese). *Psychiatria et Neurologia Japonica, 98*, 791–792.

DiGiovanni, C. (1999). Domestic terrorism with chemical or biological agents: Psychiatric aspects. *American Journal of Psychiatry 156*, 1500–1505.

Holstege, C. P., Kirk, M., & Sidell, F. R. (1997). Chemical warfare: Nerve agent poisoning. *Medical Toxicology, 13*, 923–942.

Horowitz, M., Wilner, N., & Alvarez, W. (1979). Impact of event scale: A measure of subjective stress. *Psychosomatic Medicine, 41*, 209–218.

Kadokura, M., Ogawa, Y., Shimizu, H., Ymamura, Y., Agata, T., & Ushijima, S. (2000). Posttraumatic stress disorder in victims of an attack with Sarin nerve gas on the Tokyo subway system (in Japanese). *Japanese Journal of Clinical Psychiatry, 29*, 677–683.

Maekawa, K. (1997). Acute toxicological information of Sarin poisoning in Tokyo subway. *Japanese Journal of Toxicology* (in Japanese), *10*, 38–41.

Morita, H., Yanagisawa, N., & Nakajima, T. (1995). Sarin poisoning in Matsumoto. *Lancet 346*, 290–293.

Murata, K., Araki, S., Yokoyama, K., Okumura, T., Ishimatsu, S., Takasu, N., et al. (1997). Asymptomatic sequlae to acute Sarin poisoning in the central and autonomic nervous system 6 months after the Tokyo subway attack. *Journal of Neurology 244*, 601–606.

Namba, T., Nolte, C. T., Jackrel, J., & Grob, D. (1971). Poisoning due to organophosphate insecticides. *American Journal of Medicine, 50*, 475–492.

National Police Agency & National Research Institute of Police Science, Japan (1999). *Report on victim's damage after Tokyo metro Sarin attack.* Published by author (in Japanese).

National Police Agency & National Research Institute of Police Science, Japan (2001). Report on victim's damage after Tokyo metro Sarin attack. Published by author (in Japanese).

Nishiwaki, Y., Maekawa, K., Ogawa, Y., Asukai, N., Minami, M., Omae, K. et al. (2001). Effects of Sarin on the nervous system in rescue team staff members and police officers 3 years after the Tokyo subway Sarin attack. *Environmental Health Perspectives, 109*, 1169–1173.

Okumura, T., Takasu, N., & Ishimatsu, S. (1996). Report on 640 victims of the Tokyo subway Sarin attack. *Annals of Emergency Medicine, 28*, 29–35.

St. Luke's International Hospital. (1995). Report on treatment of Sarin poisoning patients at St. Luke's International Hospital (in Japanese). *Japanese Medical Journal, 3706*, 55–56.

St. Luke's International Hospital. (1997). Report of a follow-up study: Two years after the Tokyo subway Sarin attack (in Japanese). *Japanese Medical Journal, 3828*, 42–48.

Shalev, A. Y., & Solomon, Z. (1996). The threat and fear of missile attack: Israelis in the Gulf War. In R. J. Ursano & A. E. Norwood (eds.), *Emotional aftermath of the Persian Gulf War: Veterans, families, communities, and nations* (pp. 143–160). Washington, DC: American Psychiatric Press.

Sidell, F. R. (1991). Clinical considerations in nerve agent intoxication. In S. Somami (ed.), *Chemical warfare agents* (p. 173). San Diego: Academic Press.

Streenland, K. (1996). Chronic neurological effects of organophosphate pesticides. *British Medical Journal, 312*, 1312–1313.

Weisaeth, L. (1989). Torture of a Norwegen ship's crew—The torture, stress reactions and psychiatric after-efffects. *Acta Psychiatrica Scandinavica, 80*, (Suppl. 355), 63–72.

Yamaguchi, T., & Yasuda, A. (2001). *Ophthalmologic disturbances among victims of the Tokyo metro Sarin attack.* In K. Maekawa (ed.), *Kosei-Kagaku research report: A case-control study of somatic and psychiatric effects in chronic stage on victims of the Tokyo metro Sarin attack* (in Japanese). : K. Maekawa, Tokyo.

Yokoyama, K., Araki, S., Murata, K., Nisikitani, M., Okumura, T., Ishimatsu, S. et al. (1998). Chronic neurobehavioral effects of Tokyo subway Sarin poisoning in relation to posttaumatic stress disorder. *Archives of Environmental Health, 53,* 249–256.

9

Perceived Health and Psychosocial Well-Being in the Aral Sea Area

Results from a Survey in an Area of Slow Environmental Degradation

JOOST B. W. VAN DER MEER, IAN B. SMALL,
ERIC J. CRIGHTON, and NATHAN FORD

INTRODUCTION

The Aral Sea was once the fourth-largest inland body of water in the world. Within less than one generation, its surface area shrank by half and its volume was reduced by 75%. The shoreline receded in places by more than 100 kilometers, leaving behind a thick crust of salt. This situation is the tragic sum of human interventions drastically gone awry plus subsequent neglect of national authorities and inertia of the international community. The environmental and social implications are catastrophic. The sea's destruction

JOOST B. W. VAN DER MEER AND IAN B. SMALL • Médécins sans Frontières (Holland), Aral Sea Area Program, Uzbekistan.   ERIC J. CRIGHTON • Mcmaster Institute of Environment and Health, Hamilton, Ontario, Canada.   NATHAN FORD • Médécins sans Frontières, UK Office, United Kingdom.

Toxic Turmoil: Psychological and Societal Consequences of Ecological Disasters, edited by Johan M. Havenaar, Julie G. Cwikel, and Evelyn J. Bromet. New York, Kluwer Academic/Plenum Publishers, 2002.

has affected the entire ecology of the basin and the health of the 5 million people who live there.

Médécins sans Frontières (MSF) began working in the Aral Sea area in 1997 out of concern for the health of the population and remains today the only international medical nongovernmental organization (NGO) based in the area. After an initial health assessment (Frost, 1996), a number of important perspectives were developed that became the basis for the program. It was clear that there were a number of immediate health problems that needed to be addressed in the region, such as the high rate of tuberculosis. However, the lack of understanding of the underlying causes of the poor health in the region could not be ignored. The causes for ill-health in the Aral Sea area are probably shrouded in so much uncertainty because the Aral Sea disaster falls in the category of what Glantz (1999) has defined as a creeping environmental problem (CEP), characterized as a "long-term, low-grade, and slow onset cumulative process." Usually this type of problem involves very complex environmental processes, and because of the process of relatively small, gradual changes occurring over decades, it is hard to unravel cause-effect relationships. There is a high prevalence of a number of chronic and acute diseases among the population in the region where the sea has dried up. What precisely is the relationship between the two? Is there, for instance, a link between the high rates of salts in the drinking water and kidney diseases or are dust storms linked to asthma? There were facts that needed action and questions that needed answers.

While providing medical support to the hospitals and clinics in the region, MSF also began to conduct systematic research in order to get a better understanding of how the environmental disaster impacts human health. Current research includes understanding the link between dust deposition rates and respiratory disease in children (O'Hara, Wiggs, Mamedov, Davidson, & Hubbard 2000), the high salt concentration in drinking water and hypertension, water quality and kidney diseases, and a food safety study.

The importance of psychosocial impacts has also been underlined by the World Health Organization's 1999 recommendation to "identify psychological and psychobiological mechanisms of symptom formation and determine the prevalence, impact and outcomes of health beliefs concerning unexplained symptoms of environmental syndromes" (World Health Organization, 1999, p. 9). In May and June 1999, MSF performed a population survey in three communities of Karakalpakstan (Uzbekistan), the region closest to the Aral Sea, to determine the population's perception of the health impact of the environmental disaster. The results of the survey presented in this chapter helped define a research agenda according to local priorities.

This chapter describes the work of MSF on the psychosocial impact of the Aral Sea disaster. Following a general overview of the Aral Sea disaster

and its far-reaching ecological, economical, social, and public health implications, the results of the survey on psychosocial impacts are presented. In
conclusion, the implications for research and policy in the area of psychosocial well-being are outlined.

HISTORY

The Aral Sea is a terminal lake at the edge of central Asia, fed by two
rivers, the Amu Darya and the Syr Darya. The Amu Darya River runs over
2,500 kilometers from its source in the Hindu Kush Mountains, running
between and demarcating the borders of Tajikistan and Afghanistan and,
farther along, Turkmenistan and Uzbekistan. The river eventually enters
Uzbekistan and the Aral delta. The other river, the Syr Darya, is located
farther north, beginning in the central Tien Shan Mountains and traveling
through the Fergana valley out into the steppes of Uzbekistan and Kaza-
khstan and the northern section of the Aral Sea. Both rivers provide precious
water in a parched region and are extensively irrigated along their journey.

In the 1960s, Moscow dictated that central Asia would become economically dependent on cotton monoculture—the famous "white gold." Soviet
self-sufficiency in cotton was considered a national security necessity. With
3 million soldiers needing to be equipped with uniforms, the Soviet Union
could not afford to rely on the main exporters of the time, mainly China and
the United States. However, even earlier, "the need of Russia's rapidly developing industry for cotton was a factor in the Russian government's decision to conquer Central Asia in 1864–85" (Lipovsky, 1995, p. 529). With the
demand in place, the supply had to be generated. Central Asia represented
an ideal setting with a climate conducive to growing cotton and an endless
source of exploitable labor. The only limiting factor was the natural course
of the region's water that could and would be reengineered through the
might of the Soviet system.

From Moscow's perspective, enforcing cotton monoculture would also
further settle the partly nomad population, a longtime goal of the Soviet
and tsarist regimes. Another concern for Moscow was the deliberate policy
of creating interdependence among the 15 constituent republics of the
USSR. Cotton would create central Asian dependence not only through
the imports required to maintain a functioning economy, but also on the
refining facilities for the cotton located largely outside of central Asia. In the
late 1980s, around 88% was shipped to the processing and manufacturing
industries located primarily around Moscow (Micklin, 1991). "Exploitation
by the center of the periphery's resources has resulted in systematic regional
underdevelopment in the former Soviet Union. The area most adversely
affected has been Central Asia" (Cevikoz, 1994, p. 45).

Once Moscow had set the mandate for central Asia, it employed the universal Soviet approach to resource management that was embedded deep within its economic theories. Inherent in the Soviet-communist model of development was the command economy. Centrally planned in Moscow and driven on the basis of production quotas for a 5-year span, little attention was paid to environmental costs. Such policy has been shown to be greatly flawed and eventually placed great social and economic costs on populations that found themselves living in highly contaminated environments.

It should be emphasized that the decision 40 years ago to mass-produce cotton was not a new idea. Neither were the consequences: the history of communist rule has "bequeathed a legacy of unparalleled widespread environmental degradation, impoverishment, and mismanagement. This may prove to be one of the bitterest condemnations of Soviet socialism—its wanton treatment of the environment" (Glantz, Rubinstein, & Zonn, 1994, p. 161). Indeed, it has been suggested that the consequences of draining water from the two rivers that feed the sea were well understood beforehand (Bortnik, 1999).

The Growth of Cotton and the Shrinking of the Sea

Cotton is a thirsty crop and extensive irrigation networks were developed from the two rivers. Unlined and uncovered, these systems are extremely inefficient and poorly maintained. In 1900, 1 million hectares of land were under irrigation; this had risen to 7.5 million hectares in 1992. In 1980, irrigation accounted for 84% of all water withdrawals, of which 62% was lost to evaporation and seepage into the water table, leaving only 38% to return to the rivers (Micklin, 1991). By 1990, 9% of total cultivated land was irrigated (Lerman, 1996). The rivers began to suffer from the increased irrigation. By 1978, the Syr Darya ceased to reach the Aral Sea and the Amu Darya contributed only around 5 km^3/year. Sitting in a vast desert, the terminal sea began to evaporate.

An Increasingly Inhospitable Environment

With the drying up of the sea, summer temperatures have risen by 2–3 degrees and the winter months have become colder (Zolotokrylin, 1999). From the exposed seabed, salts, possibly contaminated with agrochemicals, are whipped up by dust storms, known locally as the "dry tears of the Aral." In the 1980s, 90–140 million tons of salt-laden dust was blown off the seabed each year (Feshbach, 1992).

Vast amounts of various agrochemicals were used in the intensive cotton monoculture. Before the breakup of the former Soviet Union, around 20–25 kilograms per hectare of these chemicals were applied (Lipovsky, 1995).

The average usage in the USSR at the time was only 3 kilograms per hectare. Fertilizer use in the then Soviet Republic of Uzbekistan nearly doubled between 1965 and 1988 (Smith, 1991).

Pesticides including DDT are of particular concern. Although officially banned in the 1980s in the USSR, its use was suspected to continue into the 1990s. In almost all regions of the former USSR, DDT content in soils is about 2–7 times the maximum permissible concentration; in some regions it is 46 times higher (Glazovsky, 1995). An analysis of water samples taken between 1982 and 1985 revealed high concentrations of DDT in drainage canals. It has also been found in fish (Smith, 1991). Chemical applications have declined in recent years for economic reasons, but they will remain within the environment for years, either percolating down through the soil into groundwater or washed back into the rivers.

Due to overirrigation and the consequent rise in the water table, salts have permeated through the ground and large expanses of land have become salinized. In Uzbekistan alone, over 3 million acres of land have become so saline that they can no longer be farmed (Feshbach, 1992). The water table, which is used for human consumption, has also become highly saline. By 1989, the salt content of the Aral Sea was higher than that of the North Sea (Feshbach, 1992).

SOCIAL AND HEALTH EFFECTS

The general association between poverty and poor health is clearly linked to environmental degradation in the Aral Sea area. As a result of the continued increase in consumption and degradation of the region's natural resources, including air, land, and water, and the overallocation of resources to the cotton industry, the social and economic effects of the Aral Sea disaster are crippling.

Long considered the "fish basket" of central Asia, providing food and employment for the region and beyond, the fishing industry has collapsed. Previously between 40,000 and 60,000 tons of fish per year were taken from the Aral Sea (Glazovsky, 1995). There were over 20 different species of commercially valuable fish. Today, all but two species have died out. To keep the various canneries along the former seashore operating, fish from the Baltic were transported by rail over 3,000 kilometers to the Aral Sea area.

There were formerly 2 fishery bases, 8 fish processing plants, and 19 collective fish farms in the region employing roughly 61,000 workers (Glazovsky, 1995). Now, the few dozen fishing vessels lying wasted and rusted on the sands of the exposed seabed exhibit a stark reminder of the past. Entire communities have had to change from fishing to farming, only to see the farming become an increasingly limited means of subsistence over the years as salinization began to affect the food crops. As for the cotton industry, yields have returned to those of the 1960s due to salinization of the soil (Craumer, 1995).

As is frequently the case, women and children are suffering the most. Due to poor nutrition related to poverty and low yield of food crops, close to 98% of pregnant women are anemic (Ataniyazova, 1994). A study of mothers' milk found that almost half the samples contained DDT in concentrations of up to 0.31 mg/kg milk fat (Mnatsakanian, 1992). As a result, breastfeeding has been discouraged in some regions.

Life expectancy, one of the prime indicators of population health, has declined over the past few decades. In some villages of Karakalpakstan, life expectancy, at 64 years, is 6 years lower than that of Uzbekistan. Rates of urinary tract diseases in Karakalpakstan are among the highest of Uzbekistan, the asthma incidence is the highest of the country (CARINFONET, 1997), and esophageal cancer incidence rates are stunningly high (Zaridze, Basieva, Kabulov, Day, & Duffy, 1992). The incidence of tuberculosis, the highest in Uzbekistan, tripled between 1991 and 1996 (CARINFONET, 1997).

In 1998, MSF arrived in this region of widespread social, economic, and health problems and began to consider how best to help the population. It was evident that a psychosocial assessment would reveal not only the concerns of the population but also that those concerns might have health effects of their own. Once known and documented, these concerns are also an entry point to address and discuss health issues in an extremely complex environmental disaster. The Aral Sea environmental disaster is fairly well researched in terms of implications for birds, fish, and plankton, but is also characterized by a dearth of facts and figures on social, psychological, and public health consequences for human beings living in the area. In general, facts and figures from studies, such as the one presented here, are used by MSF to improve its programs and understanding of the context it is working in. At the same time they provide information for governmental and nongovernmental agencies and can serve to advocate toward these agencies to act within their own mandate on the findings of these studies.

MEASURING PERCEIVED HEALTH AND PSYCHOSOCIAL WELL-BEING

The psychosocial impacts of environmental disasters are defined as a "complex of distress, dysfunction and disability manifested in a wide range of psychological, social and behavioral impacts in individuals, groups and communities as a consequence of actual or perceived environmental contamination" (Taylor et al., 1991, p. 441). Reactions to stress involve the process of perceiving the threat, coping with it, and adapting to it, as well as experiencing somatic symptoms, fear, anxiety, and anger (Baum, Singer, & Baum, 1982).

This research attempted to define the relationships between perceived exposures and psychosocial outcomes in Karakalpakstan, using the above model of reactions to stress to assess psychosocial impacts. The most suitable way to disentangle some of the relationships under study is through a population-based survey. This methodology relies on respondents' perceptions as outcome measures rather than the assessment of any medically defined conditions, be it in the realm of physical or mental health. However, perceived health and medically defined conditions do overlap, as shown by studies demonstrating the association between perceived health and all-cause mortality. Perceptions about exposures may also be highly correlated with reality in situations of extensive contamination.

A questionnaire consisting of five sections was used. Standard measures, preferably tested in other cultural settings, were used as much as possible. Elliott (1992) developed the original design for use in environmental health research in Canada. The five sections address:

1. Individual perceptions and attitudes of the region and its environmental status.
2. The role of social support networks (families, neighbors, institutions) in coping.
3. Standardized measures of perceived health and psychosocial well-being including the General Health Questionnaire (GHQ-20; Goldberg, 1972), the somatic symptom checklist (SCL-90; Derogatis, Lipman, & Covi, 1973), and a subset of items from the Critical Life Events Scale (Holmes & Rahe, 1967).
4. Closed and open-ended questions assessing individual's concerns, health experiences, and perceptions of attribution (i.e., links between environment and health status) (Elliott, 1992).
5. Sociodemographic variables to check sample representation and to be included in future analyses as possible mediators of psychosocial impacts.

The questionnaire was translated from English into the local language, Karakalpak, and back-translated into English. It was pilot-tested before it was used in the main survey. All people interviewed spoke Karakalpak, although some respondents had a different mother tongue.

The study communities in the Shumanay, Kungrad, and Muynak districts in Karakalpakstan were selected based on their relative differences with regards to economic and ethnic characteristics as well as distance from the former Aral Sea coast. All people 18 years of age and older were eligible for the survey. Population lists kept by local health posts provided the sampling frame, from which a random sample was drawn with help of a computer program. Out of a total sample size of 1,113 people, 881 (79%) agreed to an interview. Fifty-four percent were female; 73% were between 18–45 years of age. The sample included 4.8% of the total population over 18 years of age in the three study sites.

The interview team consisted of 11 interviewers, 3 field coordinators, a main investigator and a project co-coordinator. With the exception of two of the field coordinators, who were previously involved in an MSF survey, all interviewers were recruited from the Karakalpakstan Academy of Sciences. All interviewers and field coordinators took part in a 5-day training program covering survey methodology and the questionnaire itself. The interviewers approached the individuals on their list, mentioned the participating organizations, and asked permission to ask some questions about the quality of life in communities in Karakalpakstan, mentioning the confidentiality of the information that the respondent would give. Verbal consent was then obtained.

RESULTS OF THE PSYCHOSOCIAL ASSESSMENT

The mean family size was 7 persons per household. Almost 18% of those interviewed reported they were "always able to make ends meet"; the general rate of unemployment was 21.9% (Table 9.1). Respondents were asked what they dislike about the place where they live (Table 9.2). Just over 40% mentioned the environment, citing "dirty water," "salty wind," and "plants won't grow." Economic and service problems (i.e., no piped water and no gas), both 10.8%, were also frequently mentioned. A little over 41% of the respondents reported environmental concerns.

The majority reported their health to be fair or poor (54.2%) for their age. Almost 46% rated their health as good or very good, the latter category being only 1% of all respondents (not shown). No respondents reported excellent health. Because of the absence of a control group it is hard to determine if the latter result is due to the environmental disaster or to cultural attitudes toward health.

Overall, findings indicate a very high degree of informal community involvement/support among residents. This is indicated by the finding that 70% reported helping or receiving help from their neighbors, and 92% reported having a close friend or relative to whom they can confide. Emotional distress was measured using the General Health Questionnaire (GHQ-20) and the somatic symptoms subscale of the SCL-90. The alpha reliability coefficient for the GHQ-20 was 0.74 (compared to .90 in the sample described by Goldberg [1972]). Two scoring methods were applied to the GHQ-20 data to determine chronic distress (Goldberg 1972; Goodchild & Duncan-Jones, 1985). Specifically, a probable case of emotional distress was

Table 9.2 Local Area Concerns

	Shumanay		Kungrad		Muynak		All sites		p-values (chi sq.)
	Number	%	Number	%	Number	%	Number	%	
Things you don't like about the place where you live									.000 (38.195)
Environmental problems	107	36.0	113	42.0	130	42.6	350	40.2	
Economic conditions	29	9.8	20	7.4	45	14.8	94	10.8	
Local services	43	14.5	14	5.2	37	12.1	94	10.8	
Climate	19	6.4	31	11.5	28	9.2	78	9.0	
Other	18	6.1	10	3.7	11	3.6	39	4.5	
No mention/don't know	81	27.3	81	30.1	54	17.7	216	24.8	
Total[a]	297	100.0	269	100.0	305	100.0	871	100.0	
Environmental concerns									.704 (.703)
Yes	116	39.3	114	42.1	129	42.4	359	41.3	
No	179	60.7	157	57.9	175	57.6	511	58.7	
Total[a]	295	100.0	271	100.0	304	100.0	870	100.0	
Perceived general health									.805 (.433)
Fair to poor	166	55.1	143	52.6	168	54.7	477	54.2	
Very good to good	135	44.9	129	47.4	139	45.3	403	45.8	
Total[a]	301	100.0	272	100.0	307	100.0	880	100.0	

[a]Deviations from the total (n = 881) caused by the exclusion from analysis of cases with missing data on characteristics concerned.

Table 9.1 Sample Characteristics

Characteristics	Shumanay (n = 301)	%	Kungrad (n = 273)	%	Muynak (n = 307)	%	All sites (n = 881)	%	Chi square	p-value
Mean age[a]	39	n.a.	39	n.a.	38	n.a.	39	n.a.	.587	.745
Female	155	51.5	149	54.6	173	56.4	477	54.1	1.474	.479
Married	217	72.6	195	71.4	213	69.4	625	71.1	.773	.680
Mean # persons/household [a]	8	n.a.	7	n.a.	7	n.a.	7	n.a.	20.583	.000
Households w/children < 5 years	149	49.5	138	50.5	181	59.0	468	53.1	6.508	.039
Mean number of years living in area [a]	29	n.a.	30	n.a.	30	n.a.	30	n.a.	.110	.946
Ethnicity										n.a.[b]
Karakalpak	79	26.2	59	21.7	159	52.0	297	33.8		
Kazakh	21	7.0	112	41.2	144	47.1	277	31.5		
Uzbek	74	24.6	92	33.8	2	0.7	168	19.1		
Turkmen	123	40.9	0	0	0	0.0	123	14.0		
Other	4	1.3	9	3.3	0	0.0	14	1.6		
Completed intermediate education	212	70.4	227	83.5	244	79.5	683	77.6	9.88	.007
Employment status									74.816	.000
Full time	151	50.3	100	36.6	112	36.5	363	41.3		
Unemployed	20	6.7	72	26.4	101	32.9	193	21.9		
Retired	54	18.0	51	18.7	52	16.9	157	17.8		
Homemaker	20	6.7	17	6.2	19	6.2	56	6.4		
Other	55	18.3	33	12.1	23	7.5	111	12.6		
Reporting being "always able to make ends meet"	56	18.7	70	25.6	31	10.2	157	17.9	23.523	.000

[a] Kruskal-Wallace non-parametric test used for age, years in area, persons in household.
[b] For ethnicity some cells are 0; chi-sq. test results are meaningless in that case, and therefore not given.

defined as scoring 4 or more (Ford, Anthony, Nestadt, & Romanoski, 1989; Goldberg 1972; Health and Welfare Canada, 1987) and 12 or more (Goodchild & Duncan-Jones, 1985). The percentage of the samples for all sites scoring 4+ was 8% in Shumanay and 7% in Kungrad and Muynak. Less than 1% of respondents had scores of 12+.

On the SCL-90 somatic symptoms subscale, respondents rate how bothered they feel by each symptom from 0, "not at all bothered" to 4, "extremely bothered." A mean score above the 0.36 cut-point indicates a probable case of emotional distress manifested in somatic symptoms. Respondents in a North American context rated how bothered they had felt by a symptom on a 5-point scale from 0, "not at all bothered" to 4, "extremely bothered." The alpha reliability coefficient for this scale was 0.81 for the original 12-item scale and 0.85 for the 16-item expanded scale. The original alpha reliability coefficient as reported by Derogatis et al. (1973) was 0.86. Mean scores were calculated on the 16-item version for the purposes of comparison with population norms. Derogatis et al. (1973) generated a normalized mean score of 0.36 for nonpatient normals on the somatic subscale.

The mean SCL score in this study was 0.47, and 48% of respondents scored above the cut-point. Shumanay had the highest proportion above the cut-point (54%), followed by Kungrad (49%) and Muynak (41%). In terms of risk factors, distress increased with distance from the sea ($p < 0.01$). The most frequently mentioned cause of somatic symptoms was specific health problems (37.3%, Table 9.3), ranging from "old age" and "pregnancy" to "poor general health" and "tuberculosis." Over 21% mentioned the environment, including "dirty air," "dirty water," and "salty water." The weather (13.7%) and lack of necessities (13.7%) were also frequently mentioned.

Eighty percent of respondents who reported concern about environmental problems (total: $n = 396$) believed that the problems might or have

Table 9.3 Respondents Registering Scores Above the Somatic Symptom Checklist (SCL) Cut-Point and the Perceived Cause

Perceived cause of problems mentioned in SCL	People above SCL cut-point[a]	
	Number	%
Specific health problems	131	37.3
Environmental problems	75	21.4
Weather	48	13.7
Lack of necessities	48	13.7
Emotional or stressful event	23	6.6
Work related	17	4.8
Other	9	2.6
Total	351	100.0

[a]Cut-point refers to a mean score above the population norm signifying a probable case of emotional distress manifested in somatic symptoms (0.36; Derogatis et al., 1973).

**Table 9.4   Perceived Links Between Environmental Problems
and People's Health and Family's Health**

Environmental problem	Perception that problems might or have affected health or family's health	
	Number	%
Water	100	31.7
Environment (general)	60	19.0
Air	59	18.7
Land	45	14.3
Vegetation[a]	19	6.0
Other[b]	32	10.2
Total (all problems)	315	100.0

[a]Category includes problems such as "trees are dying," "plants won't grow."
[b]Category includes problems such as "sodium carbonate plant nearby" and "sewer pipe near home."

affected their health or their family's health. Water quality was most frequently mentioned, followed by the environment in general and air quality (Table 9.4). Finally, a cross-tabulation of measures of perceived general
health and somatization scores with environmental concerns shows that
statistically significant differences occurred in self-perceived health and rat-
ings of the SCL between those with extreme environmental concerns and
those whose concerns are less than extreme (Table 9.5). A relatively larger

**Table 9.5   Concern About Environmental Problems ($n = 396$) and
Their Relationship to Perceived General Health and Somatic
Symptom Checklist (SCL-90) Scores**

	Slightly or moderately concerned		Extremely concerned		Total		p-value (Chi-square)
	Number	%	Number	%	Number	%	
Perceived general health[a]							.717 (.131)
Very good–good	49	36.6	74	38.5	123	37.7	
Fair–poor	85	63.4	118	61.5	203	62.3	
Total	134	100.0	192	100.0	326	100.0	
Somatic Symptom Checklist							.035
SCL[a]							(4.466)
Below cut-point[b]	64	50.4	76	38.2	140	42.9	
Above cut-point[b]	63	49.6	123	61.8	186	57.1	
Total	127	100.0	199	100.0	326	100.0	

[a]Risk ratio of those extremely concerned to be above SCL cut point versus those slightly or moderately
concerned equal 1.22, 95% confidence limit, $1.01 < RR < 1.46$.
[b]Cut-point refers to a mean score above the population norm signifying a probable case of emotional distress
manifested in somatic symptoms (0.36; Derogatis et al., 1973).

proportion of people who are "extremely concerned" about the environment rated their health as "poor." Similarly, the proportion of those with extreme environmental concerns who have an SCL-score above the cut-point is higher than those who have slight or moderate environmental concerns.

DISCUSSION

Amid many other serious problems such as high unemployment and poverty, both at least in part due to the economic decline following the receding waterline, the majority of the population is both aware and concerned about their local environmental problems and seems to display somatic symptoms related to long-term stress.

General health was perceived to be low, with over half of the respondents reporting either fair or poor health. This is poor compared to Western countries (e.g., Canada [Health and Welfare Canada, 1987]), but perceived general health is better than in Russia, where 70% of the respondents report their health as "average" or "poor" (Bobak, Pikhart, Hertxman, Rose, & Marmot, 1998). It has been suggested that dysfunctional informal social structures are partly to blame for reported poor health in Russia (Bobak et al., 1998). The high level of informal social support reported in this survey (i.e., 92% reported having someone to confide in, and almost 70% report helping or receiving help from neighbors more than once a week) may in part explain the comparatively positive subjective health evaluations in Karakalpakstan.

The level of emotional distress assessed by the GHQ-20 (7%) is low compared to studies of normal populations elsewhere: 16% in Baltimore (Shapiro, Skinner, Kramer, Steinwachs, & Regier, 1985), 10% in England (Stanley & Gibson, 1985), 30% using the CGHQ (Huppert, Gore & Elliott, 1988), and 26% in Taiwan (Cheng, 1985). After the Chernobyl nuclear accident, it was found that 65% of respondents exposed to radiation in Belarus scored above the cut-point (Havenaar et al., 1996). The findings for the Karakalpak sample suggest one of two things: either levels of emotional distress are extremely low or the GHQ-20 is perhaps not a sensitive instrument when applied in this cultural context.

The somatic symptom checklist, by contrast, indicated that almost half of the respondents were seriously distressed. Similar findings were noted among people who live near the Three Mile Island nuclear reactor following an accident (Baum, Gatchel, & Schaeffer, 1983) and people who live close to solid waste facilities (Elliott et al. 1993).

Several limitations exist within this study. First, the causal relationship of symptoms to the environmental disaster cannot be established due to the cross-sectional nature of the data. Longitudinal research is needed in the future to minimize this problem. Second, none of the instruments used to record symptoms of psychosocial stress have been validated in the cultural context of Karakalpakstan, or even central Asia. The lack of appropriate reference values makes our findings difficult to interpret. Nevertheless, being "extremely concerned" about the environment was significantly associated with high somatization scores. Finally, the sample was drawn from only three areas in Karakalpakstan and thus generalizations across the entire region cannot be made with certainty. However, we note that the sample was geographically and ethnically diverse. Despite these limitations, it is clear that many perceived that the region's environmental problems, in particular water and air pollution, affected their own and their family's health. Indeed, both water and air (dust) are suspected of being the causes of many of the region's health problems (O'Hara et al., 2000; EC-IFAS/World Bank, 1997).

Implications for Research and Policy

This survey on the psychosocial impact in three Aral Sea communities in Karakalpakstan underscores the importance of psychosocial aspects of this environmental disaster: half of the people surveyed said they are concerned about the environment. Moreover, our study also indicates that 48.8% of the respondents want to leave their homes because of the environment, and half of those want to move out of the Aral Sea area (results not shown). The issue of migration from the Aral Sea area recently reemerged with anecdotal reports of people leaving because of the severe drought of the past years that has affected the whole of central Asia. The drought resulted in further reduced crop yield and consequently threatens food and water security (quantity and quality) in the area. The prospects for the resolution of the drought remain doubtful as traditional precipitation levels are low and disputes between states sharing the same water sources preclude the release of more water from upstream. A prolonged drought could end the habitability of the area, particularly close to the former shores of the Aral Sea. Without hope, what is the potential for adaptation or even the will to cope?

The "environmental refugee" or "migrant" has become an identifiable subgroup of those fleeing from their homes, added to the long list of war, political refugees, and other migrants. At a Commonwealth of Independent States conference on refugees and migrants, held in Geneva in 1996, the estimated number of displaced people due to the environmental disaster in the Aral Sea region alone was more than 100,000 (UNHCR, 1996). Typically, refugees represent a potentially destabilizing influence either because they create new demands in the host community, or because they rebel against the forces that instigated their flight in the first place. The situation and the effects of environmental refugees in the Aral Sea area are complex, particularly when one considers that those who fled had the opportunity, skill, and wherewithal to leave and adjust to a new way of life. The concern is not just that the migrant population bears a strong grievance, but also that the population left behind has relatively fewer capacities, skills, and potential to remedy or at least adapt to the environmental and psychosocial problems that must be faced. MSF is responding to the need to understand these trends by sponsoring a demographic study on outmigration and collaborating on the assessment of the severity of the drought.

Environmental problems and economic conditions, closely interlinked in the case of the Aral Sea area disaster, are high on the list of reasons why people do not like the area where they live. The scores on somatic symptoms indicate high distress levels, suggesting that creeping environmental disasters may have an effect on psychosocial well-being. The study of the psychosocial impacts of such environmental disasters is a relatively new area and, within that, the study of psychosocial consequences of chronic disasters is virtually unknown. This study shows both that the study of the health impact of these technological or human-induced disasters should not be limited to physical health, and the study of psychosocial effects of disasters should not be limited to acute events. It is important that future research clarifies the appropriateness of present research methods and research instruments in the different context of chronic disasters. New intervention tools will also be required. Environmental disasters know no boundaries, and culturally appropriate research methods and tools will be required that are cross-culturally valid.

Psychosocial stress adds to the burden of illness of a population that already suffers high rates of somatic disorders such as anemia and tuberculosis, while the health care system can barely provide the most basic services. An increase in psychosomatic symptoms and associated health-seeking behavior has important economic considerations for the region's poorly functioning health system. Following this study, a logical next step would be to develop recommendations for intervention. To date, there are virtually no intervention tools to deal with psychosocial problems in the context of creeping environmental disasters. In the case of the Aral Sea area, the consequences of the disaster (the stressors) are omnipresent and complex. The creeping character of the disaster, in contrast to an acute event, does not produce a clear psychopathological manifestation for which interventions are available, but rather produces a complex of "vague" complaints indicating long-term stress that is hard to deal with in the health care system.

In the situation of Karakalpakstan people live in great uncertainty about what is exactly happening in their environment. This may lead to an underestimation of some health risks on one hand, and an exaggeration of different health risks on the other. In addition people have no control over their environment. The state, being a major actor to protect its citizens from adverse environmental influences, provides few or no mechanisms (laws or policies) that empower citizens to deal with environmental problems. Perhaps interventions addressing the psychosocial consequences of the environmental disaster should not necessarily be implemented at that level, but should be centered around the provision of culturally appropriate information, giving people the opportunity to make informed choices and thus enhancing the individual's sense of control.

We note that in our data, the associations of social and community networks to psychosocial impacts were nonsignificant (Crighton, van der Meer, Yagodin, & Elliott, 1999). Interventions for complex environmental disasters may have to address the community at several different levels to increase the sense of control and empower communities and individuals. Unfortunately, this approach has not been applied in disasters involving creeping environmental problems, although the experience in acute situations has shown that communication about the risks that people run—providing accurate information, even if the information is not good news—is better than doing nothing at all (Woudenberg, 1999). Research should be directed at gaining a greater understanding of how the community both expresses and copes with stress. The development of effective, context-specific, and culturally appropriate interventions needs sufficient input from the communities that are affected by the environmental disaster in order to be successful. A culturally appropriate risk communication strategy should be developed that will inform and empower individuals and communities with respect to (perceived) environmental health impacts of an environmental disaster. This may positively enhance the community's ability to cope with the impact of the disaster. Of course, further research on psychosocial impacts should be complemented by research about environmental exposure pathways that may have direct physical impacts. A concrete outcome of, among others, the survey presented in this chapter is that it helped MSF to develop an operational research agenda on environmental health.

There are a number of problems attached to developing risk communication strategies and other interventions that may help improve psychosocial well-being in the context of the Aral Sea area disaster and possibly in other complex chronic environmental disasters as well. First, because of the wealth of exposure pathways involved, and an overall lack of data, it is hard to pinpoint one specific source of pollution, thus making it difficult to advise the population on protection measures or to provide accurate information about possible exposures. Such information is required for the creation of risk reduction strategies that can be used by the population. Furthermore, it is hard to tell the population about possible risks in consumption of water and food, where the availability of both is already extremely limited—posing risks in itself. Finally, a critical gap to fill is how environmental risk is perceived in central Asia and how risks should be communicated. The considerable research on these topics derives chiefly from Western democratic nations where environmental health issues are part of open and informed debate. It is unlikely that the results of such literature can be directly applied in a setting like Karakalpakstan that is still recovering from 70 years of authoritarian Soviet rule.

In the absence of a risk communication strategy, empowering people with some simple guidelines to prevent certain potentially harmful exposures might be a feasible intervention to increase the sense of control over their own health. In the case of the Aral Sea area, for instance, one of the measures that may be advocated is showing women how to protect themselves from exposure to pesticides while picking cotton, or encouraging home chlorination to prevent infectious diseases (Semenza, Roberts, Henderson, & Rubin, 1997). Additionally, direct interventions on health problems that affect the population are necessary, even if the ills are not conventionally seen as water-based or environmentally related. An example is MSF's tuberculosis program in the Aral Sea area that addresses a major problem, both in public health terms as in the perception of the population (van der Meer, 1999). In itself, these interventions may be perceived by the population as support and have positive effects on psychosocial well-being, even of those not affected by disease. An evaluation of the effectiveness of such interventions on parameters of psychosocial well-being should be part of the interventions themselves, in addition to evaluations of these interventions on other outcomes.

Developing and evaluating such interventions could be of common interest of academia, policymakers, and NGOs working in areas of environmental disaster. However, communities like those in the Aral Sea area are becoming increasingly assessment-fatigued and frustrated with the lack of direct assistance. Research cannot stand alone. To turn research into policy and then into action, advocacy is very much the key while ensuring that populations receive humanitarian assistance as they wait for research policy and sustainable long-term solutions to catch up.

ACKNOWLEDGMENTS. We would like to thank the following people: Susan Elliott (McMaster Institute for Environmental Health) for sharing her knowledge on psychosocial impacts of environmental disasters with us and for the use of the questionnaire originally developed by her; Vadim N. Yagodin (Institute of History, Archaeology and Ethnography,

Karakalpakstan Branch of the Academy of Sciences) for sharing his knowledge about local situations and customs; Kaz de Jong (Médécins sans Frontières, Amsterdam) for some valuable comments on a previous version of the chapter; the late Demir Babanazarov, Minister of Health of the Republic of Karakalpakstan for his support and all Ministry of Health staff without whose support this survey would not have been possible; all field survey staff who worked long days in difficult circumstances; and finally, all respondents who gave their time to answer the lengthy and sometimes difficult questionnaire.

REFERENCES

Ataniyazova, O. (1994). NGO helps relieve distress of women's reproductive health in Karakalpakstan. *Surviving Together;* 37–38.

Baum, A., Gatchel, R. J., & Schaeffer, M. A. (1983). Emotional, behavioural, and psychological effects of chronic stress at Three Mile Island. *Journal of Consulting and Clinical Psychology, 51* (4); 565–572.

Baum, A., Singer, J. E., & Baum, C. S. (1982). Stress and the environment. In G. W. Evans (Ed.), *Environmental Stress* (pp. 15–44). Cambridge: Cambridge University Press.

Bobak, M., Pikhart, H., Hertxman, C., Rose, R., & Marmot, M. (1998). Socioeconomic factors, perceived control and self-reported health in Russia. A cross-sectional survey. *Social Science and Medicine, 47* (2); 269–279.

Bortnik V. (1999). Alteration of water level and salinity of the Aral Sea. In M. Glantz (Ed.), *Creeping environmental problems and sustainable development in the Aral Sea basin* (pp. 47–65). Cambridge: Cambridge University Press.

CARINFONET-WHO Information Centre for the Central Asian Republics. (1997). *Health of the population, health care and environmental health in Central Asian Republics.* CARINFONET: Bishkek.

Cheng, T. (1985). A pilot study of mental disorders in Taiwan. *Psychological Medicine, 15,* 195–203.

Craumer, P. (1995). *Rural and agricultural development in Uzbekistan, former Soviet South Project.* Great Britain: Royal Institute of International Affairs.

Crighton, E. J., van der Meer, J. B. W., Yagodin, V., & Elliott, S. (1999). *Impact of an environmental disaster on psychosocial health and well being in Karakalpakstan.* Tashkent: Medecins sans Frontieres, Aral Sea Area Program.

Derogatis, L. R., Lipman, R. S., & Covi, L. (1973). SCL-90: An outpatient psychiatric rating scale—Preliminary report. *Psychopharmacology Bulletin, 9,* 13–28.

EC-IFAS/World Bank. (1997). Aral Sea Basin Project 3.1.A. *Water quality assessment and management, executive summary—Phase one.* EC-IFAS, World Bank.

Elliott, S. J. (1992). *Psychosocial impacts in populations exposed to solid waste facilities.* Ph.D. dissertation, Department of Geography, McMaster University, Hamilton, Ontario.

Elliott, S. J., Taylor, M. S., Walter, S., Stieb, D., Frank, J., & Eyles, J. (1993). Modeling psychosocial effects of exposure to solid waste facilities. *Social Science and Medicine, 37* (6), 791–804.

Feshbach, M. (1992). *Ecocide in the USSR.* New York: HarperCollins.

Ford, D. E., Anthony, J. C., Nestadt, G. R., & Romanoski, A. J. (1989). The general health questionnaire by interview: Performance in relation to recent use of health services. *Medical Care, 27*(4), 367–375.

Frost, L. (1997). *Assessment report with recommendations for intervention.* Tashkent: Médecins Sans Frontières Aral Sea Area Programme.

Glantz, M. H. (1999). Sustainable development and creeping environmental problems in the Aral Sea region. In M. H. Glantz (Ed.), *Creeping environmental problems and sustainable development in the Aral Sea basin* (pp. 1–25). New York: Cambridge University Press.

Glantz, M. H., Rubinstein, A., & Zonn, I. (1994). Tragedy in the Aral Sea Basin: Looking back to plan ahead? In M. Hafeez (Ed.), *Central Asia its strategic importance and future prospects* (pp. 159–194). New York: St. Martin's Press.

Glazovsky, N. (1995). The Aral Sea basin. In J. Kasperson (Ed.), *Regions at risk: Comparisons of threatened environments* (pp. 92–139). New York: United Nations University Press.

Goldberg D. P. (1972). *The detection of psychiatric illness by questionnaire: A technique for the identification and assessment of non-psychotic psychiatric illness.* London: Oxford University Press.

Goodchild, M. E., & Duncan-Jones, P. (1985). Chronicity and the general health questionnaire. *British Journal of Psychiatry, 146,* 55–61.

Havenaar, J. M., van den Brink, W., van den Bout, J., Kasyanenko, A. P., Poelijoe, N. W., Wohlfarth, T. et al. (1996). Mental health problems in the Gomel region (Belarus): An analysis of risk factors in an area affected by the Chernobyl disaster. *Psychological Medicine, 26,* 845–855.

Health and Welfare Canada. (1987). *The active health report—Perspectives on Canada's health promotion survey 1985: What we think, what we know, what we do.* Ottawa: Supply and Services, Canada.

Holmes, T. H., & Rahe, R. H. (1967). The social readjustment rating scale. *Journal of Psychosomatic Research, 11,* 213–218.

Huppert, F. A., Gore, M., & Elliott, B. J. (1988). The value of an improved scoring system (CGHQ) for the general health questionnaire in a representative community sample. *Psychological Medicine, 18,* 1001–1006.

Lerman, Z. (1996). Land and water policies in Uzbekistan. *Post Soviet Geography, 37*(3), 145–174.

Lipovsky, I. (1995). The Central Asian cotton epic. *Central Asia Survey, 14* (4), 529–542.

Micklin, P. (1991). The water management crisis in Soviet Central Asia. In *The Carl Beck Papers* (p. 10). Pittsburg: University of Pittsburgh Center for Russian and East European Studies.

Mnatsakanian, R. (1992). *Environmental legacy of the former Soviet Union.* Edinburgh: Centre for Human Ecology, University of Edinburgh.

O'Hara, S., Wiggs, G. F. S., Mamedov, B., Davidson, G., & Hubbard, R. B. (2000). Exposure to airborne dust contaminated with pesticide in the Aral Sea region. *Lancet, 355,* 627–628.

Semenza, J. C., Roberts, L., Henderson, A., J. B., & Rubin, C. H. (1997). Water policy implications from a randomized intervention trial in Uzbekistan. *American Journal of Tropical Medicine and Hygiene, 59*(6), 941–946.

Shapiro, S., Skinner, E. A., Kramer, M., Steinwachs, D. M., & Regier, D. A. (1985). Measuring needs for mental health services in a general population. *Medical Care, 23* (8), 1033–1043.

Smith, D. (1991). Growing pollution and health concerns in the lower Amu Darya basin, Uzbekistan. *Soviet Geography, 32*(8), 553–565.

Stanley, B., & Gibson, A. J. (1985). The prevalence of chronic psychiatric morbidity: A community sample. *British Journal of Psychiatry, 146,* 372–376.

Taylor, M. S., Elliott, S. J., Eyles, J., Frank, J., Haight, M., Streiner, D. et al. (1991). Psychosocial impacts in populations exposed to solid waste facilities. *Social Science and Medicine, 33* (4), 441–447.

UNHCR. (1996, May 30–31). CIS conference on refugees and migrants. United Nations High Commissioner for Refugees, Geneva.

van der Meer, J. B. W. (1999). *Voices on environmental health in the Aral Sea area. Results of key informant interviews about environment, health and research.* Tashkent: Médécins sans Frontières Aral Sea Area Program.

World Health Organization (1999). Environmental health research for Europe: Third Ministerial conference on Environment and Health, London, June 16–18, 1999. Copenhagen: WHO Regional office for Europe.

Woudenberg F. (1999). Praktijk en onderzoek in de risicocommunicatie [Practice and research in risk communication]. *Tijdschrift voor Gezondheidswetenschappen, 77,* 163–168.

Zaridze, D. G., Basieva, T., Kabulov, M., Day, N. E., & Duffy, S. W. (1992). Oesophageal cancer in the Republic of Karakalpakstan. *International Journal of Epidemiology, 21*(4), 643–648.

Zolotokrylin, A. N. (1999). Climate fluctuations and changes in the Aral Sea basin within the last 50 years. In M. H. Glantz (Ed.), *Creeping environmental problems and sustainable development in the Aral Sea basin* (pp. 86–99). Cambridge: Cambridge University Press.

III

Dealing with Ecological Disaster

10

Methodological Issues in the Investigation of Chemical Accidents

HILARY M. P. FIELDER, STEPHEN R. PALMER, and
GARY COLEMAN

As many as 1,000 new chemicals enter the global market each year (Earthwatch, 1992). Public concern about potential health effects has been fueled by increasing awareness of the large amount of chemicals in production, distribution, and use, as well as the several well-documented incidents from accidental releases such as occurred at Lowermoor (Mayon-White, 1993), Bhopal (Zaidi, 1986), and Seveso (Centers for Disease Control, 1988). However, although major chemical incidents are always an ecological disaster, their impact on human health is often unknown. Disasters offer challenges to professionals—to protect the public health, to improve scientific knowledge, and to disseminate the lessons learned.

This chapter will discuss the public health investigation of chemical incidents and use case histories to illustrate some of the methodological issues in studies designed to assess associated health effects. The principles discussed are applicable to both small incidents and large-scale disasters.

HILARY M. P. FIELDER • Department of Epidemiology and Public Health, University of Wales College of Medicine, Cardiff, Wales.   STEPHEN R. PALMER • Department of Epidemiology and Public Health, University of Wales College of Medicine, Cardiff, Wales. GARY COLEMAN • WHO Collaborating Centre, University of Wales Institute, Cardiff, Wales.

Toxic Turmoil: Psychological and Societal Consequences of Ecological Disasters, edited by Johan M. Havenaar, Julie G. Cwikel, and Evelyn J. Bromet. New York, Kluwer Academic/Plenum Publishing, 2002.

EPIDEMIOLOGY OF INCIDENTS

A definition of incidents is required in order to establish their epidemiology, to enable comparisons between countries, and to promote effective cooperation in the prevention and management of incidents. The definition of an acute chemical incident requiring public health involvement developed by the International Programme on Chemical Safety (1999) is as follows:

An occurrence of public health concern caused by an acute release of a toxic or potentially toxic agent.

Level 1. An acute release with no human exposure.
Level 2. An acute release with suspected or actual exposure.
Level 3. An acute release where suspected/actual release is related to ill-health.
Level 4. An acute release giving rise to a civil defense or equivalent major emergency.

A few countries have developed or are in the process of developing surveillance of incidents using slightly different definitions. In the United States, the Agency for Toxic Substances and Diseases Registry has undertaken surveillance of chemical incidents since the late 1980s through the Hazardous Substances Emergency Events Surveillance System. Hazardous substances emergency events were defined as "uncontrolled or illegal releases or threatened releases of hazardous substances or the hazardous by-products of substances, not including events involving petroleum products exclusively. Events were included when the amount of substance that was released, or that might have been released, needed (or would have needed) to be removed, cleaned up, or neutralized according to federal, state, or local law; or when there was only a threatened release of a substance, but this threat led to an action (for example, evacuation) that could have affected the health of employees, responders, or the general public" (Agency for Toxic Substances and Disease Registry, 1996). Between 1993–1997 this system reported 24,573 incidents and a total of 23,851 people were evacuated. By 1998 surveillance was undertaken in 14 states covering a population of about 80 million.

In the United Kingdom, national surveillance began in April 1998, covering a population of nearly 60 million (National Focus, 1999.) The definition of a chemical incident used in this program was: "An acute event in which there is, or could be, exposure of the public to chemical substances, which cause, or have the potential to cause ill health." This definition was clarified further by examples of inclusion and exclusion criteria.

Examples of incidents to be excluded from national surveillance were:

1. Occupational exposure covered by the Health and Safety at Work Act 1974, where there is no potential exposure to the public, hospital staff, or emergency services, for example, a small spill at a factory in which only employees are exposed.
2. Food contamination incidents dealt with under the Food Safety Act 1990.
3. Incidents involving exposure to radiation.
4. Cases of individual exposure to domestic chemicals for example accidental childhood poisoning.
5. Incidents involving drugs and other substances of abuse.
6. Suicide attempts involving carbon monoxide, natural gas, and other chemicals.

The following incidents were included:

1. Workplace incidents resulting in off-site exposure, for example, a spill in the workplace, resulting in admission to hospital and exposure of hospital staff to the chemicals involved, or workplace exposure in which those not employed by the company responsible for the workplace are exposed.
2. Cases of nonintentional carbon monoxide poisoning where more than one person is exposed.
3. Unauthorized exposure of the public to central nervous system gas where more than one person is exposed.

In the first year, there were 10 incidents where more than 100 people were accidentally exposed to acute chemical releases and in two of these more than 100 people became ill after accidental exposure to these releases (Bowen et al., 2000). The surveillance of incidents in the United Kingdom demonstrated that communities are exposed to far more chemical incidents than are reported by the national press, and that no single agency can on its own provide a representative picture of all chemical incidents occurring in the community.

The criteria used by the UN Environmental Program in its latest listing of incidents that have involved a hazardous substance are that more than 25 people have been killed, or more than 125 people have been injured or 10 thousand people evacuated (UN Environmental Program, 1992).

Most countries do not systematically record acute chemical incidents, although some have individual databases of industrial accidents, occupational incidents, or reports from poisons information services. In most countries, therefore, it is impossible to know which are the most common chemicals likely to put the public at risk, where incidents most commonly occur, or why they occur. Chronic chemical exposures from industry and fixed sites such as incinerators or landfill cause public anxiety with ill-health often attributed to acute releases of chemicals over long periods of time. However, the true epidemiology of chemical incidents is largely unknown.

PREPAREDNESS FOR EPIDEMIOLOGICAL STUDY—THE CHEMICAL INCIDENT PLAN

There are measures that can be taken before the occurrence of an incident to facilitate subsequent investigations. All organizations responsible for management of incidents should have an agreed upon plan for serious chemical incidents, and resources should be identified for immediate use in such an emergency (International Programme on Chemical Safety, 1999). Investigation of incidents generally follows three phases: preparedness, response, and follow-up. The actions to prepare for incidents are summarized in Table 10.1.

Baseline Health Status Measurement and Information

Proving cause and effect from exposure to a chemical is difficult after an incident, and baseline population estimates of demographics, social deprivation, and health status are useful. Outline questionnaires can be prepared in advance and modified as necessary. High-definition local street maps should be stored so they can be made available quickly to show potentially exposed areas.

Staff Awareness. Advanced awareness and training of staff in accident and emergency (A&E) departments and general medical practitioners or

Table 10.1   Summary of Actions to Prepare for Incidents

National organization	Local organization
1. Appoint responsible person/agency	1. Prepare multiagency plans
2. Establish lines of accountability	2. Establish means to assess health status
3. Prepare national plans	3. Undertake community risk assessment
4. Identify likely incident sites and substances/antidotes	4. Establish necessary environmental monitoring capability
5. Train emergency response agencies	5. Establish health care capability
6. Collate and review incident reports for lessons learned	6. Undertake joint emergency training with appropriate agencies
7. Prepare/improve research instruments and disseminate	7. Establish means to evaluate response and improve plans
8. Collaborate internationally	8. Collaborate nationally

family doctors will make identifying exposed and/or affected people easier when an incident happens. Flagging the names of patients having surgeries where there is the suspicion of an incident can be used to create a case register. Biological samples, urine, and serum can be taken and stored by prior arrangement as a routine procedure when a chemical exposure is suspected.

Extra Expertise Identified. Environmental exposure measurements can be hastened by local service agreements. Without direct evidence of exposure, implicating the cause of any health effect cannot be made with certainty. Usually exposures following environmental disasters have to be estimated by surrogate measures, such as measures of distance from the incident and approximate length of time at that site.

Effective coordination and mutual trust within and between agencies improved with joint training and sharing of information derived from surveillance of incidents will be an important factor in successfully managing incidents.

Case History 1 (Lyons et al., 2000). This descriptive case study suggested the presence of an unknown chemical agent in the sewer and alerted the emergency responders to alter the operational management. The ease of establishing a case register using the A&E database made a speedy assessment possible.

On October 10, 1996, two local authority workers collapsed and died while repairing a sewage pumping chamber at Crymlyn Burrows, South Wales. Before the results of environmental sampling were available, a large number of emergency personnel, local authority, and agency staff attended the scene of the incident, assuming that the workers had died from hypoxia—the most common cause of death in sewage workers. The A&E doctor experienced upper respiratory tract symptoms when certifying death and alerted the public health department to a possible chemical incident. Over the next two days more than 83 symptomatic or concerned people attended an A&E department and 17 people were admitted to the hospital.

By prior arrangement, these people were flagged on the A&E database to form a case register and blood samples were taken, which showed that several had raised levels of creatinine phosphokinase (CPK). Because CPK levels have been shown to be higher in athletes and the physically active, a referent occupational group was recruited for comparison of symptoms and CPK levels. Headache, sore throat, shortness of breath, and weakness were found to be significantly associated with attendance at the site, and the median concentrations of CPK were higher in the cases. However, unnecessary follow-up of healthy, physically active emergency personnel with raised CPK was avoided by using the nonexposed emergency personnel's values to redefine the reference levels. The cause of death of the two men was later given by the coroner's inquest as poisoning by Freon-11.

RESPONSE PHASE AND FOLLOW-UP

Initial investigation of an incident requires the description of exposures and outcomes in terms of time, place, and person. Evaluation is considered in the preparation phase and implemented in the response phase. Many evaluations of incidents, for example, the addition of aluminum to the water supply at Camelford (Altmann et al., 1999), are hampered by lack of a case register, lack of environmental and biological monitoring, or even timely self-reported exposures. If the opportunity to collect objective data is missed during the response phase, all subsequent evaluation will be based on crude estimations and thus scientifically less rigorous. This in turn leads to anxiety as the community cannot be confidently reassured of no effect or warned about expected effects.

Further analytical study may be warranted for several reasons including:

- Identification of treatable conditions,
- Limiting and controlling further harm,
- Enhancing scientific knowledge for future use,
- Addressing public concerns,
- Answering legal challenges.

Analytical studies for the human health effects following environmental incidents divide broadly into two types—case control and cohort studies. Increasingly ethics permissions are sought to follow-up individuals, based on informed consent, as there may be health and social implications for individuals arising out of the study findings. Randomized controlled trials of further management, such as to assess the effectiveness of counseling, are not considered here.

All studies should consider biases, confounders, and effect modifiers when interpreting the findings since the association between the studied exposure and outcome can be exaggerated or masked by these factors. Age, sex, and deprivation status are determinants of most measures of health and potential confounders in epidemiological study.

Differences in response rates between exposed and unexposed groups or between case and controls can bias comparisons often away from the null, that is, more effects are identified in the exposed group as people who are ill or who are concerned tend to be the ones who respond. Another source of false positive findings is recall bias, which can sway results toward finding an association of exposure with symptoms. A study of self-reported symptoms to an emergency helpline after a water contamination incident showed that anxiety prompted people to report symptoms irrespective of any exposure to the hazard, giving a false estimate of the size of the problem (Fone, Constantine, & McCloskey, 1998). Interpreting results is, therefore, difficult in populations where there is already anxiety and concern about an association between pollution and ill-health.

Cohort Study

A cohort study design requires the definition of the population at risk from exposure or proven to have been exposed using objective measures and at least one referent group with no exposure. They are often undertaken prospectively, but can be conducted retrospectively when good records exist to define the historical cohort. Outcomes can be measured in the acute time period following exposure and at various further time intervals using routine health statistics and/or special surveys. A measure of association commonly used for cohort studies is the relative risk, which is calculated by dividing the incidence of the symptom or disease in the exposed group by the incidence of the symptom or disease in the nonexposed group. Cohort studies conducted over many years' follow-up can be very costly.

A cohort study was used to study the health of people exposed to the chemical incident at Seveso, Italy (Bertazzi et al., 1989). The advantage of this approach, involving the establishment of a cohort of exposed and nonexposed individuals, was that it avoided the possible bias caused by migration in and out of the affected area during follow-up of the incident, which would have tended to obscure any association between exposure to the dioxins and ill-health. The referent nonexposed group was chosen for its social and cultural similarity to the exposed group, which would limit biases caused by other determinants of health such as poverty and lifestyle factors. Mortality from chronic ischaemic heart disease in exposed males was shown to be raised in the 10-year period following the accident (RR = 1.6).

Case Control Studies

Case control studies begin with the identification of people with a disease or illness (cases), selecting people without the disease (controls), and comparing past exposures. Controls may be matched by characteristics such as age to the cases to eliminate confounding, or adjustment may be made for confounders during analysis. This type of study is relatively quick and inexpensive, but as data are collected retrospectively, the study is limited by the availability of unbiased historical information. A measure of association commonly used for case-control studies is the odds ratio, calculated by dividing the odds of the cases having been exposed by the odds of the controls having been exposed.

Case control studies were used to help identify the cause of asthma epidemics in Spain (Anto et al., 1989). In one study, cases were far more strongly associated with an allergic reaction to soy bean allergen compared with age and sex matched controls (OR = 61). Together with other studies, this case control study helped confirm the process of unloading of soy beans at the local harbor as a cause of asthma, and control measures could be established to prevent further epidemics.

Documentation

Full documentation of incidents, including management and epidemiological follow-up, appears to be rare and confined to only a small proportion of incidents published in peer review journals. Consequently, it is difficult to learn lessons and inform the design of subsequent investigations. Publishing validated questionnaires, for example, of self-reported water consumption after a water-borne incident, helps the next researcher. We also know that information about toxicity of chemicals is limited, with many estimates for human safety made from either small studies on healthy, young male volunteers or on animals. Any contribution to information on safety on low-dose exposures to relatively large numbers of humans of both sexes and various ages would prove very useful.

There may be a number of reasons for the lack of published studies:

- Assessment of effect requires information about population exposures and outcomes, but often the population at risk is small, and, therefore, any study will be of low-statistical power. Even though a health problem may have, in fact, resulted from an exposure, where the study is too small it may be impossible to demonstrate that the outcome was so unusual that it would have been unlikely to have resulted from chance alone.
- Often estimates of exposure only, not valid and reliable measured levels, have to be used where environmental data or biological markers are lacking.
- Risk assessments are generally calculated using occupational exposure levels, which are of limited value for children, pregnant women, the elderly, or the physically frail, and for these reasons, physiological population-based normative values may not be appropriate for monitoring specific population subgroups (Lyons et al., 2000).
- Health outcomes may not be clinically immediately obvious or may be delayed and require special tests to detect them (Altmann et al., 1999).
- Routine health statistics may not document the health effect of interest, and increased incidence of symptoms following an incident can be difficult to interpret.

- Public concern and anxiety may result in perceived health effects, and researchers are concerned about biases introduced by a sensitized population.

Researchers and publishers are understandably reluctant to publish studies that appear to lack scientific rigor even though the method used may represent the best achievable at the time, in the specific circumstances. Resources for such studies are not always easily available, and researchers may not encounter enthusiasm for their undertaking—finding evidence of health effects inevitably requires a response. However, a report on an incident and its publication allows scrutiny by others and easy accessability in order to learn how to prevent or improve the management of incidents.

Case History 2 (Lyons, Temple, Evans, Fone, & Palmer, 1999). Several lessons were learned from this study about the availability of resources and the capability to undertake an evaluation of the impact on health in a timely manner.

On February 15, 1996, the *Sea Empress* ran aground on the coast of West Wales, spilling crude and heavy oil into the sea over about 200 miles of coastline. It was the third-largest spill in the United Kingdom. Residents in coastal towns complained of relatively minor health symptoms for which a doctor's opinion is not usually sought and therefore would not be captured by routine health statistics. Therefore, a retrospective cohort study of acute physical and psychological symptoms was undertaken. The referent groups were chosen from similar communities with comparable baseline mental health measurements (SF-36) assessed before the incident.

Resources to undertake the study were not available immediately and the questionnaire was administered 7 weeks after the incident, increasing the possibility of recall bias. No direct measures of exposure were available, and the study relied on estimates based on distance. However, validated measures of anxiety and depression were included in the questionnaire, as well as a question about people's belief that their health was affected. The study found increased prevalence of symptoms including anxiety and depression in the area likely to have been exposed to the vapor. The symptoms of headaches, sore eyes, and sore throats, predicted to be associated with oil, remained independently statistically associated with exposure even after adjusting for anxiety.

THE CHRONIC PHASE: LONG-TERM EXPOSURES AND EFFECTS

Sometimes the presence of increased incidence of symptoms or clustering of diseases can cause public concern about possible exposures to chemicals. This is the opposite scenario to that where a known exposure is followed by an investigation into health effects. These symptoms or diseases can become apparent over long periods of time. One of the advantages of an investigation into outcomes following long-term exposures, including cluster research, is that the public health response can be planned and include community participation. The disadvantages are that historical environmental data and routine health statistics relating to the specific concerns are often nonexistent or inadequate to address the concerns of local populations.

Routine statistics are a useful resource to begin an investigation of a possible public health problem. Routine health statistics are derived from sources such as registers of births and deaths, family doctor records, information on hospital admissions, and special registries such as those for cancer and congenital anomalies. However, special surveys to supplement health service information are often justified on several grounds when researching environmental hazards: social influences have direct effects on well-being, routine health statistics cover only a limited range of health events, and those people most directly exposed may well be the most aware of any true damaging impact (Moffatt, Phillimore, Bhopal, & Foy, 1995).

Epidemiological studies should have the statistical power to detect an association between the exposure and the hypothesized outcome if one exists, as an inconclusive study could be viewed as a waste of resources. However, the health outcomes thought to be associated with an environmental exposure may be rare, for example, a specific congenital anomaly or childhood leukemia. Consequently, discussion with the interested parties will be necessary before agreeing to do the study, and this should cover the possibility of inconclusive results and the problems of interpretation, including the limitations of post hoc investigation of clusters.

Population exposure estimates are often made ecologically, using distance from a site as a proxy for exposure. More sophisticated computer modeling techniques have become available, but their accuracy for prediction of exposures from point sources in hilly terrain is not certain. When environmental data are lacking, reproducibility of results around multiple sites assumed to result in similar community exposures may help assess causality.

Case History 3 (Fielder, Poon-King, Palmer, Moss, & Coleman, 2000). In 1996, residents living in the wards near the Nant-y-Gwyddon landfill site were concerned that the odors from the landfill site were causing illnesses. Specific diseases that some of the residents attributed to the site included an increased number of congential malformations and specifically gastroschisis. We formed our limited number of hypotheses from these concerns and compared routinely collected health outcomes in the area close to the site with areas matched for socioeconomic deprivation. We found that the rate of reported congenital malformations was higher near the site even before the site became operational, but that there was a cluster of gastroschisis near the site.

In this study of health effects around a landfill site, instead of measuring anxiety we used the concerns to inform the study design. This study illustrated the importance of listening to community anxieties and of using available health statistics to begin addressing concerns.

CONCLUSION

Chemical incidents are common and represent a real threat to health. Public health agencies have become increasingly aware of the need to collaborate, and national and international programs have been established. Workable international definitions have been suggested but have yet to be adopted by many countries. The methodology to investigate health problems related to these incidents depends on several factors, such as time elapsed since the incidence and the availability of unambiguous information about the exposure. Table 10.2 summarizes the standard operating procedures as they are usually adopted in these investigations.

There are few reported investigations of chemical incidents in peer-reviewed literature that inform and improve future management. Very few studies document any long-term follow-up or compare different strategies to alleviate harm or suffering. Development of a consensus for accepted methods of study and standards for investigation would improve public protection.

Table 10.2 Summary of Epidemiological Investigation of Chemical Incidents

Incident known, health effects unknown
- confirm and describe by nature, time, and place
- determine chemical exposures including products of combustion and so forth
- define population at risk
- consider sampling for biomarkers of exposure
- consider surrogate measures of exposure
- consider modeling dispersion of chemicals in the environment
- identify cohort of those exposed
- follow-up for health effects and biomarkers of exposure and effect
- assess risk factors and spectrum of health effects

Health effects known, incident suspected
- confirm details reported
- develop case definitions
- define population at risk
- institute case searching
- in-depth interviews with a few cases, especially outliners
- develop hypothesis of exposure
- test by case-control study
- assess risk factors for disease

Surveillance offers the opportunity to describe the risk from chemical incidents, generate hypotheses, and test control measures. Coordination of studies and collation of results from many incidents involving smaller numbers of people exposed to the same chemical would increase the power to detect any health effects and provide useful toxicological information. Such projects could be achieved using a central agency responsible for the surveillance of chemical incidents.

REFERENCES

Agency for Toxic Substances and Disease Registry. (1996). *Annual report: Hazardous substances emergency events surveillance (HSEES)*. Atlanta: U.S. Department of Health and Human Services.

Altmann, P., Cunningham, J., Dhanesha, U., Ballard, M., Thompson, J., & Marsh, F. (1999). Disturbance of cerebral function in people exposed to drinking water contaminated with aluminium sulphate: Retrospective study of the Camelford water incident. *British Medical Journal, 319*, 807–811.

Anto, J. M., Sunyer, J., Rodrigues-Riosin, R., Suarez-Cervera, M., & Vasquez, L., & the Toxicoepidemiological Committee. (1989). Community outbreaks of asthma associated with inhalation of soybean dust. *New England Journal of Medicine, 320*, 1097–1102.

Bertazzi, P. A., Zocchetti, C., Pesatori, A. C., Guercilena, S., Sanarico, M., & Radice, L. (1989). Ten year mortality study of the population involved in the Seveso incident in 1976. *American Journal of Epidemiology, 28*, 139–157.

Bowen, H. J., Palmer, S. R., Fielder, H. M. P., Coleman, G., Routledge, P. A., & Fone, D. (2000). Community exposures to chemical incidents: Development and evaluation of the first environmental public health surveillance system in Europe. *Journal of Epidemiology and Community Health, 54* (11), 870–873.

Centers for Disease Control. (1988). Preliminary report: 2,3,7,8-tetrachlorodibenzo-*p*-dixon. Exposure to humans—Seveso, Italy. *MMWR, 37*, 733–736.

Earthwatch, United Nations Environmental Programme. (1992). Chemical pollution: A global overview. In *The International Register of Potentially Toxic Chemicals and the Global Environmental Monitoring and Assessment Research Centre* (p. 5). Geneva: UNEP.

Fielder, H. M. P., Poon-King, C. M., Palmer, S. R. P., Moss, N., & Coleman, G. (2000). Health impact assessment of residents living near the Nant-y-gwyddon landfill site. *British Medical Journal, 320*, 19–22.

Fone, D. L., Constantine, C. E., & McCloskey, B. (1998). The Worcester water incident, UK: Bias in self reported symptoms to an emergency helpline. *Journal of Epidemiology & Community Health, 52* (8), 526–527.

International Programme on Chemical Safety. (1999). Public health and chemical incidents. In *WHO Collaborating Centre for an International Clearing House for Major Chemical Incidents* (p. 12). Cardiff: UWIC.

Lyons, R. A., Temple, J. F. T., Evans, D., Fone, D. L., & Palmer, S. R. (1999). Acute health effects of the *Sea Empress* oil spill. *Journal of Epidemiology & Community Health, 53*, 306–310.

Lyons, R. A., Wright, D., Fielder, H. M. P., McCabe, M., Gunneberg, A., Nash, P. et al. (2000). Investigation of an acute chemical incident: Exposure to fluorinated hydrocarbons. *Occupational and Environmental Medicine, 57* (9), 577–581.

Mayon-White, R. T. (1993). How should another Camelford be managed? *British Medical Journal,* *307* (6901), 398–399.

Moffatt, S., Phillimore, P., Bhopal, R., & Foy, C. (1995). "If this is what it's doing to our washing, what is it doing to our lungs?" Industrial pollution and public understanding in North-East England. *Social Science and Medicine, 41* (6), 883–891.

National Focus. (1999). *National public health surveillance of chemical incidents April 1998–March 1999.* Cardiff: National Focus.

United Nations Environmental Program. (1992). *Chemical pollution: A global overview.* Geneva: The International Register of Potentially Toxic Chemicals and the Global Environment Monitoring System's Monitoring and Assessment and Research Center.

Zaidi, S. H. (1986). Bhopal and after. *American Journal of Industrial Medicine, 9,* 215–216.

11

Responding to the Psychosocial Effects of Toxic Disaster

Policy Initiatives, Constraints, and Challenges

STEVEN M. BECKER

INTRODUCTION

This chapter examines the status of efforts to address the psychosocial effects of toxic disaster. Rather than investigating particular clinical or therapeutic issues, and rather than discussing specific interventions in great detail, the chapter focuses primarily on the level of *policy*. The aim is twofold: (1) to highlight the kinds of broad initiatives that have been undertaken to address the psychosocial consequences of toxic disasters, and (2) to consider some of the difficulties and challenges affecting policy development in this area.

The chapter begins with a discussion of psychosocial interventions after chemical and radiological disasters. Included are brief reviews of several notable assistance efforts: St. Basile-le-Grand (Canada), Lowermoor (United Kingdom), and Chernobyl (Ukraine, Belarus, and Russia). The second section moves directly into the realm of policy. Here, broad initiatives for addressing the psychosocial effects of toxic disaster are examined. While the section demonstrates that some important steps have been taken in the

STEVEN M. BECKER • Schools of Public Health and Medicine, and Center for Disaster Preparedness, The University of Alabama at Birmingham, Birmingham, Alabama 35294–00220.

Toxic Turmoil: Psychological and Societal Consequences of Ecological Disasters, edited by Johan M. Havenaar, Julie G. Cwikel, and Evelyn J. Bromet. New York, Kluwer Academic/Plenum Publishers, 2002.

domain of policy, it also makes clear that overall progress has been limited. Section three asks *why* this has been the case and considers key factors that have slowed the development of policy in this area. In all, seven major impediments and constraints are identified. Finally, the concluding section discusses several steps that health and human services professionals can take to facilitate policy initiatives for addressing the psychosocial effects of toxic disaster.

BACKGROUND

More than two decades have passed since the notorious chemical contamination case in Love Canal, New York, first broke into the news headlines. The episode was pivotal in raising public awareness of toxic hazards and in creating the impetus for new environmental legislation and research. Interestingly, the case also brought with it an early recognition of the importance of psychosocial effects. Community group leader Lois Gibbs, reflecting on the events at Love Canal, argued that psychosocial assistance should be an integral part of the overall response to environmental contamination situations (Gibbs, 1982, 1998; Hess & Wandersman, 1985).

In the years since Love Canal, numerous episodes involving toxic substances have occurred around the globe. Some have involved radiation or radioactive materials, while others have involved hazardous chemicals. The 1984 chemical accident in Bhopal, India, and the 1986 Chernobyl nuclear accident in the former USSR clearly stand out because of their enormous magnitude and widespread impact. But many less well-known toxic disasters have occurred as well. Indeed, when the UN Environment Program prepared a *partial* compilation of just the *major* chemical accidents from 1970 to 1998, the list stretched to seven, single-spaced pages of small type (UNEP, 1998).

Furthermore, while strides have been made in the area of prevention, major chemical and radiological accidents continue to occur in both the developed and developing world. In 1999, for example, a criticality incident at the Tokaimura nuclear fuel facility in Japan killed 2 people and exposed dozens of others to radiation. The following year, in February 2000, a radiological accident in Samut Prakan, Thailand, killed 3 people and resulted in the hospitalization of at least 10 others who were suffering from serious radiation injuries.

PSYCHOSOCIAL INTERVENTIONS AFTER TOXIC DISASTER

Research conducted over the past two decades has confirmed that early concerns about the psychosocial consequences of toxic exposure were well founded. Studies by social and behavioral scientists have shown that toxic disasters, along with their many other impacts, have the potential to cause widespread and long-lasting psychosocial effects. (See, for example, Bowler, Mergler, Huel, & Cone, 1994; Bromet, Parkinson, & Dunn, 1990; Collins & de Carvalho, 1993; Havenaar et al., 1996, 1997; Palinkas, Downs, Petterson, & Russell, 1993.)

As awareness of the social and psychological impacts of toxic exposure has grown, psychiatrists, psychologists, counselors, applied sociologists, public health specialists, social workers, and other health and human services professionals have become increasingly involved in efforts to assist affected communities. Activities have ranged from the creation of new informational materials to the development of major projects aimed at addressing long-term economic, medical, social, and psychological aftereffects. Interventions of varying size and duration have taken place in a range of countries including Canada, Scotland, England, Israel, India, Spain, Belarus, Ukraine, Russia, Brazil, Spain, the Netherlands, Thailand, Japan, and the United States. Two such interventions—one after the cargo airplane crash in Amsterdam and another after the Bhopal chemical accident—are discussed in detail respectively in Chapters 5 and 7 of this book. In addition, several other examples will be briefly reviewed here.[1] The first—St. Basile-le-Grand—followed a major chemical fire at a warehouse in Canada. The second intervention—Lowermoor—took place in the United Kingdom. Like the St. Basile-le-Grand case, it involved a chemical release. This time, however, the medium involved was water. Finally, the third of the psychosocial interventions considered here is Chernobyl. Because of the enormous magnitude of the 1986 nuclear accident, psychosocial assistance efforts have lasted for years and represent the most extensive intervention to date after a toxic disaster.

St. Basile-le-Grand

On August 23, 1988, fire broke out in a warehouse near the center of St. Basile-le-Grand, Quebec, located 23.5 kilometers east of Montreal. The warehouse had been used to store equipment and drums of oil that were contaminated with polychlorinated biphenyls (PCBs). The intensely hot fire lasted almost 7 hours, spreading a thick cloud of noxious smoke over nearby residential areas. Roadblocks were set up and several thousand people in three downwind communities were evacuated. Protective public health measures were implemented and people were advised to wash any

---

[1]The sections on Lowermoor and Chernobyl are based on the author's fieldwork in England, Ukraine, and Belarus, while the section on the St. Basile-le-Grand is based on communications with Health Canada.

skin or hair that might have been exposed to toxic soot. In addition, women who were breastfeeding were advised to discontinue nursing until tests could verify that their milk was not contaminated (*The Gazette,* Montreal, August 24–25, 1988).

To assist the affected population, health and human services officials created a medical evaluation reception center and an information service to answer people's questions. In all, more than 3,000 people answered an exposure and symptom questionnaire and underwent physical exams and blood tests. As part of the overall response, human services professionals began an intervention to assist people from the affected areas. Practical steps were taken to ease the strain on area residents, who were away from their homes for nearly three weeks. Home visits were also made to distressed residents living near the evacuation perimeter. In addition, information and support were provided to pregnant women and other people undergoing blood and liver testing for chemical contaminants. Once the evacuation order was lifted and people returned to their homes, a six-month outreach program was conducted to help evacuees return to normal.

While a formal evaluation study of the St. Basile-le-Grand intervention was not carried out, the effort was notable for its inventiveness. For example, team members prepared *specialized materials* to help people understand and deal with the situation. Finding that very few existing disaster mental health handouts or other publications dealt with contamination hazards, team members moved quickly to create their own materials specifically related to the chemical accident. One item that was developed was a coloring book for children 6 to 10 years of age. In addition to serving an informational purpose by providing understandable explanations of terms (e.g., polychlorinated biphenyls), the coloring book was intended to help children express their fears and feelings about the situation.

For children who were slightly older—ages 9 to 12—a "mystery detective booklet" was prepared. Like the coloring book, the publication for the older children served two purposes: to help the children become familiar with terms they would encounter in connection with the accident (e.g., dioxins and furans), and to promote the expression of concerns about the episode. Other materials that were produced as part of the intervention included a publication to help adults initiate discussions of the accident with their children.

If one notable aspect of the St. Basile-le-Grand intervention was its creation of materials specifically focused on chemical contamination, another such feature was the *interdisciplinary* nature of the psychosocial assistance effort. Drawing on a range of knowledge and training from the social and behavioral sciences, the team included a sociologist, a psychologist, a specialist social worker, an educator, and a school social worker.

Lowermoor

While the St. Basile-le-Grand intervention was launched very soon after the contamination episode began and lasted for approximately 6 months, the formal assistance effort that was developed in connection with the Lowermoor chemical accident began a year after the accident and operated for about 8 months.

The Lowermoor case began in 1988 at a water treatment works in southwest England. The misdelivery of an entire tanker load of aluminum sulfate—a chemical used in limited quantities in water treatment—resulted in the accidental contamination of the drinking water supply serving 7,000 properties and 20,000 people in North Cornwall. The resulting problems were greatly compounded by multiple errors in assessing the situation, conflicting advice from authorities, considerable delays in releasing information to the public, and what many in the community saw as a slow response from central government.

In the aftermath of the contamination episode, there was general agreement that a range of acute, transient health effects (e.g., rashes, mouth ulcers, gastrointestinal disturbances) were linked to the accident. However, there was considerable, often bitter, controversy over the origins of longer-term health problems (e.g., fatigue, loss of concentration, joint pains) that a significant number of people were experiencing. The conclusion of a government-sponsored panel—that persistent symptoms were probably due to postaccident stress and anxiety rather than toxic effects—was strongly rejected by citizen groups. Meanwhile, in the aftermath of the accident, the people in the affected area suffered a variety of community-level impacts including social division, loss of trust, and social stigma.

One year after the Lowermoor accident, a part-time assistance service was created to aid people in the affected areas. In addition to a manager, five people worked in the service's office. This included one individual with formal counseling training and another with experience of trauma situations. The stated aims of the assistance effort were to provide neutral information about the contamination episode and to make available practical assistance, advice services, counseling, and referrals to conventional and alternative health care.

One interesting aspect of the intervention is that it illustrated the complexity of service delivery in the kind of charged atmosphere that often characterizes contamination situations. Because of the ambiguity, uncertainty, and controversy surrounding the Lowermoor case, the assistance service sometimes found itself the object of conflicting demands and expectations. As one staff member put it, "things got very polarized." The service intentionally took no position on whether people's health problems were due to poisoning, disaster stress, or some combination of the two. However, some in the community felt that using a service that included counseling in its range of services would be tantamount to accepting the argument that people's problems were solely psychological. Thus while the service did field approximately 100 inquiries related to the pollution incident (most of which were practical in nature), staff felt that many people may have stayed away.

Another interesting aspect of the intervention related to training issues. Those involved with the service emphasized the value of workers having a basic understanding of the technical aspects of environmental contamination situations in addition to their general human services training. A combination of the two was seen as enabling staff members to more fully understand the needs of clients in a situation of great complexity.

Chernobyl

The most extensive efforts to address psychosocial issues after a contamination disaster have been undertaken in the aftermath of the Chernobyl accident. The 1986 fire and explosion at a nuclear power plant in the former Soviet Union spread radioactive contamination over a wide geographic area. Thirty-one deaths resulted directly from the accident. In addition, the incidence of childhood thyroid cancer increased dramatically in parts of Ukraine and Belarus. (More information about the Chernobyl accident may be found in Chapter 4, this volume.)

Chernobyl has also had profound social and psychological consequences. Large-scale population relocations, continuing concerns about possible long-term health effects, and social stigma have combined to create a huge, continuing burden for individuals, families, and communities. One major effort to address such problems was launched by the UN Education, Scientific and Cultural Organization (UNESCO). Working closely with local and national governmental and nongovernmental organizations, UNESCO moved to help create a network of Community Development Centers for Social and Psychological Rehabilitation in Ukraine, Belarus and Russia. Three such "Trust" Centers were opened in each country, for a total of nine centers. One center was set up to serve Chernobyl power plant staff and their families. Other centers were sited so as to be able to assist former Chernobyl cleanup workers and their families, evacuees, and people still living in contaminated zones. In some cases, centers were specially built to serve evacuees from highly contaminated areas. Finally, a center was also set up adjacent to the Clinic of Nuclear Medicine near Minsk, Belarus. Every year, thousands of children go to the medical clinic to be tested for radiation-related illnesses, and treatment is provided to some of Chernobyl's worst-affected victims. The goal in setting up a

center right on the grounds of the medical clinic was to be able to provide an integrated approach to service delivery, combining medical screening and care, education, and psychological support for children (UNESCO,
1996).

While arrangements vary somewhat from location to location, the staff
for each of the nine Centers for Social and Psychological Rehabilitation typically includes a manager, social workers, psychologists, teachers, day care
workers, activities organizers, and accounting, administrative, and support
staff. Although UNESCO's role in the program has come to an end, the
centers continue to receive some assistance from the UN Development
Program. UN agencies have worked with West European universities to provide center staff members with additional intensive training in social work,
psychology, and related fields. In addition, staff members at the centers
have also participated in training focused specifically on radiation, health
and environmental issues, and on the various problems resulting from the
Chernobyl accident.

Utilizing both staff and volunteers, the centers have been able to sustain a high level of activity. While still devoting considerable attention to
Chernobyl and its aftereffects, the centers have also, over time, developed
into full-fledged community facilities that provide assistance to the broader
population. This is intended both to meet the broad range of social needs in
countries of the former USSR and to place Chernobyl-related services in a
more comprehensive framework. Among the services offered are individual
and family counseling, support groups, day care, play therapy and art therapy, a variety of workshops and classes, information services, and radiation
and ecology education. Thousands of people have made use of the services
provided by the centers since their opening in 1993–1994.

Each of the interventions reviewed above offers important lessons for
psychosocial assistance efforts after toxic disaster. The six-month-long intervention at St. Basile-le-Grand called attention to the usefulness of having specialized materials specifically related to toxic contamination situations. In
addition, the Canadian case provided a useful example of interdisciplinary
cooperation in addressing social and psychological effects. The Lowermoor
intervention helped to show that the highly controversial and conflicted
nature of contamination situations can easily spill over in a way that touches
assistance projects. Finally, the UNESCO Chernobyl intervention is significant because it shows that after a major toxic disaster, the need for social
and psychological assistance can be extensive and long lasting. Furthermore,
it reminds us of the potential administrative, political, and organizational
complexity of service provision after a large-scale ecological disaster. The
project involved creating centers in three countries and required the cooperation of actors at the local, state, national, and international levels.

Likewise, it required collaboration between governmental and nongovernmental actors.

ADDRESSING THE PSYCHOSOCIAL EFFECTS OF TOXIC DISASTER: POLICY INITIATIVES

Clearly, then, a great deal has been learned from the interventions described above and from other community assistance efforts that have been carried out after toxic disasters. Yet interventions, by their very nature, are focused on *specific* cases. To achieve improvements that are more far-reaching and more long lasting requires action in the domain of *policy*. It is only through the development and implementation of *general* policies and programs that experience gained in particular interventions can be translated into overall improvements in planning, training, preparedness, and response.

IFRC

Since the mid-1990s, several efforts to translate specific experiences into more general policy initiatives have been inaugurated.[2] One such effort, at the international level, was undertaken in 1995 by the International Federation of the Red Cross and Red Crescent Societies (IFRC). Reflecting on its growing experience with technological disasters, the IFRC prepared a policy document on chemical and nuclear accidents. The document was actually the culmination of a study initiated in 1989 in response to a resolution adopted at the IFRC's 25th International Conference in 1986.

Titled "The Role of the Red Cross and Red Crescent Societies in Response to Technological Disasters," the 1996 report noted that chemical and nuclear disasters present special challenges. "Although every disaster . . . is unique in itself, technological disasters may create an extra dimension." Among other things, these disasters can happen everywhere and at any time; communities far from the site of the accident can be affected; and they have the potential to cause long-term environmental contamination. The report also specifically identified the need to have psychosocial support

---

[2] The discussions of IFRC-CHARP, the Psychosocial Support Program, and the UNESCO Trust Centers are based on the author's fieldwork in Ukraine and Belarus and on communications with the Red Cross, the United Nations Development Program/UN Chernobyl Project, and the United Nations Education, Scientific and Cultural Organization. The discussion of the ATSDR Psychological Effects Project is based on communications with ATSDR and on the agency publications cited in the text.

available. "Experiences from Chernobyl and other technological disasters have shown that psychosocial support . . . is also of tremendous importance." Among other things, the IFRC policy document recommended the creation of a Reference Center for Technological Disasters. The purpose of the center would be to collect and distribute information on prevention and relief related to chemical and nuclear accidents (IFRC, 1996).

More recently, the IFRC has moved to translate knowledge gained through its extensive Chernobyl assistance projects into more general policy insights. Since 1990, the IFRC has operated the Chernobyl Humanitarian Assistance and Rehabilitation Program (CHARP). After initially working to distribute dosimeters and food monitors, CHARP created six mobile diagnostic laboratories. The mobile labs operate in the most affected regions, providing medical examinations and distributing health information. Most recently, the focus has been on medical screening of subpopulations that are at high risk for thyroid cancer and other pathologies. Between CHARP's inception and the end of 1999, more than 400,000 people affected by Chernobyl had been screened by the mobile diagnostic laboratories.

Beginning in 1997, CHARP added a Psychosocial Support Program (PSP) to its range of activities. The PSP helps people manage the considerable day-to-day problems and stresses that result from living in contaminated areas. Evaluations of the overall CHARP program were carried out in 1993, 1996, and 1999, and evaluations of the PSP are also anticipated. The IFRC will use findings from these evaluations, plus the more general experience gained in relation to Chernobyl, to inform future policy development (IFRC, 2000).

UNESCO, too, has been moving to translate the specifics of its Chernobyl experience into more general policy formulations. For example, a preliminary evaluation study of the work of the Trust Centers was carried out under UNESCO's auspices. Various meetings have also been conducted to learn from the work of the centers. At a May 1998 conference, specialists from all of the centers gathered to exchange information and share views. In addition, UNESCO is currently preparing a comprehensive report on the Trust Centers project and its general lessons for policy.

In addition to the IFRC and UNESCO activities, a third significant initiative—this one at the national level—was begun at the Agency for Toxic Substances and Disease Registry (ATSDR) in the United States.

ATSDR Psychological Effects Project

In the aftermath of the Love Canal episode in New York and a major industrial fire in Elizabethtown, New Jersey, concern about the threat of hazardous substances grew dramatically in the United States In 1980, Congress passed the Comprehensive Environmental Response, Compensation, and Liability Act (also known as Superfund). Part of this law created the ATSDR. The agency's mandate was broadened in later legislation, and today its responsibilities include keeping a comprehensive inventory of health information on hazardous substances, maintaining toxicological databases, providing medical assistance during hazardous materials emergencies, examining the links between hazardous substance exposure and illness, conducting public health assessments at National Priorities List hazardous waste sites, educating health professionals about the toxic effects of hazardous substances, and maintaining a registry of serious diseases and illnesses and registries of people environmentally exposed to hazardous substances. Based in Atlanta, ATSDR is part of the U.S. Public Health Service (ATSDR, 1997).

In response to a growing understanding of psychological issues after toxic disaster, and as part of its overall effort to protect public health from the threat of hazardous substances, ATSDR launched the Psychological Effects Project in 1996–1997. The aim of the program is to better understand the psychological stresses associated with hazardous substance exposure and to help "prevent or mitigate adverse effects on psychologic health that may occur as a result of living near a hazardous waste site or being exposed to a hazardous substance." The Psychological Effects Project has had several significant accomplishments to date. In 1997, the project organized a workshop on the feasibility of measuring stress related to hazardous waste. The aims were to "develop scientifically sound guidance to evaluate stress occurring in communities affected by hazardous waste sites and releases" and facilitate "the development and implementation of a community-focused framework to intervene directly in such situations" (ATSDR, 1997, p. 62; 2000).

Also on February 3–7, 1997, staff members developed a module on the psychological effects associated with living near a hazardous waste site, which was created to help train state, local, and federal field staff. Other training sessions for health professionals have also been held more recently. For example, a training workshop for physicians was conducted in Cincinnati in February 2000. Plans are also being made to develop a handbook on psychological issues and hazardous substances and to offer training to health, environmental, and other personnel who work with contaminated communities.

In addition, Psychological Effects Project staff members have been directly involved in community assistance efforts. When residents of an Alabama apartment community had to be permanently relocated as a result of contamination from multiple chemicals, the overall ATSDR assistance effort included a workshop on stress and stress management as it relates to toxic agents. In another case—this one in Mississippi—ATSDR staff provided training to social workers so that they could more effectively assist people who had been displaced because of methylparathion in their homes. Information generated by the Psychological Effects Project is expected to be factored into overall ATSDR policy for managing toxic contamination situations.

THE BIG PICTURE: A PAUCITY OF POLICY INITIATIVES

There is no doubt that initiatives such as these represent significant steps forward. Indeed, they represent the cutting edge of efforts to develop general policies for addressing the psychosocial effects of toxic disaster. At the same time, however, the IFRC and UNESCO policy efforts, as opposed to the specific Chernobyl interventions, are still at a relatively early stage of development. And in the case of the ATSDR initiative, limited staff and resources have kept implementation relatively modest in scope.

Looking more generally at the overall picture, there have been surprisingly few moves to craft general policies for addressing the psychosocial dimensions of toxic disaster. This is true whether one is speaking of (1) the development of totally new policies, (2) steps to systematically integrate psychosocial issues into existing policies for chemical and nuclear accident management, or (3) measures to incorporate toxics-related issues into existing disaster mental health policies. Formal initiatives in this area have been largely conspicuous by their absence, and most agencies—local, state, national, or international—remain unaware of, and ill-prepared to address, the special challenges connected with the psychosocial effects of contamination.

In the United States, for example, state and local committees set up under the Emergency Planning and Community Right-to-Know Act rarely include more than the most cursory attention to psychosocial effects when preparing chemical accident response plans. Likewise, government-sponsored training exercises for nuclear and chemical accident management are generally devoid of social and behavioral issues. Even when psychological issues are given some attention, the focus is almost entirely on immediate effects. The kinds of widespread, long-term impacts seen after Chernobyl and other toxic disasters are simply not addressed. Furthermore, precious little detailed guidance—national or international—has been developed for addressing the specific psychosocial challenges posed by contamination situations. In sum, the assessment made by Unger, Wandersman, and Hallman (1992) still largely applies: "Systematic local, state, and national policies do not generally exist for dealing with the psychosocial consequences of toxic emergencies."

CONSTRAINTS AND IMPEDIMENTS

Why, when there is a large body of literature demonstrating the widespread and long-lasting psychosocial effects of toxic disasters, has relatively little happened in terms of formal policy development? Why, when there have been numerous toxic disasters and repeated calls for the creation of programs to address the psychosocial effects of contamination, has there been such modest progress? To answer these questions it is necessary to take account of several policy-relevant factors: the characteristics and dynamics of toxic disasters, the broader policy environment, and the nature of the agenda-setting process in public policy. When these considerations are taken into account, at least seven factors that have constrained and impeded policy development in this area become apparent.

Invisibility

The job of getting an issue onto the policy agenda can be made more difficult when a problem is invisible. As public policy analyst James E. Anderson (1994, p. 87) notes: "The nature and scope of some public problems may be difficult to specify because they are diffuse or 'invisible.' Because measurement may be quite imprecise, policymakers may be uncertain about the magnitude of the problem and in turn about effective solutions, or even whether there is a need for governmental action."

The social and psychological impacts of toxic disaster are difficult to see. Therefore, they are less likely to attract the kind of attention that visible, physical damage tends to draw. For the media, psychosocial effects provide few dramatic pictures; for legislators, they offer few "photo ops" with which to impress constituents; and for decision makers, the invisibility of psychosocial effects may make them seem "less serious" or "less important" than other, more visible kinds of damage. The invisibility of the problem makes it less likely to be acted upon.

Lack of a Consistent Constituency

Issues that have an active and continuing constituency are more likely to find a place on the policy agenda. As political scientist Charles O. Jones has noted:

> Implicit in the discussion of "public problems" is the notion of aggregation .... Also implied is a degree of organization. That is, if aggregates are going to have "consequences systematically cared for," they are going to have to organize for action. Immediately one can see some important factors which may determine what happens in policymaking. For example, the number of people affected, the extent to which they aggregate, and the degree and type of organization all may influence the policy process and the particular outcome in regard to the problems being acted on. (1997, p. 28)

Having a consistent, organized constituency can call attention to an issue, support or pressure decision makers to act on it, work to ensure that adequate resources are allocated, and take steps to keep the issue in the limelight.

In general, policy initiatives to address the psychosocial effects of toxic disaster lack such an active, continuing constituency. First, when people are affected by a contamination episode, they are likely to be preoccupied with immediate problems associated with that particular case, rather than having the opportunity to demand broader policy changes. Second, widely publicized toxic disasters only occur intermittently and in scattered locations, so there is not a steady source of pressure for the development of psychosocial assistance policies. A particular toxic disaster may act as a "focusing event" for a time, but such events "only rarely carry a subject to policy agenda prominence by themselves" (Kingdon, 1995, p. 98). In the absence of sustained follow-up, the policy impact is likely to be transient. As time passes, the issue may drop off the agenda or be displaced by other concerns. "Issues," notes Eyestone, "are frequently displaced before they achieve a definitive resolution. When one issue pushes another off the public agenda, the impetus to action is cut short" (1982, p. 22).

Just as psychosocial assistance programs and policies lack a continuing constituency among affected individuals, the same has also been true in the professional human services community. Relatively few social workers, psychologists, psychiatrists, and sociologists, even those involved in disaster issues, have had experience or involvement with toxic disasters. Furthermore, most human services professionals who have had experience with contamination cases have been focused primarily on clinical issues or service delivery. Few in the professional community have devoted attention to key program and policy issues related to toxic disaster.

Unclear Responsibility

The matter of who should be responsible for developing toxic disaster psychosocial assistance policy is not clearly defined because of fragmented responsibilities for chemical and nuclear accidents. Within the UN system, for example, many chemical accident issues are dealt with by the UN Environment Program, while nuclear accident issues fall under the International Atomic Energy Agency. Meanwhile, natural disaster and complex disaster assistance is normally handled by an entirely different body, the Department of Humanitarian Affairs. And in the case of Chernobyl assistance, it was UNESCO that initially assumed the lead role. The same sort of fragmentation can also be seen at the national or state level. It is typical for different agencies to handle nuclear and chemical accidents, and responsibility for short-term disaster mental health assistance is usually found still elsewhere.

In such a situation, it is not always clear what agency should be responsible for addressing the kinds of long-term psychological impacts seen after toxic disasters. To make matters worse, it is even less clear whose job it is to tackle such contamination-related social problems as community division, community conflict, and social stigma. In such a situation, it is relatively easy for policy development related to the psychosocial effects of toxic disaster to fall between the cracks. The issue may be ignored because it is seen as "being taken care of somewhere else" or because it is thought to be another agency or department's responsibility (Kingdon, 1995).

Professional Orientations

Although awareness of the role of psychosocial issues in toxic disasters has increased in recent years, such issues do not have a high profile. This is true with respect to the general public, but perhaps more significantly, it is also true in relation to most emergency planning and disaster management organizations. In part this stems from professional orientations and training: only a minority of decision makers in the emergency planning and disaster management fields have had significant exposure to social and behavioral issues. The same is true with respect to agencies that deal specifically with chemical or nuclear accidents. Decision makers in such regulatory, environmental health and other organizations are usually more familiar with traditional physical science and engineering issues than with social and psychological considerations related to toxic exposure. Thus, the psychosocial component is less likely to be incorporated into training, exercises, guidance, and policy.

Views of Prevention Programs

A significant emphasis of psychosocial assistance after toxic disaster is on prevention. The idea is to intervene early to avoid more serious problems from developing. But in general, it is harder to secure funding for prevention-oriented programs than for programs intended to fix damage after the fact. As Jansson (1994, p. 145) notes, "decision makers often perceive 'preventive programs' negatively." They "may not want to divert scarce resources to persons currently lacking a problem" when there are immediate problems to be addressed.

Organizational Issues

Along with whatever other primary goals they have, organizations typically try to invest their limited resources in a manner that ensures growth and success. All other things being equal, organizations prefer to allocate their scarce resources, energies, and personnel to issues or domains that are likely to bring substantial benefit to the organization. Issues or policy areas that are seen as risky or unlikely to bring benefit to an agency are less likely to be taken up.

For several reasons, some agencies could view involvement in the issue of psychosocial assistance after toxic disasters as having drawbacks from an organizational standpoint. First, as a rule, decision makers tend to try to avoid issues that risk embroiling an agency in conflict unless there is a very good reason for doing so. Toxic disasters are emotionally charged and highly contentious situations. In a context where arguments over physical versus psychological causation of health problems feels like a "life and death" issue for people, policy development that would involve an agency in many such situations could easily make the agency controversial or unpopular. Under some circumstances, the organization or policy could become a lightning rod for people's anger and discontent. Thus, for some agencies, involvement in the area of toxic disaster psychosocial assistance could be seen as risky.

Second, because the psychosocial effects of toxic disaster can be very long-lived, becoming involved could also be seen as representing an open-ended commitment. For an organization operating with limited resources, this, too, could be viewed as risky unless some significant political or organizational benefit could result.

Third, while it is difficult to see or measure the successes of programs intended to provide psychosocial assistance after toxic disaster, failures can easily be attributed to an organization. It is hard to see psychosocial impacts that are averted, but easy to see those that are not. In such a situation, agencies may also be reticent about becoming involved.

More generally, these sorts of organizational considerations—a conflict-ridden environment, potentially open-ended commitment, limited payoffs, and a potentially significant risk of failure—may make involvement unattractive for some agencies. Without some very good reason for wanting to be involved (e.g., public pressure, statutory requirement), agencies might simply prefer not to engage themselves in policy issues related to psychosocial assistance after toxic disaster.

Knowledge Gaps

While a great deal is now understood about the psychological sequelae of toxic disaster, many gaps remain in our understanding of how best to address such problems as long-term stress and contamination-related stigma. Adding to such research gaps is the fact that few evaluation studies of toxic disaster interventions have been conducted. While work is being carried out in connection with the Chernobyl Trust Centers and the IFRC Psychosocial Support Program, a majority of interventions have gone completely unstudied. Indeed, most toxic disaster interventions have not even had basic descriptions of their activities written up for the published literature. One possible explanation is that the immediate demands of service delivery leave little time for such data gathering and analysis. Insufficient funding, staffing and resources may be another contributing factor. But the net effect is that valuable information is being lost. Such gaps not only call out for additional research, they also make the development of current policy more difficult.

CONCLUSION

Although a wealth of experience has been gained from specific interventions, the constraints and impediments identified above have had an inhibiting effect on efforts to translate that experience into policy. Despite a considerable body of research on the effects of toxic disasters, and despite repeated calls for enhanced capability to tackle such effects, the disaster response infrastructure has yet to develop systematic policies to address the psychosocial impacts of contamination. Indeed, given the innovative interventions and assistance efforts undertaken over the past 10 years, surprisingly little progress has been made in the domain of general policy.

This is not the end of the story, however, for the policy process is open and amenable to change. In this regard, there are several important practical steps that health and human services professionals can take to improve the situation (Becker, 1997, 2001). Psychiatrists, psychologists, social workers, counselors, applied sociologists, and others in human services fields can become more directly involved in bodies responsible for toxic disaster preparedness and response. To date, the involvement of social and behavioral health professionals in such planning mechanisms has been minimal. Greater involvement would increase awareness of the importance of psychosocial issues in toxic disaster planning and help call attention to the special challenges posed by contamination situations. In the United States, for example, human services professionals could work more closely with the network of State Emergency Response Commissions (SERCs) and Local Emergency Planning Committees (LEPCs) that were mandated under chemical accidents legislation adopted in 1986.

Human services professionals can also contribute to the writing and implementation of nuclear and chemical accident training exercises. As noted earlier in the chapter, such exercises are generally devoid of social and behavioral issues. Even when psychological issues are given some attention, they tend either to be "assumed away" or focused almost entirely on immediate effects. Little consideration is given to the kinds of widespread, long-term impacts seen after Chernobyl and other toxic disasters. By contributing to exercise development, and by incorporating psychosocial issues, social and behavioral health professionals can help to make training more robust and realistic.

Finally, in addition to direct involvement with chemical and nuclear accident training exercises and response plan development, human services professionals can work to improve research and education on the social and behavioral dimensions of toxic disaster (Becker, 2000). Continuing education modules and workshops could enhance understanding of the issues among other professions and within the human services themselves. Likewise, evaluation studies of past or present psychosocial interventions would be valuable. These and related actions would help raise the profile of psychosocial issues and ease the way toward effective policy development.

REFERENCES

Anderson, J. E. (1994). *Public policymaking: An introduction*, 2nd edition. Boston: Houghton Mifflin.

ATSDR. (1997). *Agency profile and annual report, fiscal year 1997*. Atlanta: Agency for Toxic Substances and Disease Registry.

ATSDR. (2000). *Report of the expert panel workshop on the psychological responses to hazardous substances*. Atlanta: Agency for Toxic Substances and Disease Registry.

Becker, S. M. (1997). Psychosocial assistance after environmental accidents: A policy perspective. *Environmental Health Perspectives, 105*(S6), 1557–1563.

Becker, S. M. (2000). Environmental disaster education at the university level: An integrative approach. *Safety Science, 35*, 95–104.

Becker, S. M. (2001). Psychosocial effects of radiation accidents. In I. Gusev, A. Guskova, F. A. Mettler, Jr. (Eds.), *Medical management of radiation accidents*, 2nd ed. (pp. 519–525). Boca Raton: CRC Press.

Bowler, R. M., Mergler, D., Huel, G., & Cone, J. E. (1994). Psychological, psychosocial, and psychophysiological seqeulae in a community affected by a railroad chemical disaster. *Journal of Traumatic Stress, 7*, 601–624.

Bromet, E. J., Parkinson, D. K., Dunn, L. O. (1990). Long-term mental health consequences of the accident at Three Mile Island. *International Journal of Mental Health, 19*, 48–60.

Collins, D. L., & de Carvalho, A. B. (1993). Chronic stress from the Goiania CS-137 radiation accident. *Behavioral Medicine, 18*, 149–157.

Eyestone, R. (1982). Why some issues are ignored. In James E. Anderson, ed., *Cases in Public Policy-Making* (2nd ed., chap. 2). New York: Holt Rinehart & Winston.

Gibbs, L. M. (1982, August 24). *Community response to an emergency situation: Psychological destruction and the Love Canal*. Paper presented at the meeting of the American Psychological Association.

Gibbs, L. M. (1998). *Love Canal: The story continues*. Stony Creek, CT: New Society Publishers.

Havenaar, J. M., Rumyantzeva, G. M., van den Brink, W., Poelijoe, N. W., van den Bout, J., et al. (1997). Long-term mental health effects of the Chernobyl disaster: An epidemiologic survey of two former Soviet regions. *American Journal of Psychiatry, 154*, 1605–1607.

Havenaar, J. M., van den Brink, W., Kasyanenko, A. P., van den Bout, J., Meijler-Iljina, L., Poelijoe, N. W. (1996). Mental health problems in the Gomel region (Belarus): An analysis of risk factors in an area affected by the Chernobyl disaster. *Psychological Meicine*, *26*, 845–855.

Hess, R. E., & Wandersman, A. (1985). What can we learn from Love Canal?: A conversation with Lois Gibbs and Richard Valinsky. *Prevention in Human Services*, *4*, 111–123.

IFRC. (1996). International Federation of the Red Cross. Annex III: The Role of the Red Cross and Red Crescent Societies in Response to Technological Disasters. *International Review of the Red Cross*, *310*, 55–130.

IFRC. (2000). *Chernobyl Humanitarian Assistance and Rehabilitation Programme (CHARP): A brief outline of the activities*. International Federation of the Red Cross and Red Crescent Societies.

Jannson, B. S. (1994). *Social policy: From theory to practice*. 2nd ed. Pacific Grove, CA: Brooks Cole.

Jones, C. O. (1977). *An introduction to the study of public policy*. 2nd ed. North Scituate, MA: Duxbury Press.

Kingdon, J. W. (1995). *Agendas, alternatives, and public policies*. 2nd ed. New York: HarperCollins College Publishers.

Palinkas, L. A., Downs, M. A., Petterson, J. S., Russell, J. (1993). Social, cultural, and psychological impacts of the Exxon *Valdez* oil spill. *Human Organization*, *52*, 1–13.

UNEP (1998). *List of selected accidents involving hazardous substances, 1970–1998*. Paris: United Nations Environment Programme.

UNESCO. (1996). *Community development centres for social and psychological rehabilitation in Belarus, Russia and Ukraine: Achievements and prospects*. Paris: United Nations Educational, Scientific and Cultural Organisation Chernobyl Programme.

Unger, D. G., Wandersman, A., & Hallman, W. (1992). Living near a hazardous waste facility: Coping with individual and family distress. *American Journal of Orthopsychiatry*, *62*, 55–70.

12

Voices from the Inside
Psychological Responses to Toxic Disasters

ANNE SPECKHARD

INTRODUCTION

We flew over the oil spill three or four days after the event. It was so overwhelming. It shocks your mind. And then the implications that you begin to see. It's forever. This doesn't go away. It's not like a bone break that heals. The smell in the first few days—It was just the light ends of hydrocarbons, like gasoline, but very heavy. We flew very low over the oil spill. We got sick, toxic from the smell, raging headaches. When it hit the shore there was mousse—wave beaten oil. It was rotting vegetation, carrion and petroleum all wound together. It smelled of petroleum and of rotting flesh. It had none of that nice clean marine smell that the ocean usually has. The smell would stick in your nostrils. You could never get away from it. We couldn't take showers. It was on your hands. We were just living with it. It would just stick in your senses. (Page S, an ecologist 12 years after the Valdez *oil spill)*

March 24, 1989. Super tanker Exxon *Valdez* strays out of her shipping lane onto a reef in Prince William Sound. Eleven million gallons of unrefined crude oil spill into the pristine Alaskan coast poisoning delicate ecosystems and killing thousands of animals.

ANNE SPECKHARD • Vesalius College, Free University of Brussels. 1150 Brussels, Belgium.

Toxic Turmoil: Psychological and Societal Consequences of Ecological Disasters, edited by Johan M. Havenaar, Julie G. Cwikel, and Evelyn J. Bromet. New York, Kluwer Academic/Plenum Publishing, 2002.

COMPREHENDING ECOLOGICAL DISASTER

At times words, especially scientific words, used to describe the psychological effects of ecological disasters fall short of getting to the heart of the matter. Sometimes scientific words can give no real voice to the pain felt by those who suffer when an untouched land is forever spoiled, when oil weighs heavy on the wings of struggling wildlife, when radiation threatens the health of hundreds of thousands of children, when mothers are afraid to breastfeed, or even to bear their own children for fear of toxins released into their surroundings. These are tragic events beyond words, or are they?

This chapter seeks to give voice to the experiences of real people struggling to comprehend and come to terms with ecological disaster. It takes the insider's point of view: from the simple villager struggling to comprehend invisible toxins to the journalist striving to retain objectivity and professionalism in the midst of chaos and danger, to the bureaucrat and healer, each laboring to make sense and find a healing journey out of the stormy eye of ecological disaster. It's a journey that begins with the shock of recognition: the awakening comprehension that life has suddenly changed, perhaps forever. It follows real voices through their struggles with recognition, denial, fear, dread, anger, and grief. It follows from dysfunction to coping, in and through the paths tread by those who suffer when ecological disaster robs them of what they hold most dear. Perhaps in these voices we too can find comprehension.

EYEWITNESS AND EARLY ACCOUNTS

The Chernobyl Disaster

> *The former USSR government decided not to tell anything about Chernobyl because they were afraid of panic and also because it was a Soviet tradition not to tell anything significant. They were afraid of losing control over the people. If they tell the truth they have to tell the truth in other cases as well. It is the way the Soviet government functioned. Some educated people learned about Soviet actions from the Western radio, but it was like a game. Crowds of people didn't know anything. It seems to me that the Soviet government was in a phase of dissociation; they couldn't accept the reality of what had happened and kept waiting for maybe the problem will solve itself. It is usual for our mentality. (Belarusian psychologist 15 years after the disaster)*

Early morning April 26, 1986. The fourth reactor of the Chernobyl nuclear power plant blows up, releasing a radioactive cloud that moves over northern Ukraine and southern Belarus, heading toward Moscow. While the people of the former Soviet Union sleep, grave decisions are made about what to do and who to tell. Emergency weather planes are sent to seed the cloud. Radioactive rain falls over the Gomel region of Belarus, contaminating the southeastern region of the country. Radioactive fallout is measured as far away as Sweden and months later microdoses of radioactivity are detected in crops in France and Italy and in fish in North America. The first news of the disaster amazingly does not come from Moscow but from Swedish scientists who detect atmospheric hints of the accident.

Journalist Observers

An ecological disaster can be on the one hand impossible to miss, or on the other hand covered up. In between, are those disasters that are not obvious at first, appearing as ordinary accidents or daily routine until contamination is discovered. Philip Castle, an Australian journalist, recalls such an incident:

> I attended a story many years ago involving a fairly serious truck accident in which there was a nasty "toxic" spill that subsequently caught fire. There were a number of quite stupid aspects to that spill such as the warnings about the contents of the truck were written on the truck's side in Italian, I think. It took some time for that to be translated. The firefighters, as they are prone to do, doused everything in water, which was apparently the worst thing to do because the chemicals reacted to water and gave off even more toxic fumes. (I think they were swimming pool chemicals). In addition the rather large truck had other items in its load including dog food, which had spilled onto the roadway and down the side of a bridge. Some passing motorists "took" some of the scattered contents, which of course were contaminated and I had to write another story trying to get them to return them. Yes, as you might guess the toxic waste was washed off the bridge straight into the river below. It happened on the outskirts of our national capital Canberra in the early 1980s. I wonder whether we have learnt anything since?

Rumors/Cover-Ups

In some instances contamination is rumored, but not substantiated by the authorities, leaving those exposed to the disaster to draw their own conclusions and sort out their anxieties over subsequent illnesses.

> I saw the plane crash down. I was with the fire brigade. I worked at the site for a week. It was the first time for that kind of work. It was not fun, but it wasn't the hardest part. It was something awful, but you can live with it. Its over, you've pictured it. The hardest part was two years later when colleagues became sick. One got cancer, one got skin problems, all kinds of diseases. There are people living in the area with the same complaints. Most of the complaints are tiredness. There was a school close by. After the crash, children played on the

*playground with the same dust and some are sick. I wasn't feeling well. Later
I was diagnosed with fibromyalgia. The only thing in common was we were at
the same place at same time.*

*It's 9 years since the crash. We worked two years to get them to admit it.
There was an investigation, a political investigation, that revealed there was
uranium (in the cargo of the plane) and it was burned. It was a step closer to
the truth. I've heard so many stories. Everyone tells another. It's awful, the pain
and not getting the answers. We want to get better. A lawsuit is not the issue.
We just want to know why we are all sick. It takes those doctors from medical
research two years, three years, to get the right answers, but last week there was a
news report about the depleted uranium in Bosnia. They came up with answers
in only two weeks. Why is one research taking two years and one can be complete
in two weeks? And why do they say there was nothing there. Those soldiers are
sick too. I don't know why they say it can't be the uranium, they don't know.
They should admit, we don't know. (Emergency worker 9 years after the Bijlmer
crash).*

October 4, 1992, the Bijlmer Plane Crash. An El Al plane crashes in the
Bijlmer district of Amsterdam. Rumors circulate that lethal substances including uranium and precursors to chemical warfare have been strewn over
the crash site. An air traffic controller testifies at a public inquiry that he
had been instructed shortly after the crash to keep such information "under
his hat." The authorities never substantiate the rumors. However, many residents of the area and rescue workers who had not been warned to take
extra precautions during the cleanup are later haunted by concerns over
toxic exposure.

INITIAL REACTIONS

Learning of an Ecological Disaster

The high impact phase typical of most disasters usually includes sensory
overload from the flood, fire, hurricane, tornado, or whatever has been
experienced. This aspect may be completely absent in an ecological disaster:
nothing to see, feel, or hear (Havenaar & van den Brink, 1997). Instead, a
different type of nerve-racking stressor replaces sensory overload: horrifying
information followed by the dread of contamination and its potential life-
threatening consequences.

When information is the main stressor, there is a particularly strong responsibility put upon authorities and news persons to report accurately from
the onset and to be aware of their power to form attitudes. The media is
tremendously influential in shaping early attitudes about toxic exposure,

attitudes that may be difficult to subsequently change. Journalist Robert Frank points out that in a disaster situation people often:

> Only recall from the peak moment, in the peak intensity, and far less attention is paid to the more accurate picture that emerges over time. It has [a] terrible effect on the persons who are the object of the coverage, these intense moments. It creates a predisposition to think a certain way before the facts are fully presented and afterward then only to listen and retain those that confirm what was previously believed. This puts a tremendous onus on news people to get the story right rather than get it quickly. It demands a requirement for self-discipline, which is present in the vast majority of cases. It is however, very, very seductive to news workers to appear knowledgeable when you are not.

Cwikel, Havenaar, and Bromet write in Chapter 3, "The media can play a pivotal role in either providing responsible information on the situation or inflating rumors that increase anxiety." As journalist and advocate for news persons traumatized by disaster, Robert Frank points out, "The rule about crises is that the first thing you hear is usually wrong."

Lies, Coverups, and Loss of Trust

> I was living in Russia as a student when the Chernobyl disaster occurred. Immediately after the explosion there was no news from the Soviet government. The only news that was coming into the country was from foreign presses. BBC was reporting off of other services and reporting it as a horrendous calamity affecting the health of thousands. The soviet press was completely silent. It was an eerie feeling. We did not know whether to evacuate or not. (British student)

Ivan Ivanovich, Chernobyl cleanup worker speaks of this "unforgivable pause" by the Soviet government in failing to give information to their citizens and to those sent to contain the disaster.

> While the authorities still kept silent the special groups had already been at work in the region of the catastrophe. They moved people out, blockaded the contaminated territory, built multi-kilometer obstructions around it, and organized a patrol service and checkpoint admission regimen. In the first days they were responsible for guarding the territory, gathering things, deactivating the land and burying villages.

The government was not equipped for such a large-scale disaster and issued no protective clothing or equipment to the thousands of workers who were sent naïvely and unprotected into the contaminated area. No one was briefed about radioactivity. As workers fell ill, information circulated through unofficial channels about radioactive contamination and the invisible horror they had been sent to fight. The cleanup workers, referred to as "liquidators," went into the Chernobyl zone on active duty, with medical records showing good health ahead of time. Now, Ivan Ivanovich mourns his ill and dead colleagues.

There was a very great deal of stress when we saw the truth of what was going on. The dosimeters showed the truth. We had a wonderful doctor. When he saw the dosimeter it blew his mind.[1]

  Over the 13 years since the disaster there has become a rise in all possible diseases, including oncological and psychic, among those who lived in the contaminated area or happened to be there because of their job. In my group of liquidators, more than 192 veterans of the invisible war (i.e., against radiation) have already died, 167 are invalids and 162 are mentally deficient (incapacitated due to contamination or traumatic stress and thus unable to work and function normally).

Shattered Assumptions

Natural disasters often pull communities together as they struggle to recover from the ill fate that befell the community. Technological disasters differ in that the element of human failure that has caused the disaster often leads to feelings of anger and blame. Societal divisions arise between those responsible for the accident, its prevention, or cleanup; those who control information and resources; and those who see themselves as victimized by their exposure to it (Green, 1998). These situations create distrust and disintegration of community bonds and shatter assumptions of a safe world (Janoff-Bulman, 1992). As a result community strengths and cohesiveness that are often present following a natural disaster are frequently not present following a technological disaster.

Community Disintegration

After the spill the fishermen's lives were completely upended. Fishing was stopped that summer. No one would buy the fish because they would be contaminated. Alaska ordered the fishing in this area to be stopped. One of the fisheries collapsed biologically. We know it was oil because nowhere else did it collapse. Some of the fish came back, but they were sickly, had viruses, and the roe concentrations were less than normal. Some of the fishermen are very concerned. Some are angry. Some give up hope, think it will never get better, and sell, at great losses. There is a lawsuit that Exxon lost, with punitive damages set at five billion dollars. Exxon has appealed it, but some of the fishermen, some of the litigants, are older and have died. There are many who are still outraged by the whole thing. (Bud, a scientist 12 years after the Valdez *oil spill)*

---

[1] The literal translation of this remark is that his "roof went off," which a Russian speaker would recognize as it blew his mind.

When the disaster is of the magnitude that people lose homes, jobs, or livelihoods, community and even legal battles often ensue over who should be responsible to pay for these losses. Those in positions of authority and scientists are often called upon to make public statements, to pinpoint exact causes of illness and pathways of toxins in the environment and within the human organism. This is difficult and often contentious and provokes anxiety for the ordinary citizen who is trying to sort out his own responses to the risks. Journalist Robert Frank points out: "Ordinary people do not understand statistical risk. They just want zero percent risk, which of course is not possible in the real world."

Consumers in Belgium learned in 1999 that they had been exposed to dioxin in animal products raised on contaminated feed. For one mother this led to a collapse in trust of public authorities. She recounts her anger.

The problem with the dioxin scare was finding out that the authorities were aware of the problem before there was public disclosure. I think they knew for about a month without doing anything. It was not simply a day or two before the first advice was given and the decision was made to take products off the shelves. First they took the chickens, then the eggs and then the dairy products. I was trying to diet at the time. I was on a protein diet so I was eating more eggs than normal. I was quiet disturbed to learn about the dioxin. It's a carcinogen. It creates a lot of mistrust of the authorities. Now when there is a question about the safety of beef products, I just don't even eat it, even though all the claims by the authorities are that it is safe. There's no reason to trust them.

Another woman recounts her family's believed exposure in England to BSE or mad cow disease that has been linked to Jacob Creutzfeldt disease in humans. She too no longer trusts authorities when it comes to public statements about the safety of foods despite increased surveillance and public awareness since the BSE outbreaks in Europe.

My mother-in-law died of Jacob Creutzfeldt disease. It was awful. It's probably the worst combination of Alzheimer's, Parkinson's and Lou Gerig's disease rolled into one. We don't absolutely know if she got it from contaminated beef, but we do know that we were all in London during the time when it was said to be the time of highest exposure. We were living there and she came to visit. Of course we took her out to eat often, and I remember treating her at the steak houses. We had no idea that the beef was dangerous. Now I can't help but think that she became infected from those meals. I don't remember what my husband and I ate but we don't eat beef at all anymore and we certainly don't feed it to our son. No one can convince us of its safety anymore.

There are many situations following technological disasters in which it is impossible to sort out the interaction of stress, toxic exposure, and the incentives caused by secondary gains upon reported illness patterns. A re-current theme in interviews with victims of toxic disasters is their frustration in their interactions with the authorities to get the help they feel they need. Their self-help and advocacy efforts begin to feel like exercises in frustration, with the victims finding themselves receiving accusations from those they believe should be helping them. Those who become ill may find themselves isolated and without pity, accused of psychosomatic reactions, and those who advocate for the ill are told that they are causing stress by bringing attention to and attributing illnesses to the disaster.

Losing homes, jobs, or the capacity to function well can all be components of the losses wrought by toxic disasters. News persons who cover these disasters are also not immune; they too can become victims of contamination exposure and traumatic stress.

> *I have talked with members of the news media from all over the world. I am not a mental health practioner but I see what appears to be the aftermath of traumatic stress. Covering a news story where you are not a victim yourself, but a dispassionate observer, you can be traumatized. Traumatic stress plays a very significant role in the lives of news people, especially those who have to get in close, and process imagery. I have talked to news people who have daily waking dreams from being involved in a story. I know news people who have left their jobs as a result of trauma, a photographer who could have won a prize for his photo, but couldn't bear to see the image again. If they are affected by the traumas they are covering; anger, blame and numbing can be the aftermath. Trauma should not be the factor in limiting news. (Journalist Robert Frank)*

Journalist Philip Castle also relates how his colleagues became ill:

> *I attended (the toxic spill) as a reporter and many were affected by the smoke fumes and a number of the people who came close to it were hospitalized. I received some minor symptoms (I think) but the photographer I was working with was affected for years afterwards and some of the rescue workers never returned to work. None of us realized at the time how poisonous the fumes were.*

Family Stress/Disintegration

The emotional aftermath of ecological disasters places particular stress on families who may be suffering from fears over exposure to contaminants, evacuation, job loss, uncertainty, illnesses, and from being involved in the cleanup. Adults and children have differing needs. Likewise, men and women frequently grieve and deal with stress differently, and these differences can cause family conflicts (Levenson, Carstensen, & Gottman, 1994).

Boys and girls likewise often show gender-specific responses to traumatic stress (Perry, Pollard, Blakley, Baker, & Vigilante, 1995) with boys being more prone to acting out and girls to dissociative defenses. One couple involved with the *Valdez* oil spill describe how their marriage disintegrated:

Bud became angry and I became injured, and that was really a bad combination. When I would cry Bud would just flip out. He was grieving through anger. He was struggling with everything he had to make it different and even he, with all his maleness, couldn't make it different. I grieved crying. We both were powerless. It was not about that we did not love each other. That's the tragedy of this whole thing. (Page)

In the spill-affected area, there was a six times higher divorce rate afterwards. Our experience was not unusual. (Bud)

Confusion, Health Rumors, Unofficial Channels, and Changes in Behavior

Technological disasters are by definition situations when the unexpected and unthinkable has occurred, and as such, there is frequently no prepared response. Information seeking, a common route to reducing stress and positive coping, is often frustrated after an ecological disaster by confusion, lack of public disclosure, and multiple conflicting answers. Likewise any information about health risks, no matter how low, can lead to increased anxieties. Public officials often find themselves ill-informed and are slow to act. Corporate executives may be bound by liability concerns, and experts notoriously disagree. This also leads to aggravation, despair, and increased anxieties. Within the vacuum of public disclosure trust in authorities is damaged. In this situation, rumors and unofficial sources often gain importance as potentially credible sources of information, and unofficial channels often become as important as official channels of information.

You know our government failed to give us iodine tablets right after the explosion. When people heard about it, it was already too late, but people did not understand this. They didn't have iodine tablets but they knew that iodine was supposed to protect the thyroid. So they took antiseptic iodine and swabbed it across their throats, making a huge mark across their necks. It was so stupid, but they believed it would protect them. These were fairly educated people doing this. You know the radioactive iodide was already gone by that time. Its half-life is only fourteen days. So it was pure stupidity. (Belarusian woman 14 years after Chernobyl)

LONG-TERM RESPONSES

Health Worries: Stress, Dread, Illness and Psychosomatic Responses

I got a rash on my hands that wouldn't go away. We didn't even know to cover up. My hands were in it, I don't know if it was stress, or direct contact. It took months for that rash to clear up. (Page, ecologist—Valdez oil spill)

After a disaster, increased awareness of disease often heightens as anxieties focus on the possible consequences of exposure. Detection efforts are often stepped up, which can cause reporting of even normally occurring illness to be increased and attributed wrongly to toxic exposure. Official responses such as evacuation, increased reporting of potential health risks from exposure, or the failure to take protective actions can increase factors such as anxiety and stress, which in turn can cause increases in reported illness rates. Anxiety, somatization, subclinical depression, and elevations in stress-mediated health conditions are common.

Psychosomatic illness versus real damage from toxins is a thorny issue following most technological disasters. Frequently, patients, their health care providers, and even researchers disagree about causes, effects, and what to do, which creates stress for all. This leads to accusations and recriminations between victims, authorities, and those held responsible for the disaster and its consequences.

Social Alienation, Genetic Damage, and Reproductive Concerns

I was pregnant when Chernobyl exploded. We lived in Kiev, which was very close by and down river from the plant. We had no idea it had happened until days later. It was sunny weather so we were outside, exposed. But later we learned. At that time, everyone was panicking, sending their children away. You couldn't even get close to a train at the station. It was the most horrible moment for me. I didn't know what to do. Everyone said to have an abortion. Most pregnant women aborted but I decided against. Later children who were exposed started having problems. Some got thyroid cancer. It was awful. Children were born with defects. I was nearly out of my mind the entire pregnancy. I look at my son and think I can't believe this happened to us. I hope he never becomes ill from it. He is my only son. I will never have another pregnancy. I'm too afraid to even think about it. (Ukrainian mother 14 years after Chernobyl)

Potential parents and pregnant and nursing mothers are especially vulnerable to distress from toxic exposure, fearing chromosomal damage and the effects of toxins on fetal development. After Chernobyl, 75% of a sample of liquidators were found to have suffered impotence at various times in the 13 years following the disaster (V. Vishnevskaya, personal communication). Whether this was physiological and or psychological in origin could not be determined, but the researcher noted that many of the liquidators feared fathering children with genetic defects due to their exposure and that frequently potential partners shunned them for the same reasons.[2]

Researchers analyzing Danish national register data stated that fear of radiation after Chernobyl probably caused more fetal deaths than the radioactivity itself (Knudsen, 1991). Abortions carry with them their own potential consequences for post-traumatic stress responses, especially among women wanting the pregnancy or having already formed an attachment to the fetus (Mufel, Speckhard, & Sivuha, 2001; Speckhard & Rue, 1992). Hence, genetic counseling is helpful after toxic disasters to fight misinformation and rumors that may lead to poor decision making and unnecessary abortions.

Scientific Advances for Biological and Chemical Threats

The scientific ability to genetically alter living organisms and the potential for chemical and bioterrorism also raise new fears for society. Those who fear exposure to such toxins are faced with the challenges of trying to understand their altered health, getting help with problems that are difficult to diagnose and treat, and the stigma of exposure. Recently, an outbreak of anthrax contamination in the United States (following the September 11, 2001, terrorist attacks), involving relatively few Americans, demonstrated the way in which millions of people could abruptly begin to fear biological or chemical attack and worry over how best to respond. Gas masks swiftly found a ready market among worried Americans and others around the world. Likewise medical, mental health, and security professionals realized how unprepared society is for chemical and bioterrorism and how anxiety over such events can suddenly lead to increased health and security problems. An American diplomat posted in the U.S. Embassy in Brussels recounts his fears:

> Did you hear that we received an anthrax letter yesterday? It was filled with brown powder. They've already sealed the room, but we are hoping it will be a false case. I already can't sleep. This is getting worse each day. The stress levels are overwhelming.

The psychological aftermath of exposure to chemical warfare may endure for significant time periods. American military personnel who were

---

[2]This is not an entirely unfounded fear as genetic mutations in the offspring of Chernobyl liquidators conceived after the explosion as compared to siblings conceived prior to Chernobyl have been indicated by researchers (Weinberg, Korol, & Kirzhner, 2001).

recruited in their youth into top-secret mustard gas tests suffered psychological trauma from their ordeals even decades afterward (Green, Lindy & Grace, 1994). Likewise, Lifton (1967) immortalized the post-traumatic concerns of Hiroshima victims who long after the nuclear blasts evidenced psychological damage, even without having suffered radiation illnesses.

Hysteria and overreactions to chemical and bioterrorism spread quickly and are difficult to contain. A former Soviet Union diplomat commented on his country's response to the anthrax attacks:

> As far as I know we are not even a target to such activities and our embassy is not anywhere near NATO headquarters but already we received a directive from our country to measure everyone for gas masks, including the children. I cannot imagine why we need them, but we will have them. We have to laugh at such things or we will lose our minds from stress.

When a toxin is invisible, difficult to identify, or is potentially arriving from terrorist sources, rumors often abound. A U.S. diplomat's wife recalls such a reaction following the September terrorist attacks on America:

> Today my husband called from the embassy in a panic. He said there was a security advisory stating that anthrax had been put inside The Economist. After I was in the bathroom with latex gloves attempting to wrap it up so nothing could spread. Of course I couldn't stop myself from breathing while I worked. Later he called to say it was discovered to be a hoax. That was pretty scary. It got my pulse up.

The issues of secrecy and denial by authorities that surround weaponry and acts of war create difficulties for those who worry about chemical exposure. Today the military and civilians worry over illnesses from Agent Orange, Gulf War syndrome, and depleted uranium. Many feel that their governments limit information that is necessary to guard one's health. Likewise, increasingly military and civilian populations fear threats of biological and chemical toxins from terrorist activities. As the capability increases to invent biological weapons, along with the technology to hide and transport them, and genetic alterations abound, these worries are only likely to expand to even larger groups.

Posttraumatic Stress

The magnitude of the losses, perceived threat to self, to others, and even to the earth itself from toxic contamination can be horrific enough to create posttraumatic stress responses (Bromet, 1989; Bromet, Carlson, Goidgaber & Gluzman, 1998; Green, et al., 1994; Havenaar & van den Brink, 1997). In these persons the whole picture of posttraumatic stress disorder (PTSD) (American Psychiatric Association, 1994) may ensue or only portions of it: flashbacks, intrusions, hyperarousal, avoidance, psychic numbing, dissociation, the inability to function in significant roles, and so on.

Hyperarousal, Posttraumatic Recall, and Avoidance

I forgot to tell you about "Chernobyl rain"—we call the very rare rain with sun Chernobyl rain because it is the same type of rain we had right after the explosion, when no one knew to stay inside away from the radioactive fallout. Whenever that rain comes I become upset and agitated and I can't stop thinking of all the things that can come from Chernobyl. We were outside on those days and who knows what will happen to us now? Can I have normal children, will we live very long? (Belarusian woman 15 years after Chernobyl)

Ecological disasters often differ from typical posttraumatic stressors (Baum, Fleming, & Davidson, 1983; Havenaar & van den Brink, 1997) in that the main stressor may contain only horrifying information. When this is the case, the traumatic event is frequently benignly experienced at first and only later becomes embedded with an overlay of horrifying information that redefines it as terrifying and life-threatening.[3] As a result of the delay in experiencing the event as traumatic, there is often also a significant difference in how victims experience the time distortions and the concurrent hyperarousal states typical of PTSD. This was found to be true in a sample of Chernobyl liquidators. They met paper and pencil criteria for PTSD but did not evidence typical hyperarousal states when tested with physiological measures, which raised the question of whether horrifying information alone is capable of acting as a traumatic stressor capable of engendering PTSD (Pitman, Orr, Forgue, DeJong, & Claiborn, 1987; Tarabrina et al., 1993).

In considering this question, it is important to note that the dread and anxiety that occur upon learning that one has potentially been exposed to toxins and the terror of what that contamination may bring often create atypical time distortions and hyperarousal states that more often look *forward* than backward. Hence, the intrusive thoughts and the horror that

---

[3] The idea of an event being experienced at first benignly only later to be reexperienced in the mind as a trauma due to receipt of new horrifying information has been found with other events as well. For instance, Speckhard (1996) reported on women who at first experienced their abortions benignly only later to report posttraumatic responses upon learning of subsequent infertility, seeing pictures of aborted fetuses, viewing a sonogram of a subsequent pregnancy, and so forth. These were each events that retroactively redefined the abortion as a death event or brought to it elements of horror and inescapability, or otherwise caused it to be redefined as traumatic.

constantly intrude into consciousness may consist of typical flashbacks of the event itself, such as horrifying memories of being exposed to contaminants. Or they may just as likely be such that the person flashes into an internally created "experience" of horror that is *yet to come:* cancer, death, loss of loved ones, genetic mutations, infertility, evacuation, loss of home, job, community, and so forth. With these posttraumatic intrusions the mind is flooded with anxious images and horror-filled fears of the *future* consequences of contamination. The body enters into a state of hyperarousal similar to a flashback, and this state is as difficult to calm as a typical flashback until it is somehow contained, avoided, or otherwise shut down. All of the defenses of PTSD—avoidance, psychic numbing, and so forth—are necessary to try to contain the emotional fallout of these *future-oriented thought intrusions,* which are triggered by reminders of what occurred and by what may yet come from the disaster. These time distortions and their concurrent hyperarousal states are more aptly named "flash-forwards" than flashbacks (Speckhard, 2001). Interestingly, a Soviet researcher also noted differences in posttraumatic time distortions among victims of the Chernobyl disaster (Kronick, Akhmerov & Speckhard, 2001). Thus it appears that horrifying information alone is capable of engendering true PTSD, but significant differences may occur in the time orientation of intrusive thoughts and their resultant hyperarousal states.

Avoidance, Despair, Cynicism, and Dissociative Responses

I am a person who can follow rules, especially if I think they will protect me. At first I tried to do everything they said. We took our shoes off before coming in the door and washed all the dust from them so that we wouldn't bring the contamination into our homes. We kept the windows shut all day, even though it was hot and stuffy inside. But as the rules increased I began to see that it was impossible to do everything they said. How could I keep the cat from coming in and going out? How could I live in a room where I never opened the windows? It was too hard and I gave up and stopped listening. Maybe I endangered my health, because now I have thyroid problems and I am part of a research study where they keep observing it to see if it will become cancer. But I could not do everything they told us to do. Now I don't even react when I hear the news every spring about Chernobyl exploding again. There is nothing I can do. (Belarusian woman 14 years after Chernobyl)

Despair is sometimes shared between those involved in advocacy and those exposed to the disaster. Journalist Svetlana Alexievich (1999), who chronicled the suffering of Belarussians following the Chernobyl disaster, reported her own feelings of despair when confronted with what she called the Belarusian "cult of helplessness." Likewise, community advocate Louis Bertholet speaks about sharing sorrow and feelings of helplessness with the people living near the Bijlmer crash:

> *There is a family of four who live on the fourth floor of one of the high-rise apartments so typical for this multicultural quarter of town. On the day of the crash this part of the apartment was constantly in the smoke. You just could not escape it. Smoke entered their apartments; they walked in full smoke when they left their houses. The house was filled with friends who later on have become ill as well. In time the health problems for the family started with vague complaints, difficult to diagnose. It became increasingly more difficult to go to work every day. The terrible coldness of the bureaucracy is stunning. All four of the family is out of a job, they live on the poverty line. The mother who has been mentally very strong, helps where possible, is the listening ear to many apartment dwellers around her, cannot see the suffering of her children anymore. When I came to her to let off steam and of course to be a listening ear, she said to me: "Look, Louis, I bought a large plant forcing bed (45 cm × 120 cm) for on the balcony. When I die put me in it and bury me in it. It's my size and it is cheap and good for a dehumanized being. This must be my coffin." It breaks your heart, I'll tell you.*

Dread and hyperarousal can continue for years. A common theme repeated by victims of ecological disasters around the world is the shattered trust and fear that human failure or carelessness will result in a repetition of the disaster. To many the second-worst thing after their own health concerns is the horror that it can happen again. A Hungarian man recalls the poisoning of the River Tiza:

> *Last January we had the worst environmental disaster in the world, second only maybe to the accident at Chernobyl. There was a mining accident in Romania, upstream that leaked cyanide into our river. It killed all the living things in the river, everything. Every single fish was killed. It will take years before they will be replenished to how they once were. The people could no longer fish and the drinking water supply was not safe so they had to have water trucked into the villages. It was horrible. River Tiza feeds into the Danube, the main river for our capital Budapest. Thankfully the cyanide was diluted before it got to River Danube. The area around River Tisza is known for tourism but this accident hit hard on the tourism industry. No one wanted to travel there. The accident happened because a mining dam burst in Romania. The worst thing about it is that the mining continues in Romania and it can happen again, anytime.*

Grief and Complicated Mourning

> *The sorrow did not end. Last week I was down in Seward (Alaska). We were out on the coast again. I couldn't stop crying. It's been 12 years now, but it's still real hard. I lost trust in things that have always been a part of my life, things that are integral to my life and suddenly gone. (Page, an ecologist working on the Valdez oil spill, 12 years after)*

Almost all disasters create grief and losses. Grief that is tangled up with post-traumatic responses can be buried deeply, only to resurface when triggered by reminders of the trauma, even years later. Likewise, the changes made by ecological disasters frequently endure beyond the lifetimes of those who witnessed them. This is a sobering realization for many.

REACTIONS TO OFFICIAL RESPONSES

Cleanup Efforts, Frustration, Exhaustion, and Bureaucratic Conflicts

It was such a frustrating thing, nothing you could do. There were rivers of oil floating off shore, fisherman were driving their boats with nets trying to break it up into smaller pieces. But when their nets got the oil on them they started to sink and they had to radio for help. What should we do, cut our nets? The coast guard got on the radio and I'll never forget his voice. He said, "I don't know." That was the heart of it. It was so big, bigger than any of us. No one knew what to do. It was truly Pandora's box.

It was long hours, day and day after for months on the spill. Personal lives began to crumble. It was one emergency after another, nonstop emergencies. People had differences about how to do things. We had to separate them. One guy in the field quit on the spot. (Bud, 12 years after Valdez *oil spill)*

The rescue and cleanup workers brought into a ecological disaster often become victims as well, by virtue of their exposure to toxins or simply by shattering assumptions about a world they believed to be more orderly and protected than what they experienced within the disaster.

Interventions

The dull pain of an ecological disaster that is too big to understand, that could not be contained by humans and whose consequences are yet unknown, finds a container in the human psyche. If it is overwhelmingly traumatic it gets locked inside, walled off from consciousness, and becomes the slow burn of anxiety, triggered by distressing questions, illnesses, painful reminders of what happened and what might still occur. Each person must find their own way of unlocking and working through these painful emotional responses to disaster. For some this occurs through self-help efforts, such as journaling.

I had to get the hell out of Seward. I started writing the day after I got out of the oil spill. Writing was therapeutic. The words just kept flowing out of my fingers. I have never written before and never used writing as a healing tool, but it seemed to serve a purpose. During that time I couldn't concentrate. My brain had gone away. This is a very scary thing to someone who earns her living with her brain. I didn't know if I was going to get my brain back. There were months in there where to be able to sit down and write a report, or read a scientific paper, anything professional—I couldn't think logically. My short-term memory was shot. My boss said, "Page do whatever you need to do to get well. We need you long-term." This man saved my life. (Page, after the Valdez oil spill, Spencer, 1990)

Rebuilding the Community

The mothers in our clinic were apathetic and became upset when we asked about their perceptions of the effects of radiation on their children's health. They tried not to discuss it. It took time to gain their trust, to help them understand that we were not just researchers asking questions and then going to disappear. When they understood that we wanted to help them and that we were willing to help them have a voice with the local authorities to do whatever they can to improve their children's health, then they became interested. The mothers want help; they just don't know how to get it. They almost all agreed to return for monthly discussion groups. (Belarusian psychologist working in a Gomel health clinic 14 years later)

Understanding and kind responses by others can go a long way to help ease the pain and give a respite for dealing with the emotions that may have been too overwhelming to process during the disaster (Esveenko, Kravchenko, Nadolskaya, & Korchevaya, 1999). On the other hand advocacy efforts must walk a fine line between empowering those exposed to a toxic disaster and not inflaming fears. Frequently giving information about risks, even small risks, can inflame fears.

Public education also has the potential to be therapeutic. Victims of technological disasters are often distrustful, frightened, tired, and disheartened. They want trustworthy information and they want to protect themselves, but in ways that are not too overwhelming. Social alienation and cynicism can be altered if community leaders find creative ways to foster increased social bonding and joint social activism. Despairing cynicism needs to be replaced with honest appraisals of self and others. Likewise shattered assumptions that have broken into shards of a world that is no longer safe and authorities that are no longer protective can over time be replaced by a sense of communal assertiveness for safeguards and by sensitivity in the community about the needs of others similarly hurt. If public officials desire to do so, they can build community forums to honestly inquire into what went wrong and to discuss community efforts to safeguard the future. Internet bulletin boards, chat rooms, and Web pages give the possibility of quickly disseminating information to many people who can access the information conveniently, in privacy and paced according to their needs.

Trauma victims are often greatly aided by knowing that they are not alone in their post-traumatic responses to a disaster. Education that puts risks into perspective and outlines typical stress responses is very useful in the short term. A woman who attended a disaster stress debriefing after the September terrorist attacks on America states:

> It was really good to discuss the usual symptoms after this kind of event. I was alone afterward and I thought I was going crazy. My heart was racing so fast. Also it helped to realize that the risks I take driving my car are probably greater than the risks of dying in a chemical attack. I'm still driving so maybe I can calm down a bit.

Large-Scale Interventions

When large groups of people have been affected, such as in the Chernobyl disaster, creative approaches must be developed to reach large numbers of people. "Lifeline," a computer program developed by a former Soviet-era researcher (Kronik, 1993), was used with Ukrainian children to help them adjust to their post-traumatic responses to Chernobyl. In this program schoolchildren worked on computers with a trained professional to assess and change the effects of their experience upon their expectations of their futures. Cognitive and behavioral changes were suggested within the framework of perceiving one's "lifeline" with very good success in altering post-traumatic responses. The children often began with dark views of their life experiences and future, but improved quickly when their attention was directed toward new possibilities other than the dire health worries that dominated their thoughts (Kronik, Akhmerov, & Speckhard, 1999).

CONCLUSION

Those who work with victims of toxic disasters face unique challenges. There are still many unanswered questions about toxic exposure and the need to construct trustworthy disease models. Yet technological advances and their consequent threats hurdle ahead. Psychologists must keep up and develop models that address both fears and reality, something that can be hard to discern when information is not readily available and when stress interacts with toxic challenges to the body. Likewise large-scale disasters demand responses that abandon the luxuries of one-on-one care in favor of strategies that are low cost, reach many, and are effective.

When authorities lose their credibility, others are quick to step in to the gap, filling the need for information, especially in these days of Internet access when truth and rumor can quickly be spread the world over. Useful community forums for discussion and activism can also be built using new technology, including Internet discussion groups where real people's voices can both be heard and responded to. Likewise, mental health professionals would do well to offer their expertise to news professionals and authorities to help them form truthful messages that do not over incite anxieties and may even be able to soothe and contain fears. They can also be on hand to assist those in the front lines to deal with their own responses to such disasters.

As the field runs alongside technology to address the new challenges of toxic nightmares both from accidents and malignant intent, it is crucial to remember that in constructing models and designing responses, it is the victim's voice that is important to hear. True understanding can only occur when one takes the time to listen to the inside story.

REFERENCES

Alexievich, S. (1999). *Voices from Chernobyl: Chronicle of the future*. London: Aurum Press.

American Psychiatric Association. (1994). *Diagnostic and statistical manual of mental disorders* (4th ed.). Washington, DC: Author.

Baum, A., Fleming, R., & Davidson, L. M. (1983). Natural disaster and technological catastrophe. *Environment and Behaviour 15*, 333–353.

Bromet, E. J. (1989). The nature and effects of technological failures. In R. Gist & B. Lubin (Eds.), *Psychosocial effects of disaster* (pp. 120–139). New York: Wiley.

Bromet, E. J., Carlson, G., Goidgaber, D., & Gluzman, S. (1998). Health effects of the Chernobyl catastrophe on mothers and children. In B. L. Green (Chair), *Toxic contamination: The interface of psychological and physical health effects*. Symposium conducted at the 14th annual meeting of the International Society for Traumatic Stress Studies, Washington, DC.

Cwikel, J., Abdelgani, A., Goldsmith, J. R, Quastel, M., & Yevelson, I. I. (1997). Two-year follow up study of stress-related disorders among immigrants to Israel from the Chernobyl area. *Environmental Health Perspectives, 105*, (Suppl. 6), 1545–1550.

Esveenko, V., Kravchenko, V., Nadolskaya, M., & Korchevaya, G. (1999). *Chernobyl nuclear disaster effect on the Belarusian population: A pilot survey report*. Unpublished research document available from the author.

Green, B. L. (1998). Psychological responses to disasters: Conceptualization and identification of high-risk survivors. *Psychiatry and Clinical Neurosciences, 52* (Suppl.), S67–S73.

Green, B. L., Lindy, J. D., & Grace, M. C. (1994). Psychological effects of toxic contamination. In R. J. Ursano, B. G. McCaughey, & C. S. Fullerton (Eds.), *Individual and community responses to trauma and disaster: The structure of human chaos* (pp. 154–176). Cambridge: Cambridge University Press.

Havenaar, J. M., and van den Brink, W. (1997). Psychological factors affecting health after toxicological disasters. *Clinical Psychology Review, 17*(4), 359–374.

Janoff-Bulman, R. (1992). *Shattered assumptions: Towards a new psychology of trauma*. New York: Free Press.

Knudsen, L. B. (1991). Legally induced abortions in Denmark after Chernobyl. *Biomedicine and Pharmocotherapy, 45*, 229–231.

Kronik, A. A. (1993). *LifeLine i drugie novye metody psikhologii zhiznennogo puti [LifeLine and Others New Methods of Psycho-Biographical Analysis]*. Moscow: Progress-Culture.

Kronik, A. A., Akhmerov, R. A., & Speckhard, A. C. (1999). Trauma & disaster as life disrupters: A computer assisted model of psychotherapy applied to adolescent victims of the Chernobyl disaster. *Professional Psychology: Research and Practice, 30*(6), 586–599.

Levenson, R. W., Carstensen, L. L., & Gottman, J. M. (1994, July). Influence of age and gender on affect, physiology, and their interrelations: A study of long-term marriages. *Journal of Personality & Social Psychology, 67*(1), 56–68.

Lifton, R. (1967). *Death in life*. New York: Touchstone Book, Simon & Schuster.

Mufel, N., Speckhard, A. C., & Sivuha, S. (2002) Predictors of posttraumatic stress disorder following abortion in a former Soviet Union country. *Journal of Pre- and Perixotal Psychology*.

Perry, B. D., Pollard, R. A., Blakley, T. L., Baker, W. L., & Vigilante, D. (1995). Childhood trauma, the neurobiology of adaption and use-dependent development of the brain: How states become traits. *Infant Mental Health Journal, 16*(4):271–291.

Pitman, R. K, Orr, S. P., Forgue, D. F., DeJong, J. B., & Claiborn, J. M. (1987). Psychophysiologic assessment of posttraumatic stress disorder imagery in Vietnam combat veterans. *Archives of General Psychiatry, 44*(11), 970–975.

Speckhard, A. C. (1996). Traumatic death in pregnancy: The significance of meaning & attachment. In C. Figley, B. Bride, & N. Mazza (Eds.), *Death & trauma: The traumatology of surviving* (pp. 67–100). Philadelphia: Taylor & Francis.

Speckhard, A. C. (2001). Mental health effects of technological disaster: The psychological aftermath of toxic contamination. In N. Berkowitz (Ed.), *Chernobyl: The event and the aftermath* (pp. 13–45). Madison, WI: Friends of Chernobyl Centers, U.S.

Speckhard, A., & Rue, V. (1992). Post abortion syndrome: An emerging public health concern. *Journal of Social Issues, 48*(3), 95–120.

Spencer, P. (1990). *White silk & black tar: A journal of the Alaska oil spill*. Minneapolis: Bergamot Books.

Tarabrina, N. V., Lazebnaya, E. O., Zelonova, M. E., Lasko, N. B., Orr, S. P., & Pitman, R. K. (1993). *Psychophysiological responses of Chernobyl liquidators during script-driven imagery*. International Society for Traumatic Stress Studies Annual Meeting, San Antonio, Texas.

Weinberg H. S., Korol A. B., & Kirzhner V. M. (2001, May). Very high mutation rate in offspring of Chernobyl accident liquidators. *Proceedings of the Royal Society of London series B-Biological Sciences, 268*(1471), 1001–1005.

13

Disasters and the Selection of Public Mental Health Priorities

A Perspective from Developing Countries

JOOP DE JONG

INTRODUCTION

Disasters, like wars, earthquakes, floods, cyclones, landslides, technological accidents, and urban fires, occur all over the world. Asia leads the rest of the world, averaging 197 disasters per year, followed by the Americas at 111 disasters, Europe at 77, Africa at 61, and Oceania at 18. Although some developed countries, such as the United States, are quite vulnerable to disasters, developing countries are disproportionately exposed (Somasundaram, Norris, Asukai, Srinivasa Murthy, & Shalev, 2002).

DeGirolamo and McFarlane (1996) estimated that the ratio of disaster victims in developing countries to disaster victims in developed countries is 166:1. The ratio of morbidity and mortality following disasters in developing countries to developed countries is 10:1. There is every reason to believe that this imbalance will only get worse in the foreseeable future. Increasing industrialization, urbanization, decaying infrastructures, and deforestation are among the factors that place many of the world's countries at increased or increasing risk (Quarantelli, 1994). Psychological problems tend to affect

JOOP DE JONG • Transcultural Psychosocial Organization (TPO), 1016 EE and Vrije Universiteit, Amsterdam, The Netherlands.

Toxic Turmoil: Psychological and Societal Consequences of Ecological Disasters, edited by Johan M. Havenaar, Julie G. Cwikel, and Evelyn J. Bromet. New York, Kluwer Academic/Plenum Publishers, 2002.

some 30–40% of the disaster population within the first year. After two years, levels are generally lower, but some posttraumatic sequelae become chronic (Raphael, 1986).

Over the past 30 years, I have worked in a variety of countries hit by disasters. After being exposed to the cyclone in east Pakistan in 1970 while doing research on reproductive health, I worked among returned refugees in Bangladesh after it became independent from Pakistan. I then worked as an expert in public health and tropical medicine among refugees and war-afflicted populations in West and Central Africa. After specializing in psychiatry and psychotherapy, I worked for 4 years in postwar Guinea-Bissau, combining clinical and social psychiatric work with epidemiological and psychiatric anthropological research (de Jong, 1987, 1996). At the request of collaborators in developing countries, I developed a large international non-governmental organization (NGO), the Transcultural Psychosocial Organi-zation (TPO), also known as Peace of Mind. This WHO-collaborating center implements public mental health programs in Algeria, Burundi, Cambodia, Congo, Eritrea, Ethiopia, Gaza, India (Tibetans), Indonesia, Kosovo, Mozambique, Namibia, Nepal, Uganda, Sri Lanka, Sudan, and Surinam. In some countries, the public mental health programs evolved into a local NGO (e.g., Cambodia, India). In other countries, TPO assisted local organi-zations with training, research, or management expertise (e.g., Algeria, Congo, Nepal, and Gaza) (de Jong, 2000, 2002a, 2002b). In addition, together with the Vrije Universiteit in Amsterdam, TPO develops concepts and service delivery models and conducts epidemiological research among immigrants and refugees in the Netherlands (cf. de Jong & van den Berg, 1996). Although TPO also became somewhat involved in Central America in the period after Hurricane Mitch, this chapter especially draws from my experience with the consequences of human-made disasters, such as armed conflicts.

TPO spends about 20% of its human power and funding on qualitative research and on psychiatric epidemiological and cost-effectiveness research. For example, using culturally sensitive measures to assess posttrauma psy-chopathology, we found that in a random sample of postconflict survivors in Algeria, Cambodia, Ethiopia, and Gaza, 47% of those who experienced violence, showed evidence of psychopathology compared to 24% percent of the nontraumatized sample. Of those who experienced violence, the lifetime prevalence was 30% for posttraumatic stress disorder (PTSD), 14% for de-pressive disorder, 27% for anxiety disorder, and 5% for somatoform disorder. Thirteen percent of the traumatized sample met criteria for two disorders, and 7% for three or four disorders. Comorbidity of PTSD and other anxi-ety disorders had the highest prevalence in all samples except Gaza (PTSD and depression). Eighty percent of the respondents with PTSD experienced other psychiataric disorders (de Jong, Komproe, and Van Ommeren, 2002).

PUBLIC MENTAL HEALTH CRITERIA

The development of psychosocial and mental health services for adults and children living in disaster situations should be based on public mental health considerations. The selection of treatment priorities in a society coping with the massive consequences of natural, industrial, or human-made disasters would ideally take place with the help of the public mental health criteria mentioned in this chapter. The criteria for the selection of interventions are similar to the criteria for the selection of training priorities: interventions require training, and training will be guided by the selection of interventions. This chapter will mention 7 criteria. It will explain the rationale for each criterion and mention some methods one can use to apply the criteria in the field. It will conclude by stating that handling criteria is always a subjective and judgmental process. Policy considerations, discipline, and professional expertise will influence the weight that we attribute to the different criteria.

Criterion 1: Role of Epidemiology and Community Concern in Ascertaining Prevalence of Health and Mental Health Problems, Risk Factors, and Disaster Characteristics

In public health, prevalence is considered the evaluated component of need. Evaluated need represents professional judgment about people's health status and their need for medical or psychosocial care. It is closely related to the kind and amount of treatment that will be provided after a person or patient has presented to a care provider. Whereas the prevalence criterion addresses the *evaluated* component of need, *community concern* is related to *perceived* need by communities, families, and individuals.

How does one assess prevalence? The *prevalence* of a problem is preferably determined with the help of a culturally sensitive epidemiological survey. Epidemiology is the study of the distribution and determinants of disorders in populations. It is an important discipline in understanding the magnitude of and risk factors for morbidity, including psychological morbidity, such as post-traumatic stress syndromes (PTSS), providing a methodology for investigating the relative contribution of exposure and individual vulnerability (cf. de Girolamo & McFarlane cited in Marsella, Borneman, Ekblad, & Orley, 1996). The rate of disorder in the population affected by a disaster is often referred to in disaster studies as the *impact ratio*, that is, the proportion of the population that is affected. The extent to which the level of exposure is a risk factor for disorder can be demonstrated by comparing prevalence rates to intensity of exposure, whether radioactive pollution, hazardous chemicals, or war-induced trauma, in cases and noncases. In contrast, the role of vulnerability factors is examined by distinguishing the characteristics of individuals who do and do not develop morbidity, given similar levels of exposure. One of the challenges of epidemiology is to develop appropriate measures that will identify individuals who, once exposed, go on to develop a disorder from those who have not. Epidemiology is therefore valuable in the design of treatment services after large-scale traumatic events because it provides prevalence estimates that help define the size of the affected populations and help us in planning services.

Studies conducted within a significant period of time after the trauma also provide essential information about the chronicity of symptoms and disability that can result from type-II trauma or continuous traumatic stress. According to Raphael (1986), disasters that are human induced and that are accompanied by high shock and destruction lead to persistent levels of impairment. Disability is a critical issue for treatment, since we should not assume that interventions will automatically modify survivors' ability to work or function within families. One study showed that, 30 years after the Second World War, former American prisoners of war (POWs) had an increased risk of mortality from tuberculosis and accidents (Keehn, 1980). Experience in Europe has shown that the long-term sequelae of war traumas have long been underestimated. For example, one study showed that 45 years after the Second World War 56% of a sample of Dutch Second World War–resistance veterans were suffering from PTSD. Only 4% were totally free of PTSD symptoms (Op den Velde et al., 1993). Research on American Vietnam War veterans also demonstrated a link between exposure to severe stress and the onset of coronary disease (Boscarino & Chang, 1999). Vietnam veterans with a diagnosis of PTSD were found to be more than 10 times more likely to be not working than veterans without PTSD. Veterans with PTSD were also earning 22% less per hour than their counterparts without PTSD (Fairbank, Ebert, & Johnson, 1999). One may conclude that chronicity and disability are critical issues in arguing for service provision and for secondary and tertiary prevention. Studying chronicity, disability, and moderating factors shows which people belong to high-risk vulnerable groups and therefore need special attention regarding secondary and tertiary prevention.

PTSD is one of the highest prevalent disorders after a natural or human-made disaster. In four post-conflict situations, TPO found that conflict-related events after the age of 12 year were related to PTSD in all samples. This type of event acts like a universal cause for PTSD. Torture was associated with the presence of PTSD in 3 out of 4 samples, and psychiatric history and quality of housing in 2 out of 4 samples (de Jong, Komproe, and van Ommeren, 2002).

In our research, we prefer the concept of PTSS because it allows for the inclusion of culture-specific traumatic stress reactions beyond the possibly

Western-bound construct of PTSD (de Jong, 2002a). One of the issues to which epidemiological research contributes is the relationship between PTSS and comorbid disorders. Although various disorders predispose individuals to PTSS, the boundaries between mood disorders and anxiety disorders are of primary interest. Because these boundaries are known to be vague among non-Western populations, and because there is overlap with the symptoms of somatization, dissociation, and PTSS, this is an important question to answer. Therefore, studying the prevalence of comorbidity is another way of identifying high-risk groups.

Ideally, an epidemiological survey should include a study on help-seeking behavior. Studying help-seeking behavior provides information about service utilization. For example, do people in the affected setting tend to use professional or indigenous (traditional) services to deal with emotional problems? If not, how are emotional problems handled, if at all? By studying help-seekers themselves, we can determine the distribution of stress reactions and psychopathology in individuals presenting to different health care sectors. As valuable as such studies can be, it is important to recognize that only 10% of the traumatized population may look for help (cf. Brom et al. 1993). This 10% is low in comparison with the results of epidemiological studies showing a 47% rate of psychopathology following major conflicts (de Jong, Komproe, and van Ommeren, 2002). In addition, even in outside disaster situations, more than 25% of the population has suffered from a psychiatric disorder in the past year. The problem of low service utilization is compounded in disaster areas where the infrastructure may be destroyed or in war-affected areas, where "treatment" in the Western sense is often absent. Therefore, while studying help-seeking behavior contributes to the planning process for which services should or could be provided by, for example, health workers, teachers, local healers, or relief workers, it is not an appropriate source of information on prevalence of psychopathology following disasters.

Finally, as noted above, epidemiological research can generate information on risk factors and protective factors by studying sociodemographic and economic variables, gender, coping style, social network, and structural and functional social support. Modification of these factors is an important objective of an effective intervention and prevention program. We emphasize that identifying protective factors is as important for epidemiology as identifying risk factors.

Over the past years, a new approach to measuring health status has been developed. This method quantifies not merely the number of deaths but also the impact of premature death and disability on a population, and combines these into a single unit of measurement of the overall "burden of disease," or global burden of disease, on the population. These new measurements have shown that while psychiatric conditions like depression, alcohol dependence, bipolar disorder, and schizophrenia are responsible for little more than 1% of deaths, they account for almost 11% of disease burden worldwide (Murray & Lopez, 1996). To measure the global burden of disease, an internationally standardized form has been developed, called the disability adjusted life year (DALY). The DALY expresses years of life lost to premature death and years lived with a disability of specified severity and duration. Specifically, *one DALY is one lost year of healthy life*. The DALY is intended to be a transparent tool to enhance dialogue on the major health challenges facing humanity. To calculate DALYs for a given condition in a population, years of life lost (YLLs) and years lived with disability (YLDs) of known severity and duration for that condition have to be estimated and then the total is summed. Over the coming decades, the complexity of collecting data in postdisaster areas will undoubtedly be a major obstacle to measuring DALYs in those areas. Measuring premature death caused by catastrophe is difficult because census data in developing and war-torn countries are known to be unreliable. Moreover, when massive populations show extremely high levels of anxiety and depression, it is methodologically difficult to distinguish psychiatric cases from noncases in cross-cultural settings. One can also question the use of diagnosing a mental disorder when most people show high levels of anxiety, depression, and stress. Moreover, measuring disability related to specific disorders is hard to assess when most people suffer from extreme poverty, malnutrition, fallout, landmine accident, or war acts. This makes it hard to disentangle the relative contribution to disability of anomalies such as anemia, parasites, chronic infectious disease, physical handicaps, or mental disorder. If one day we are able to tackle these methodological problems, one would expect that all of these risk factors related to disasters would lead to extremely high figures of DALYs in comparison to other areas worldwide.

Community Concern. Whereas the *prevalence* criterion addresses the *evaluated* component of need, *community concern* is related to *perceived* need by communities, families, and individuals. Community concern and perceived need are largely social phenomena that can be explained by social structure and health beliefs. Community concern is increasingly regarded as a very important criterion, because addressing the needs of the people is related to community involvement, community empowerment, and sustainability. Community concern and perceived need will help us to better understand help-seeking or care-seeking and adherence to an intervention program or treatment (Andersen, 1995). Community concern is also related to the perceived cause of a disaster. According to Bolin (1985), human-caused events (including technological disasters and complex emergencies) such as dam collapses and industrial accidents, represent in the eyes of victims a callousness, carelessness, intentionality, or insensitivity on part of the others.

How can one assess community concern? Measuring community concern is best approached using qualitative and operational research methods. Qualitative approaches are characterized by (1) an emphasis on providing a comprehensive (or holistic) understanding of phenomena; (2) the description of social phenomena from the perspective of those being studied; (3) and a research strategy that is flexible and interactive (Bryman 1992; Hudelson 1994). Agger defends the scientific rigor of qualitative research by referring to concepts as triangulation, comprehensiveness, negative case analysis, and transferability.

TPO uses a combination of the following multimethod approaches:

1. *Snowball Sampling.* Snowball sampling is used to select key informants. Multiflex snowball sampling involves the selection of samples utilizing "insider" knowledge and referral chains among subjects who possess common traits (Kaplan, Korf, & Sterk, 1987). A subject, selected on the basis of a particular trait, is asked to identify others sharing that trait. From the set of those nominated, a simple random selection is made. In this way a number of key informants are identified. The method is especially useful with regard to "hidden" problems a program has to address or should have addressed, such as rape of women, perpetrators of violence such as boy-soldiers, stigmatizing neuropsychiatric disorders, substance abuse, seropositivity, or prostitution.

2. *Key Informant Interviews.* Key informants are chosen for their knowledge or insight about a community, preferably with a snowball sampling method. The interviews are carried out by one or two key program individuals, one of them preferably being a "professional stranger" such as an anthropologist. Key informants are selected on the following criteria:

- They are representative of the various ethnic groups and both genders.
- They hold a position of respect and trust.
- They have lived in the community for a considerable length of time.
- They have functions.

They have functions that bring them into contact with many people within the community or with a particular section of it. Examples include shopkeepers, teachers, religious leaders, local healers, traditional birth attendants (TBAs), members of political or women's organizations, or health workers. Key informants can be interviewed either individually or in focus groups. The information about key informants that is important to record includes demographic data, duration of stay in the community, and their qualifications as a key informant. It is important that they understand that the interviewers are interested in their own opinions and that it is not necessary to mention their name for the purpose of the interview. In some cultures there may be a formal or informal religious, political, or traditional leader who speaks for the group, and the others may conform to his or her ideas (i.e., group think). Group think can reflect the strict hierarchy within a culture or family or mistrust that is often rampant in postdisaster situations (de Jong, 1987). If it occurs during the first focus group, it is better to organize individual key informant interviews.

3. *Focus Groups.* The method consists of open yet guided group interviews with 5–10 persons to obtain qualitative information on priorities, needs, and attitudes (Krueger, 1994). We also use focus groups for a variety of other reasons. They can be used, for example, as an orientation toward positive coping strategies, toward newly arisen problems in the area, for the evaluation of a program, for possible shifts in program priorities, or for the assessment of community dynamics. Focus groups are organized on the macro-, the meso-, and the micro-level. The *macro-level* is the society-at-large and the culture in which people live. The *meso-level* is the community. The *micro-level* is the level of the individual and the family. In other words, the focus groups range from ministries, regional and district officials, to community leaders and families in the postdisaster context.

4. *Interviews of Parents.* When the family, or children, are the target of the assessment, this method is mainly used to evaluate the outcomes initiated by the project. The parents supply information on a chosen priority or target during a household survey or in a health or educational facility.

5. *Participant Observation and Phenomenological Narratives.* Participant observation is the preferred research technique of many anthropologists. A narrative is obtained in a sequence of steps that can be summarized as follows. The first part consists of an autobiographically oriented story. The technique used resembles the personal interview taught to journalists, medical doctors, and ethnographers. This part of the narrative or life history should be as broad as possible. The interviewer then asks more specific questions. Respondents are next asked to theorize about their lives and their "problem." Subsequently, the researcher must utilize guidelines to identify which data are worth further consideration, paying attention to primacy (what comes first in a story), uniqueness (what stands out in a story), omission (what seems to be missing from the story), distortion and isolation (what does not follow logically in the story), and incompletion (when the story fails to end in a satisfying way). In this stage, patterns of meaning and experience are sought and an analytic abstraction of the case is written.

6. *Community Meetings.* Organizing a meeting with the community is done in accordance with local ways of gathering a community, paying attention to representativeness of, for example, age, gender, and ethnicity.

The methods briefly described above are used in an eclectic way on different levels. For example, narratives and individual key informant interviews are used with individuals and families. On the community and societal levels, one may organize focus groups to develop an inventory of priorities and responses of officials regarding the consequences of disaster on each administrative level. One may conduct more specific focus groups if there are rumors or stories about certain problems. For example, a focus group could be composed of traditional birth attendants in cases of fear of increases in congenital deformities, or in cases of sexual violence or rape. Another example is a focus group composed of adolescents if they cannot express certain preoccupations in the presence of the elderly.

Community concern can be hard to assess in postwar circumstances. Victims may have been so seriously deprived of basic human needs such as shelter, water, or food for a considerable amount of time that these issues form the whole gestalt of any interview. Or they may be so accustomed or conditioned to ask for material help from (non)governmental organizations that bringing forward any other issue does not come to their minds. They may also be so accustomed to the effects of traumatic stress that a distortion of the population norm has taken place with regard to normality and deviancy. For example, during focus groups discussions in a war-ridden area in East Africa, the mothers stated that their children were not affected by the war. Since the results seemed hard to believe, the focus group discussions were repeated. It turned out that almost all children had night terrors and that all children up to the age of 12 were wetting their bed, whereas in that area being potty trained at the age of 1 year is not exceptional.

The assessment of community concern mostly starts during the project preparation phase. It is an integral part of (rapid) appraisal methods and is reflected in a project proposal or policy document. Throughout the development of a service delivery program, community concern is measured during the repetitive cycle that characterizes multiannual programs heading for sustainability. In addition to the aforementioned techniques, such as focus groups or key informant interviews, community concern can be assessed by looking at the type of problems that people present to community services or health services in the affected areas. Another indication for community concern are the requests being transmitted by community leaders. These requests can be forwarded by district or provincial authorities to the government and subsequently to international agencies or organizations.

Community concern and epidemiology are complementary (Table 13.1). That is, the presentation of specific problems provides insight into concerns that correspond to or enrich the results of the epidemiologic study or the research on help-seeking behavior. As noted above, assessing community concern reflects the perceived psychosocial well-being of a population. In contrast, epidemiological studies provide quantitative,

Table 13.1 Complementarity of the Epidemiologic and Community Concern Approaches

Prevalence	Community concern
Driven by epidemiology	Driven by social science
Assesses disorder and its distribution:	Assesses perceived concerns, idioms
e.g., depression, anxiety, alcoholism, PTSS	if distress, folk illnesses
Estimates morbidity, mortality, disability	Estimates suffering
Meant to increase health	Meant to increase well-being,
	community involvement, &
	empowerment & sustainability
Technique: quantitative cross-culturally	Technique: qualitative: grounded
reliable and validated psychodiagnostic	theory, multimethod (rapid appraisals,
and psychometric instruments	focus groups, key informant interviews,
	in-depth interviews)
Cross-sectional, rarely longitudinal	Throughout the program cycles
One survey may take considerable time	One assessment plus reporting may
	take 2–8 weeks
Etic-emic*	Emic*

*The emic approach studies behavior from within the system, the etic approach from a position outside the system (cf. Berry, 1969).

public health, or health systems data. Before starting any service delivery, one would ideally like to do a survey on the prevalence of disorders. This information also serves to refine the components of training programs and to further develop training materials. However, it is important to note that current requirements for cross-cultural validity and translation of instruments is so time consuming that a reliable epidemiological study in developing countries may take 2 to 5 years. Most programs in (post)conflict situations—but also in peacetime—do not have that amount of time. Within TPO, this means that community concern has been our major criterion for setting up a program although over the years, we have added epidemiological research when it is feasible to do so.

Criterion 2: Predictability, Rapidity of Onset, Duration of the Crisis, and Severity of the Problems

Predictability, rapidity of onset, and duration of the crisis are important attributes of a disaster (Somasundaram et al., 2002). They determine whether people were able to prepare themselves and whether the threat persists. For example, flash floods and earthquakes often occur with very little warning, whereas there is often a substantial warning period before riverine floods and hurricanes. Warning systems and the mass evacuations they allow have saved countless lives and prevented an even greater number of physical injuries. Given that personal injury, threat to life, and bereavement are among the strongest predictors of postdisaster psychological distress, we may also infer that warning, preparedness, and evacuation greatly reduce the trauma potential of disaster agents. The superiority of their warning systems may be among the strongest advantages that more developed countries have over less developed countries. However, more gradual onset and predictability do not necessarily translate to greater preparedness or trauma reduction because potential victims do not always believe or heed such warnings even if they receive them.

The duration of the crisis is an important variable in relation to morbidity and mortality. After the nuclear power plant accidents at Three Mile Island and Chornobyl, residents remained fearful about the long-term effects of exposure to radiation and the possibility of future accidents. In postconflict situations, prolonged chronic stress causes cumulative strain, manifesting itself in different types of problems that present service providers over time (Baron, Buus Jensen, & de Jong, 2002; de Jong, 2001).

Seriousness. Immediately following a disaster, general distress and minor psychological disorders can affect almost the entire population. In a later phase, a majority of the people usually recover without professional support (Green et al., 2002).

Because distress and minor psychological disorder are ubiquitous, they are a priority early on. However, their management needs to be balanced with the needs of victims with more severe psychiatric reactions. Because most programs struggle with a discrepancy between a need for services and a lack of funding, one has to weigh the seriousness of a mental disorder among a minority of the population against the enormous amount of distress among a majority that is usually short lived. This choice is in fact complicated when one considers that failure to treat distress in the early stages can potentially lead to more serious psychopathology in the future. Often the distress is expressed in persistent somatic symptoms, including chronic pain, gastrointestinal disorders, headaches, and seizures (Friedman & Schnurr, 1995). Service providers have to disentangle the contribution of somatic disorder and psychological distress causing these somatic complaints. Another compounding factor is that a program may decide to focus on a problem that is considered important, whereas the local cultural setting dictates another priority. For example, when TPO visited Honduras after hurricane Mitch, it became clear that the effect of the hurricane in rates of PTSD was offset by the much more traumatizing and omnipresent domestic violence.

Another source of confusion in considering the seriousness of a disorder is that subgroups among the population may show a different response when mental health services are offered. For example, when setting up mental health care services in Cambodia, we found that in areas with high concentrations of returnees from the Thai border camps, the consumption of mental health care services was many times higher than in areas that had never known any allopathic mental health care service over and above the services that were delivered by the local healers and monks. The reason for the difference was that, although both groups regarded mental disorder as a serious condition, only the returnees from the border camps knew from their previous experience in Thailand that such a thing as allopathic treatment for mental disorder exists (Somasundaram, van der Put, Eisenbruch, & de Jong, 1999).

Criterion 3: Adequacy of Resources

Susceptibility to Management, Treatability, or Feasibility. The criterion of susceptibility to management, treatability, or clinical improvement is important both with regard to the question of whether people with certain problems get support from their environment and whether there are sufficient resources in terms of personnel, time, and funds to treat specific problems. For example, in some areas of Africa and Asia, the prevalence of epilepsy is as high as 3.7–4.9% and it is often treated in psychiatric and primary health care services (Adamolekum, 1995). In addition, especially in situations of massive stress, a large number of people show symptoms of dissociation varying from individual possession as an "idiom of distress" to classical fugue states and epidemics of mass psychogenic illness with or without psychogenic fits (de Jong, 1987; van Ommeren et al., 2001). In low-income countries, one often still sees the classical phenomena described by Janet in the Salpêtrière. While setting up services, one has to consider which health care sector is best equipped to deal with the high prevalence of all kinds of convulsions, whether of neurologic or dissociative origin (conversion or hysteria). Offering treatment to those with epilepsy is a feasible option. A total of 95% of a sample of West African patients with generalized epileptic convulsions were correctly diagnosed and treated with phenobarbital by primary health care workers who received a couple of hours of training; the average seizure frequency decreased from 16 to 0.34 per month (de Jong, 1996). On the other hand, dealing with the equally highly prevalent dissociative states often requires sophisticated and scarce psychotherapeutic skills. In many cultures, adequate management for both groups implies triage of the epileptic patients and referral of those with dissociative states to the local healers or possession cults.

A similar problem exists with regard to the treatment of complex PTSD as a result of type-II trauma in war-affected areas. In the West, the psychotherapy of complex PTSD requires a long-term commitment from both therapist and client. In most war-affected areas, psychotherapists are less available, and long-term therapy is mostly alien to the local culture. This is one reason why mental health care professionals often have to resort to short therapies, limiting themselves to the stabilization phase of the three-phase model of Janet, for example (Meichenbaum, 1997; van der Kolk, McFarlane, & Weisaeth, 1996). It is obvious that on the previous criterion of seriousness, the neuropsychiatric consequences of HIV or an increase of neoplasms would receive high priority, but that on the criterion of treatability one can often do little more than assist people in the process of dying. This applies especially to developing countries and countries in transition. One of the impediments to the treatment of various types of illnesses is that modern and often complex types of psychotherapy, such as cognitive-behavioral therapies, are extremely hard to apply in non-Western settings (de Jong, 2000). In addition, their appropriateness has not been established.

Knowledge, Skills, and Availability of (Mental) Health Care Professionals. Before setting up a multidisciplinary, multisector intervention program, one needs to enumerate the number and types of mental health care professionals, general health workers, and other possible trainees from sectors such as education or social services available. The assessment can be done with the help of an instrument such as the Health Staff Interview, a 30-minute semi-structured interview developed by the WHO, which can be adapted to local circumstances (de Jong, 1987, p. 156). Any assessment should answer questions regarding (1) the ability to handle different types of psychosocial and mental health problems, (2) normal duties and responsibilities, (3) the kind of problems providers come across in their work, and (4) the kind of training and supervision that are needed. It should also determine (5) the extent to which the trainees themselves have been traumatized by the disaster. Training should address their traumatic experiences, and (6) after the training a second assessment should be carried out to determine whether the trainees are able to deal with the traumas of others. Group and individual debriefing, (peer) supervision, and job rotation are useful measures to prevent burnout.

Criterion 4: Sustainability

The sustainability of a program will depend primarily on the institutional capacity and the creation of enough human resource capacity to continue the interventions. In our view, sustainability has to be a top priority from the very beginning of any project or program. It implies reflection on the continuation of cost-effective service delivery, on the quality of management, and on future means to guarantee funding for the interventions. In the context of an NGO like TPO, it means that in an early stage, projects are often quite dependent on headquarters. But in subsequent years this dependence is transformed into a situation of interdependence or autonomy.

The following aspects are important with regard to sustainability:

1. One has to be aware of the paradox that a large amount of external funding in a postdisaster setting may hinder future sustainability. Ideally one should find a balance between external and local resources. The larger the discrepancy between these two sources of income, the harder it is to build up a sustainable program. Being poor may create an inverse relationship between initial external funding and long-term sustainability. In general mental health activities are hard to fund among marginalized people living in peripheral areas of host countries.

2. A program is made vulnerable by the source of its fundings. For example, the Tibetan government in exile in Darhamsala depends almost entirely on donor funds and therefore is extremely catious about creating positions it has to sustain. On the other hand, the rebel movement in South Sudan requested TPO to set up a program. It is run by refugees that are trained by our program among the Sudanese in north Uganda. But the past human rights record of the rebel movements in South Sudan makes the program vulnerable if major political changes do occur among the competing rebel factions and funds subsequently may be withdrawn.

3. Most donors increasingly require that programs should be demand driven and that priorities should be determined by the target groups. On the other hand, donors often have their own agenda following the whims of political decision makers requiring a shift in priorities that often endangers the continuation of a program. Receivers of funds may therefore try to make themselves less vulnerable by looking for multiple donors and creating a buffer, which in turn may evoke distrust among donors.

4. Work in (post)conflict areas implies crisis interventions and ad hoc interventions when violence flares up. This may happen at the expense of rational project design, of developing preventative action, of a larger coverage of populations, of acculturation of services, or of adequate monitoring due to the volatile situation. It requires that a program be flexible and yet maintain the goal of becoming sustainable.

5. Becoming sustainable often requires working in collaboration with local authorities, the government, or a UN agency. This may imply adaptation of management and accountancy structures; incorporation in government structures that may not be able to pay salaries or that may change their health priorities; or being obliged to survive as a vertical mental health program because horizontal integrated public health programs only exist on paper or in people's minds.

6. To guarantee continuation of the activities in countries with limited numbers of professionals, the program should train as many paraprofessionals as possible from the affected community. (It is obvious that this type of empowerment also has a preventive effect on the community.) In an early stage, one has to reflect on the career development of these trainees. This enhances the attraction to continue to work with the program and can prevent a brain drain to other organizations, departments, or countries. It can be done for example by certification of the trainees or by training some psychiatrists or psychologists abroad.

7. Sustainability is also important with regard to the provision of psychotropic drugs. As mentioned before, postdisaster populations often contain individuals with serious psychiatric disorder or epilepsy that present to the mental health services. When setting up a program, it has to be remembered that these patients need to continue their medication after resettlement or returning to their homesteads.

8. Another aspect promoting the sustainability of a program is to take a politically neutral stance when implementing the program (see "Political Acceptability"). This chapter clearly shows that this requires quite some flexibility and a need to be able to *reculer pour mieux sauter* from all the people involved.

Criterion 5: Political and Ethical Acceptability

Political Acceptability. It is important to evaluate the (hidden) agenda of policymakers and their opinion of the possible implications of the work. For example, in epidemiologic research, it is important to measure traumatic stressors and life events before and during the preimpact, the impact, and the postimpact phases in order to measure the effect of these independent variables on psychosocial well-being and psychopathology. The results of this type of research play a central role in designing culturally appropriate interventions. However, the same data can also be used for other purposes, such as for community rallies to sensitize administrators regarding restoration or compensation, or for human rights workers to advocate against repressive government practices at home or in a guest country. Governments may therefore be ambivalent toward this kind of psychosocial and research activity. On the one hand, the activities may result in safer environments, or they may stimulate democracy, respect for human rights, and psychosocial support. On the other hand, governments may be afraid of being exposed as lax or repressive. For example, TPO supported an Asian NGO involved in human rights to develop a psychosocial program. Although the director of the program stayed in hiding during the prodemocracy movement in the early 1990s, I was surprised to see that he was treated as an honorable person by high government officials within his community. The explanation appeared to be that the officials welcomed the human rights activists in case they themselves would be imprisoned, thus needing the benefits of the human rights organization.

Ethical Acceptability. The possible harm that might be inflicted on others should be considered. For example, in acute situations, data should be gathered only when they help to develop appropriate programs and not solely for research ends. Another example is carrying out research that lacks cultural sensitivity. All too often scholars are eager to collect psychodiagnostic or psychometric data to be published without questioning whether the data will help in formulating preventive or curative interventions for the affected population.

Another sensitive issue is the psychological impact of interviewing survivors of disasters or human rights abuse. We regard an interview, both during the preassessment of a program and as part of an epidemiologic survey, as an intervention in itself. Clinicians who treat torture victims have described the emotional upset associated with recalling a torture experience (Allodi, 1991; Kolb & Multipassi, 1982). Tulving (cf. Mollica, 1994) notes that an open-ended interview using free recall elicits the greatest emotional distress and poorest recall. Neutral retrieval cues, such as a list of possible events, produce more accurate responses and much less emotional distress. A considerable proportion of the individuals who are interviewed feel relieved to have an opportunity to talk about their trauma experience. Westermeyer (1989) stated that asking about traumatic events does not create distress; rather it elicits distress that is already present. Still, one should take into account that an interview may cause such upset and that counseling may be required immediately.

Taking these precautions into account, why do we regard an interview as an intervention? In circumstances of massive traumatization, survivors tend to create their "conspiracy of silence" because they do not want to embarrass others with their traumatic past, because everybody is occupied with surviving, or because the culture does not facilitate the disclosure of a traumatic past. Therefore, interviewees often perceive an interview as a unique event enabling them to share their problems and feeling recognized in their suffering. It also offers them the possibility of giving a testimonial about their plight. The urge to be heard may create a dilemma for the interviewer. Knowing that neutral cues and a moderate amount of empathy creates less distress for the inteviewee and may run counter to the need to disclose the past. Methodologically this dilemma also poses a problem. An interview format may impose time limitations, and allowing time for specific events may create memory bias. On the other hand, probing beyond the structured format may elicit culture-specific expressions of distress, emotion words, or metaphors, which are important to enrich the questionnaire when using a "grounded theory" approach (Strauss, 1987) or when trying to prevent the "category fallacy" (Kleinman, 1977). To handle these ethical dilemmas requires careful preparation of interviewers in role plays.

Western-style informed consent with signatures on an elaborate consent form has to be discussed thoroughly before being applied. As Bromet (1995) argued after the Chornobyl accident, such forms may be perceived with distrust and suspicion. Sometimes local people will not reveal much because of fear that the interviewer will gossip about what they have said in the interview. The procedure may evoke fear, such as of being disowned by one's country, as we discovered in countries such as Cambodia, Ethiopia, or Gaza. One way of solving this problem is verbal informed consent, preferably in the presence of a family member or friend (cf. ICH/CPMP, 1997).

Another ethical consideration is the above-mentioned sustainability of the project. Psychosocial and mental health assistance requires a long-term commitment. In low-income countries, it may take 4–7 years before local trainers are trained and before they are able to then train and supervise enough secondary- and tertiary-level staff to ensure continuity of the work.

Criterion 6: Cultural Sensitivity

Culture defines reality for its members. It defines the purpose of the life of the individual and the group and prescribes and sanctions proper behavior. The beliefs, values, and behaviors of a culture provide its members with personal and social meaning, learned through tradition and transmitted from generation to generation. Culture serves two functions. It is *integrative*, that is, it represents the beliefs and values that provide individuals with a sense of identity. It is also *functional*, meaning it furnishes the rules for behavior that enable the group to survive and provide for its welfare, while supporting an individual's sense of self-worth and belonging. These two functions are analogous to the warp and woof of a tapestry (Kagawa-Singer & Chi-Yung Chung, 1994). The weaving technique is universal, but the patterns that emerge from each culture are particular. A thread can be taken out and compared cross-culturally, but its function can only be understood within the cultural fabric from which it came.

As a result, each aspect of a public mental health intervention has to be tested for its cultural assumptions and consequences. For example, Green (1993) has suggested eight generic dimensions of trauma: (1) threat to life and limb; (2) severe physical harm or injury; (3) receipt of intentional injury/harm; (4) exposure to the grotesque; (5) violent/sudden loss of a loved one; (6) witnessing or learning of violence to a loved one; (7) learning of exposure to a noxious agent; (8) causing death or severe harm to another. Some of these dimensions (e.g., 1–3) can be regarded as universal stressors, but even then culture is an important moderator. For example, in Bangladesh, 90% of rural respondents ($N = 48$) reported that they prayed to Allah as a precautionary measure to mitigate the effects of an impending cyclone (WHO, 1989). Some of the universal stressors are perceived differently in specific cultures. For example, in Uganda we found that group rape of abducted women can be dealt with by a collective purification ritual under the aegis of the elders, whereas in Algeria, Cambodia, Nepal, or Namibia the shame caused by rape can lead to suicide or marginalization of the victim. Surprisingly, even in the latter cultures we found that most women are willing to talk about rape in an interview situation, and it appeared that the shame of the interviewers in hearing about the rape was greater than the shame of the survivors. Violence in the family is regarded as a serious consequence of continuous traumatic stress in many cultures, but some cultures are lenient toward battery violence, whereas in other cultures it is found to be unacceptable (cf. Finkler, 1997). Loss of an older loved person (dimensions 5 and 6) who has children and some accumulated wealth can be acceptable in African animist cultures, since the person will travel to the reign of the ancestors. On the other hand, although some Westerners think that parents suffer less in cultures with high exposure to child mortality, the death of a child in the same culture is considered to be a disaster. An individual who is a perpetrator (dimension 8) may be regarded as a hero if he or she is a (child) soldier in countries such as Liberia, Sierra Leone, or in the Middle East.

Even exposure to the grotesque can be mediated by religious convictions such as the role of karma in Buddhism in Asia. These culturally determined subjective components are important in determining subsequent psychopathology. Therefore, the development of scales to quantify the severity of traumatic exposure is a complex issue necessitating collaboration with cultural informants and social scientists.

The role of culture is equally important in the design of any psychosocial, psychotherapeutic, or psychiatric intervention, be it curative or preventative. This means that local mental health care professionals—especially if they were trained abroad—should "indigenize" their knowledge and expertise in order to provide services. In my opinion Western mental health care professionals who are equipped with the best of intentions but without work experience in low-income countries or without extensive transcultural experience should be extremely cautious in offering their Western culture-bound expertise in disaster-ridden areas elsewhere. This caution also applies to evaluating disasters in settings where there is no local research tradition under the assumption that "Western" scientific methods can be universally applied.

Criterion 7: Effectiveness

There are at least four reasons to do research on the effectiveness of mental health programming in low-income countries affected by disasters.

First, thus far there is no empirical research establishing the effectiveness of care for traumatized people in disaster situations. (There are no published results on effectiveness studies on mental health.) Given the current trend among international aid donors to fund, albeit modest, mental health care, it is pertinent to establish effectiveness information. If we do not develop information on what works and what does not work, it would be unethical to continue carrying out such programs. Without such information, program donors are likely to move their focus to other issues. On the other hand, if proven cost and time effective, the interventions could be of great importance in the large-scale mental health care of natural, industrial, and human disaster. The feasibility of different interventions is an important issue considering the realities of day-to-day running of community mental health services in troubled regions of the world.

Second, the proposed research is important because with effectiveness information, programs can be adapted to become more effective. For example, we know little about the typical course of recovery or about the influence of culture and societal structures on the recovery process (Somasundaram et al., 2002).

Third, we need to develop information on effectiveness because it is theoretically possible that the current programs are doing harm. By focusing on the vulnerability of traumatized individuals, programs may cause unnecessary distress and helplessness. Mental health programs may create sick-roles among traumatized people, with the result that survivors undervalue their own capacities for recovery. If the programs under scrutiny have these negative side effects, they will need to be reframed or even closed.

Fourth, almost all research on trauma has been conducted in the West. However, as mentioned earlier, most trauma survivors live in low-income countries.

WEIGHING THE SEVEN CRITERIA

Early in the chapter, I mentioned that the application of the seven criteria is always subjective and judgmental. Which factor gets more weight depends on one's discipline or policy. For example, an epidemiologist or a World Bank expert may decide that DALYs and prevalence figures are the real hard data and therefore should get more emphasis. A field expert or gender specialist may feel that community concern and cultural sensitivity are all that count because the only way of achieving a sustainable program is by empowering the people who will ultimately carry the program themselves. A mental health professional may want to focus on seriousness, treatability, and (cost-)effectiveness. A human rights activist may focus on political and ethical acceptability because these are considered the roots of evil. However, in my view a serious community oriented psychosocial and public mental health care program has to consider all the factors mentioned in this chapter. The aim of this chapter is to help professionals understand what is foremost in the minds of different collaborating partners.

REFERENCES

Adamolekum, B. (1995). The aetiologies of epilepsy in tropical Africa. *Tropical Geographic Medicine, 47*(3), 115–117.

Allodi, F. (1991) Assessment and treatment of torture victims: A critical review. *Journal of Nervous and Mental Disease, 170*(1), 4–11.

Andersen, R. M. (1995). Revisiting the behavioral model and access to medical care: Does it matter? *Journal of Health and Social Behavior, 36*, 1–10.

Baron, N., Buus Jensen, S., & de Jong, J. (2002). The mental health of refugees and internally displaced people. In B. Green, M. Friedman, J. de Jong, T. Keane, & S. Solomon (eds.) (2000). *Trauma in War and Peace: Prevention, Practice, and Policy.* New York: Kluwer/Plenum.

Berry, J. W. (1969) On cross-cultural comparability. *International Journal of Psychology, 4,* 119–128.

Bolin, R. (1985). Disaster characteristics and psychosocial impacts. In B. Sowder (Ed.), *Disasters and mental health: Selected contemporary perspectives* (pp. 3–28). Rockville, MD: National Institute of Mental Health.

Boscarino, J. A., & Chang, J. (1999). Electrocardiogram abnormalities among men with stress-related psychiatric disorders: Implications for coronary heart disease and clinical research. *Annals of Behavioral Medicine, 21*(3), 227–234.

Brom, D., Kfir, R., & Dasberg, H. (1994, November 23). *A controlled double-blind study on the offspring of Holocaust survivors.* Poster presented at the annual conference of the Society of Traumatic Stress Studies, Chicago.

Bromet, E. J. (1995). Methodological issues in designing research on community-wide disasters with special reference to Chernobyl. In S. E. Hobfoll & M. W. de Vries (Eds.), *Extreme stress and communities: Impact and intervention* (pp. 267–283). Dordrecht: Kluwer.

Bryman, A. (1992). *Quantity and quality in social research.* London: Routledge.

Cohen, R. E., & Ahearn, F. L. (1991). *Handbook of mental health care for disaster victims.* London: Johns Hopkins University Press.

de Girolamo, G., & McFarlane, A. C. (1996). The epidemiology of PTSD: A comprehensive overview of the international literature. In A. J. Marsella, M. J. Friedman, E. T. Gerrity, & R. M. Scurfield. *Ethnocultural aspects of posttraumatic stress disorder* (pp. 35–36). Washington DC: American Psychological Association.

de Jong, J.T.V.M. (1987). *A descent into African psychiatry.* Amsterdam: Royal Tropical Institute.

de Jong, J.T.V.M. (1996). A Comprehensive public mental health programme in Guinea-Bissau: A useful model for African, Asian and Latin-American countries. *Psychological Medicine 26,* 97–108.

de Jong, J.T.V.M. (2000). Psychiatric problems related to persecution and refugee status. In F. Henn, N. Sartorius, H. Helmchen, & H. Lauter (Eds.), *Contemporary psychiatry*, Vol. 2 (pp. 279–299). Berlin: Springer.

de Jong, Joop, J.T.V.M. (2002a.) Public mental health, traumatic stress and human rights violations in low-income countries: A culturally appropriate model in times of conflict, disaster and peace. In J.T.V.M de Jong (Ed.), *Trauma, war, and violence: Public mental health in socio-cultural context.* New York: Kluwer/Plenum.

de Jong, J.T.V.M. (Ed.) (2002b). *Trauma, war, and violence: Public mental health in socio-cultural context.* New York: Kluwer/Plenum.

de Jong, J. T.V.M., & van den Berg, M. (Eds.). (1996). Transculturele psychiatrie & psychotherapie [Transcultural psychiatry & psychotherapy]. *Handboek voor hulpverlening en beleid [Handbook of Transcultural Psychiatry & Psychotherapy].* Lisse: Swets & Zeitlinger Publishers.

de Jong, J.T.V.M., Komproe, I. H., van Ommeren. (2002). *Psychiatric disorders, comorbidity and disability in 4 postconflict settings.* Manuscript submitted for publication.

de Jong, J.T.V.M., Komproe, I. H., van Ommeren, M., El Masri, M., Mesfin, A., Khaled, N. et al., (2001). Lifetime events and post-traumatic stress disorder in 4 post-conflict settings. *JAMA, 286*(5), 555–562.

Fairbank, J. A., Ebert, L., & Johnson, G. A. (1999). Socioeconomic consequences of traumatic stress. In P. A. Saigh & J. D. Bremner (Eds.), *Posttraumatic stress disorder: A comprehensive text.* Boston: Allyn & Bacon.

Finkler, K. (1997). Gender, domestic violence and sickness in Mexico. *Social Science and Medicine, 45*(8), 1147–1160.

Friedman, M. J., & Schnurr, P. P. (1995). The relationship between trauma, post-traumatic stress disorder, and physical health. In M. J. Friedman, D. S. Charney, & A. Y. Deutch (Eds.), *Neurobiological and clinical consequences of stress: From normal adaptation to post-traumatic stress disorder.* Philadelphia, PA: Lippincott-Raven Publishers.

Green, B. L. (1993). Identifying survivors at risk: Trauma and stressors at cross events. In J. P. Wilson & B. Raphael (Eds.), *International handbook of traumatic stress syndromes* (pp. 135–144). New York: Plenum.

Green, B. L., Friedman, M., de Jong, J.T.V.M., Solomon, S., Keane, T., Fairbank, J. A. et al., (2002). *Trauma in war and peace: Prevention, practice, and policy.* New York: Kluwer/Plenum.

Hudelson, P. M. (1994). *Qualitative research for health programmes.* Geneva: World Health Organization.

ICH/CPMP. (1997). *Guideline for good clinical practice including the Declaration of Helsinki and the Belmont Report.* London: ICH.

Kagawa-Singer, M., & Chi-Yung Chung, R. (1994). A paradigm for culturally based care in ethnic minority populations. *Journal of Community Psychology 22,* 192–208.

Kaplan, C. D., Korf, D., & Sterk, C. (1987). Temporal and social contexts of heroin-using populations. *Journal of Nervous and Mental Disease, 175*(9), 566–574.

Keehn, R. J. (1980). Follow-up studies of World War II and Korean conflict prisoners. *American Journal of Epidemiology, 111,* 194–211

Kleinman, A. (1977). Depression, somatization and the new cross-cultural psychiatry. *Social Science and Medicine, 11,* 3–10.

Kolb, L. L., & Multipassi, L. R. (1982). The conditioned emotional response: A subclass of the chronic and delayed post-traumatic stress disorder. *Psychiatric Annals, 12,* 979–987.

Krueger, R. A. (1994). Focus groups: A practical guide for applied research. UK: Sage Publication.

Marsella, A. J., Borneman, T., Ekblad, S., & Orley, J. (1994). *Amidst peril and pain.* Washington DC: American Psychological Association.

Meichenbaum, D. (1997). *Treating post-traumatic stress disorder. A handbook and practice manual for therapy.* New York: Wiley.

Mollica, R. (1994). Southeast Asian refugees: Migration history and mental health issues. In A. J. Marsella, T. Borneman, S. Ekblad, & J. Orley (Eds.), *Amidst peril and pain: The mental health and well-being of the world's refugees* (pp. 83–100). Washington, DC: American Psychological Association.

Murray, C., & Lopez, A. D. (1996). *The global burden of disease.* Geneva: World Health Organization.

Op den Velde, W., Hovens, J. E., Falger, P. R., de Groen, J. H. M., van Duijn, H., Lasschuit, L. J. et al. (1993). PTSD in Dutch resistance veterans from World War II. In J. P. Wilson & B. Raphael (Eds.), *International handbook of traumatic stress syndromes* (pp. 219–230). New York: Plenum.

Quarantelli, E. (1994). *Future disaster trends and policy implications for developing countries* Newark, DE: Disaster Research Center.

Raphael, B. (1986). When disaster strikes. London: Huichinson.

Somasundaram, D., van der Put, W. A. M., Eisenbruch, M., de Jong, J.T.V.M. (1999). Starting mental health services in Cambodia. *Social Science and Medicine 48*(8), 1029–1042.

Somasundaram, D., Norris, F. H., Asukai, N., Srinivasa Murthy, R., & Shalev, A. (2002). Natural and technological disasters. In B. Green, M. Friedman, J. de Jong, T. Keane, & S. Solomon (Eds.), *Trauma in war and peace: Prevention, practice and policy.* New York: Plenum Kluwer.

Strauss, A. (1987). *Qualitative analysis for social scientists.* Cambridge, Eng.: Cambridge University Press.

van der Kolk, B., McFarlane, A., & Weisaeth, L. (1996). *Traumatic stress. The effects of overwhelming experience on mind, body and society.* New York: Guilford.

van Ommeren, M., Sharma, B., Komproe, I., Poudyal, B., Sharma G. K., Cardeòa, E., & de Jong, J.T.V.M. (2001). Trauma and loss as determinants of medically unexplained epidemic illness in a Bhutanese refugee camp. *Psychological Medicine, 31*(7), 1259–1267.

Westermeyer, J. (1989). *Psychiatric care of migrants: A clinical guide.* Washington, DC: American Psychiatric Press.

World Health Organization (WHO). (1989). *Managing the psychosocial consequences of disasters.* Geneva: WHO.

14

Epilogue

Lessons Learned and Unresolved Issues

JOHAN M. HAVENAAR, JULIE G. CWIKEL, and
EVELYN J. BROMET

INTRODUCTION

This book has compiled a set of diverse experiences that have occurred in the
wake of past ecological disasters. Our key purpose is to draw lessons for the
future and to identify areas where further research is needed. We hope that
the knowledge base encompassed within this volume will heighten awareness among professionals and authorities that environmental catastrophes
are, unfortunately, not uncommon occurrences, and furthermore, that an
ecological disaster may evolve from what seems to be an environmentally
limited human-made or natural catastrophe. Regardless of the realities of a
situation, once information emerges that hazardous substances have been
released into the environment during an accident, the aftermath is likely
to turn "toxic" in the psychological and societal senses. Subsequent events

JOHAN M. HAVENAAR • University Medical Center and Altrecht Institute for Mental Health
Care, Utrecht, The Netherlands.   JULIE G. CWIKEL • Department of Social Work and
Center for Women's Health Studies and Promotion, Ben Gurion University of the Negev, Beer
Sheva, Israel.   EVELYN J. BROMET • Department of Psychiatry and Behavioral Science,
State University of New York at Stony Brook, New York 11794-8790.

Toxic Turmoil: Psychological and Societal Consequences of Ecological Disasters, edited by Johan M.
Havenaar, Julie G. Cwikel, and Evelyn J. Bromet. New York, Kluwer Academic/Plenum
Publishers, 2002.

tend to be dominated by this information, especially when the information is inconsistent or contradictory, as is often the case. In short, an information disaster may follow from what started as a concrete physical catastrophe. Throughout the book, examples are given of how the quality and timeliness of information and the way it is presented are crucial in determining outcome. We therefore hope that the experience gathered in this book will contribute to the quality of future interventions, especially those relating to the dissemination of information.

As is documented in the various chapters of the book, ecological disasters are typically followed by a complex web of psychological and physical health consequences, both in the short and long run. In many cases, the psychological consequences outweigh the physical ones, and in practically all cases, there is debate about how to disentangle the physical and psychological sequelae. As illustrated by the Chernobyl experience, concern over possible physical health consequences may modify people's awareness of symptoms and the likelihood that people will interpret any somatic symptom as caused by the exposure (Bromet, Goldgaber, & Gluzman, in press; Havenaar, De Wilde, van den Bout, Drottz-Sjöberg, & van den Brink, in press). One important lesson from the case reports in this book is that the health effects of these disasters are far more than the sum of their physical or psychological health effects, including post-traumatic stress disorders. In addition, medically unexplained symptoms or syndromes may be the most prominent negative health outcome. The reports also indicate that the symptom presentations may be accompanied by a marked shift in illness behaviors, perceived health care needs (e.g., demand for check-ups or examinations), and health care utilization that can overtax the public health system. Further research is needed to document such changes and to investigate their underlying dynamics. Wessely suggests in Chapter 6 that one approach to a better understanding of the occurrence and persistence of these phenomena will come from the social sciences and not just from epidemiology or laboratory-based research methods. Barsky and Borus (1999) note that a critical set of psychosocial factors underlie the tendency to develop such symptoms, including the belief that one is sick, the act of becoming a patient, and chronic stress.

Can these complex medically unexplained health effects be prevented? Once they occur, how can they be assessed and dealt with in the most effective way so as to prevent them from becoming chronic and recurrent? Prevention, assessment, and management of health problems are linked to the preparedness, early intervention, and long-term intervention phases of a disaster. During each phase, both physical and psychological mechanisms will be at work simultaneously. The situation is made more complex by the many different parties that are involved: the victims of the exposures, rescue workers, health care professionals, news reporters, representatives of different agencies and government authorities, and finally the public at large. All of these groups will have their own views of what has happened and will have implicit expectations of what should be done next. As Kleber, Figley, and Gersons (1995) point out in a previous volume in this series, the impact of disasters (by definition) exceeds the level of the individual and involves processes at group and societal levels.

This observation, in combination with the ubiquitous nature of these events and the complex interactions occurring between psychological and physical sequelae, prompted us to take a public health perspective on these events rather than a purely psychological one. In this respect, this book differs from most of the previous disaster literature that has focused on psychological dynamics, either at the level of the individual or of the community. The public health approach is further characterized by its emphasis on preventive and organizational approaches within the dynamic of the interaction between the individual and environment, as opposed to the predominant treatment approach taken previously. In the model described in Chapter 3, perception of the individual and community risk inherent in the disaster plays a central role. In Chapter 13, this theme is further elaborated by showing the importance of public perception of an event. In de Jong's opinion, and backed by the examples in the book, concern over the potential long-term health consequences of a disaster is one of the central public health issues. This also means that personal narratives deserve careful attention by professionals. Lay perspectives, being so central to the perception of the threat as well as the valuation of the response, have to be taken seriously. In Chapter 12, Speckhard's verbatim accounts of persons who have undergone toxic exposures vividly portrays this aspect. Therefore, another major lesson that can be learned from this collection of case examples is to move beyond a purely professional or organizational approach and include a "consumer's perspective." Just as in any contemporary approach to improving quality of care, we should strive to integrate these different perspectives if we wish to enhance the quality of our disaster management (Donabedian, 1980; Øvretveit, 1998, p. 240).

In this chapter, we will summarize the lessons encountered in the different chapters of this book. We will do this for each phase of the disaster separately (i.e., preparedness, immediate response, and long-term response), taking into account the different points of view of victims, professionals, authorities, and the general public. This approach will also help us identify where the gaps in our knowledge are and which should be given priority in future research.

QUALITY OF INTERVENTIONS IN ECOLOGICAL DISASTERS

The Preparedness Phase

Preparing the Public. If there is one important message this book carries it is that the perception of what happened is the central link in the chain of events following a toxic exposure. Preparing people for what they might expect may be possible in residential areas near hazardous industrial sites. This practice has been implemented in several places around the world. For example, residents of housing areas in the vicinity of major industrial areas in Rotterdam were given information leaflets about chemical facilities and emergency procedures in their neighborhood. Unfortunately, many accidents happen when and where they are least expected, and little preparation is possible.

The group that perhaps plays the most visible, if not the most influential role, in relation to general public preparedness is the media. They need to be informed about the risk to themselves and the population, as well as the risk their very messages can carry. In the aftermath of the Bijlmer airplane crash (Chapter 5), the importance of visual images and sound bites was clearly shown. Likewise, for weeks after the World Trade Center tragedy, television images of the airplanes crashing into the towers and their subsequent collapse were repeatedly broadcast together with snapshots of distraught relatives and interviews with sobbing survivors. These powerful images replayed by the media represent a kind of recurrent traumatic flashback at a societal level. Perhaps they can be partly understood to reflect the traumatization of the news people themselves, not just the public's desire to again watch the unfolding of horrible events. Educating the news people how to act responsibly in order to protect their own and the public's mental health is an issue that deserves attention. Two recent responses deserve mention. The International Society for Traumatic Stress Studies joined forces with the Dart Center for Journalism and Trauma at the University of Washington to educate journalists about trauma and post-traumatic responses. Newscoverage Unlimited, a newly founded organization, was established to aid news people who have experienced trauma as part of their work. Both organizations work to train news people to recognize post-traumatic effects and minimize traumatic news coverage (Dart Center for Journalism & Trauma, 2000).

Preparing the Professionals. There are many national and local opportunities for enhancing preparedness for ecological incidents. Fielder, Palmer, and Coleman summarized many in Chapter 10 (see Table 10.1). They range from preparing multiagency disaster plans to organizing sampling frames and reference data in areas where such events are likely to occur. Unfortunately, the funding for such preventive data collection is limited.

Another important and very practical lesson in relation to immediate intervention is to prepare the rescue teams who are the first to enter the contaminated grounds. The experience in Japan (cf. Chapter 8) showed that in their zeal to rescue as many people as possible, many emergency workers who rushed in after the terrorist attack became victims of the nerve gas themselves. This is a common occurrence that can at least be partly prevented by instructing rescue personnel on safety procedures in such cases. Most important, the preparation of rescue workers must include information on what they can expect in terms of psychological traumatization and the best way to cope with this. Disaster teams should therefore also include professionals from the mental health field.

After the World Trade Center collapse, the Red Cross called upon psychologists and other mental health professionals to offer counseling on site. All licensed professionals were eligible to help, but few were specifically trained in disaster or trauma relief. As similar events may happen in the future it is important that rescue workers and mental health teams be educated beforehand on how best to contribute to early interventions. Mental health professionals working with victims and their families in the wake of the World Trade Center tragedy struggled to cope with the same psychological problems as others in the community (Keyes, 2001).

In setting up mental health delivery systems, helping the helpers must be facilitated in community crisis situations (Cwikel, Kacen, & Slonim-Nevo, 1993; Talbot, Manton, & Dunn, 1992). Those that are knowledgeable about research can also play a role in designing studies that can shed light on the subsequent psychological as well as physical health consequences of these events. The importance of including comparison populations in the research design cannot be overstated, as it affords the possibility of making causal inferences about disaster-related health effects.

A third group of professionals who must be targeted in the prevention phase is medical doctors, especially those working in primary care and emergency medicine. Murthy described in Chapter 7 how medical personnel were trained in the psychological aftereffects of the Bhopal disaster. These professionals can play a key role either in suppressing or amplifying the signals of concern arising from the population (Kasperson et al., 1988). Training physicians in behavioral medicine and models of stress and health is essential if they are to deal skillfully with the psychological concerns of exposed populations.

Organizational Aspects of Preparedness. Impressive progress has been made in the area of general contingency planning by authorities at various levels. Again and again, however, these plans exist mainly on paper. Exercises involving police, fire departments, and health care institutions are rarely conducted. Certainly most contingency plans are not equipped to deal with major toxicological accidents or attacks. At the policy level, as Chapter 11 demonstrates, relatively little work has been done to increase preparedness. Following the wave of anthrax-infected envelopes that were mailed throughout the United States and Europe in the period after the World Trade Center collapse, substantial funds were appropriated to the U.S. Centers for Disease Control and Prevention to develop community wide bioterrorism detection and response programs. This directive may lead to better community preparedness for all types of ecological disasters.

Our knowledge of the specifications of such plans is limited. One official representative of the Ministry of Health of the Netherlands who participated in a conference on the consequences of ecological disasters aptly put it: "Tell me what legislation is needed or what agency I should set up." At this stage it would not be easy to formulate such laws or tasks. Clearly more work is needed in this area.

The Immediate Response Phase

The Immediate Impact on Those Directly Involved. Ecological disasters do not always have an acute phase as is shown, for example, by the Aral Sea drough (Chapter 9). For this type of event, Bertazzi (1989) has coined the term "diluted disasters." If there is an acute phase, the victims are usually too overwhelmed to make sense of what is happening. There may be devastation, and there may be dense smoke and putrid smells. During these peak moments, initial impressions often tend to have the deepest impact. As one journalist said about the early moments after a disaster: "They have a profound effect on the persons who are in the middle of these events and, if they are journalists, they will create a disposition to interpret the events and to act accordingly before the facts are fully presented." This may not only create immediate danger as people rush in unprotected, but it will also influence the way the journalists will interpret the events from then on and how they will describe it afterward.

In every disaster situation, the immediate need for practical and emotional support is readily observable. Unfortunately, the disaster literature on this point is not very clear. We have little information on the kinds of interventions that will be effective or even if an immediate intervention by mental health professionals is needed. The fact is that at this moment, there is considerable debate among mental health specialists about whether immediate support, such as the emotional debriefing programs that are now regularly implemented after traumatic events, are indeed helpful (see below). Even if people feel the need for such care at this time, they might prefer support from peers and family members.

The Role of the Professional in the Early Phase. From the perspective of the medical professional, two angles are important—dealing with the physical consequences and dealing with the psychological effects. In the immediate phase of a toxic disaster, it is of utmost importance that environmental measurements, such as air and soil samples, and biophysical measures, including blood samples, are taken as soon as possible. This is not only important for identifying immediate risks to rescue workers and bystanders, but pinpointing exposures occurring in the immediate aftermath is also important for understanding the health problems that are manifested at later phases. Long-term storage of such samples is therefore advised.

Besides providing direct relief, psychologists and other mental health workers may be involved in the early stages by organizing support services, such as crisis counseling or emotional debriefing, as well as community education programs, individual and family outreach, and recovery counseling (Lebedun & Wilson, 1989). The World Health Organization's Division of Mental Health provides training material and professional services for disasters, although not specifically tailored to this type of disaster (World Health Organization, 1992). Other specific materials are also available from international agencies (see Danieli, Rodley, & Weisaeth, 1996 for available resources). Aside from direct crisis intervention, the role of the mental health professionals may include public education and media responses, bolstering indigenous support networks, supporting family members who have lost a loved one, and, as noted above, working with the Red Cross and other relief organizations to provide psychological first aid (Green & Lindy, 1994).

New forms of psychological and pharmacotherapeutic treatments are being developed and tested with survivors of trauma (Brady, 1997). Even though a number of specific treatments have been designated as "probably effective" by the American Psychological Association (Chambles, Baker, Beaucon, Bentler, Calhoun, & Crits-Christoph, 1998), the empirical evidence for these prevention and intervention strategies is fragile. Indeed, some studies have even shown detrimental effects (Bowman, 1999). Yzermans and Gersons (Chapter 5) describe how leaflets informing the public of possible "normal psychotraumatic responses" were distributed in apartment buildings neighboring the destroyed building, an intervention that does not appear to have resulted in a diminished rate of PTSD. Another important conclusion noted by Asukai and Maekawa (Chapter 8) and by de Jong (Chapter 13) is that Western-style trauma treatments may have questionable validity in non-Western countries such as Japan or Africa.

What the Authorities Should Do. One valuable recommendation is to establish a central information center in the wake of an ecological disaster, preferably keeping it open for quite some time. Such a center was established a year after the El Al airplane crashed into a housing block in Amsterdam, as described in Chapter 5. The Chernobyl accident and other nuclear spills such as those in Winfield (UK) and Hanford (U.S.) clearly show that covering up and misleading the public will have a boomerang effect in the long run (Brewin, 1993; Young & Launer, 1991). A straightforward approach involving timely and accurate information seems to be the best way to handle this type of crisis, although examples of successful information management are few and far between.

In the aftermath of ecological disasters, health registers or other forms of monitoring are usually set up. As Bromet and Litcher point out in Chapter 4, it is of utmost importance that these should include mental as well as physical health effects. The advantage of such a registry may be that it can form a basis for monitoring health over the long term and facilitate identification of late onset cases with mental or physical disorders, hence curtailing discussions in later phases about who was and who was not a "victim." We note, however, that establishing a registry can also have negative effects by fostering a victim mentality that can lead to medicalization and iatrogenic health problems. Indeed, when it is conducted without a clear focus on specific outcomes, health monitoring programs can create false expectations and promote preoccupation with physical sensation. As the Bijlmer experience shows (Chapter 5), this is especially likely if it is not known what health effects to look for and if no adequate reference data are available. The experiences following the Seveso incident (Bertazzi, 1989) and the Chernobyl disaster (Havenaar et al., 1997) seem to support this.

Long-Term Response

Living with the Long-Term Effects of Ecological Disaster. A worst-case scenario of an ecological disaster is described by van der Meer, Small, Crighton, and Ford (Chapter 9) in their account of the situation near the Aral Sea in Karalpakstan, Uzbekistan. It exemplifies some of the nightmarish consequences of these events: a decline in population size through emigration and decreased number of births, sometimes referred to as "sociodemographic pessimism," and widespread illness and decline in well-being throughout the affected population. Once this stage is reached, it may be nearly impossible to mount adequate countermeasures. The most active and vital elements of the population have left or are trying to leave the area, while those staying behind lose hope and slump into protracted psychological and economic depression.

As was pointed out in the chapters by Cwikel, Havenaar, and Bromet (Chapter 3), Asukai and Maekawa (Chapter 8), and Speckhard (Chapter 12), social stigma can be one of the most negative long-term consequences. This stigmatization of survivors has never been reported after natural disasters, but may be compared to what survivors of the atomic bombing of Hiroshima and Nagasaki, or veterans from the Vietnam War, have experienced. Unfortunately, very little is known about the mechanisms that perpetuate it. Stigmatization may promote or sustain a "victim identity" and foster social malfunction and illness behavior, such as somatization and substance abuse. For young people particularly, social stigmatization may mean being less eligible as a marriage partner and living with a constant concern about the health of their children and of future generations.

The Long-Term Professional Response. As the impact an ecological disaster stretches over time, the attention tends to shift from emergency medicine to the need for mental health professionals. The follow-up of Gulf War veterans and population groups affected by the Chernobyl disaster has shown that the discussion about the role of physical and psychological factors in producing the health effects may go on for many years. From the point of view of the affected populations, both issues should be taken seriously. Demonstrating causality is often complicated partly because of the many methodological pitfalls involved in this type of investigation.

A related problem is how to translate uncertain or contradictory research findings to the people who have been exposed and who are worried about the risks. An illustration of this is the continuous stream of findings of genetic damage in children and liquidators exposed to low levels of irradiation at dosages most radiobiologists would expect to be relatively harmless (Shigematsu, Chikako, Kamada, Akiyama, & Sasaki, 1993; Weinberg et al., 2001; Emerit et al., 1997).

What is so problematic about these reports is that it is hard to establish a causal link with ionizing radiation, and even harder to relate them to specific clinical outcomes. What is the responsible message to tell an exposed person when laboratory evidence of DNA damage is found after exposure to ionizing radiation? Will it translate into a 1%, 5%, 10% greater risk of cancer or other illness or none at all? Informing exposed persons about a presumed health effect without adequate scientific knowledge may cause more iatrogenic psychological distress than the actual biological risk. We lack good clinical guidelines to deal with these issues.

The contradictory long-term findings about mental and physical health mirror the chaos that ensues from the very beginning of these events. The scientific ambivalence that arises may result in the delay or rejection from publication of important findings. However, the research difficulties inherent in proving causality should not lull concerned health care professionals into apathy or complacency about continuing to follow up on exposed populations (Steingraber, 1998).

Maintaining the Attention of Official Agencies. Chapter 5, 7, and 8 show that in the immediate phase, government agencies tend to become flexible and generous in providing solutions and adapting rules and regulations to the extraordinary circumstance. After a year or so, however, they tend to revert to business as usual. They are not prepared to deal with long-term consequences, such as the financial problems that are the result of unemployment due to direct or indirect effects of the disaster (e.g., decline in tourism in areas hit by an oil spill or, in agricultural production, in areas that are no longer considered safe to grow food. By the time these problems come to the foreground, most relief workers have left and other priorities demand immediate attention. An information center, such as those established by UNESCO in some of the villages near Chernobyl, that can continue to inform the public about newly emerging facts related to the exposure, can also serve as a communication medium to inform authorities about new problems arising in the affected communities.

The media also play an important role in keeping agency officials and health professionals aware of new health problems that arise. In Ukraine, for example, news articles appear regularly on the health consequences of the accident.

CONCLUSION

This Epilogue was composed in the weeks following the World Trade Center (WTC) collapse, during a period when the public reaction in the world reflects what is common after ecological disasters. There is the perception that life as we knew it can never be the same. The attacks with anthrax that have followed since September 11 have confirmed most people's feelings that events are divided into two distinct periods of time—before WTC and after. This distinction implies that after WTC, it is impossible to recapture the sense of security and invincibility that surrounded us like a blanket of forgetfulness. We are all struggling to understand how a small group of "rogue" terrorists could have acquired western technology and cultural patterns so thoroughly as to be able to use them as lethal weapons of mass destruction.

During this period, it is possible to observe a collection of public responses that echo many of the issues raised in this book. They include such aspects as the fear of future attacks, fear of formerly neutral stimulae, such as any white powder appearing unexpectedly, and disagreement among agencies, for example on how best to protect postal workers from becoming contaminated with anthrax. Typical for this type of occurrence is that the psychological and societal effects resulting from the fear for exposure is far greater than the effects of the exposure itself. For people affected by ecological disasters and terrorism elsewhere, many of these issues have been part of everyday life for years.

Reporting physical symptoms in the aftermath of an ecological disaster is governed by a complex combination of cultural, psychological, social, and physiological factors. Female gender, chronic anxiety, and previous traumatization are among the individual factors that lead people to focus on environmental damage and physical cues for changes in health status. High-stress environments, the presence of plausible causal attributions or secondary gain, and the absence of distracting stimuli are among the social factors that can influence the spread of symptom reports (Bresnitz & Eshel, 1983; Pennebaker, 1994). In trying to cope with a communal stressor, people take their emotional cues about how to react from others in their environment, including what they see in the media.

The chapters in this book suggest that catastrophes involving toxic exposures create subpopulations who live in conditions of chronic threat. These populations may remain in the areas where these accidents occur, or as was the case with Chernobyl, they may scatter throughout the world. What is clear from the various chapters in this book is that as time passes, the affected populations often become even more symptomatic and more hyper-vigilant about their health and well-being. The physical health effects often do not appear for years, as is the case with exposures involving ionizing radiation. Post-traumatic stress symptoms, once they arise, are persistent and associated with a wide variety of comorbid physical and psychiatric syndromes.

The public health perspective shows us how each phase of a disaster and each player in disease onset (host; agent; environment) intertwines. Underneath it all is perception—by the sufferers, the health care providers, the government agency officials, and the media—and it is these perceptions that drive the magnitude, persistence, evolution, and even the risk and protective factors that are identified after major ecological catastrophes. We need a comprehensive, longitudinal, long-term approach that combines physical and mental health evaluations to further our understanding of the consequences and the relative effectiveness of different interventions as these tragedies occur.

In conclusion, as recent events have shown, government and public reactions to ecological disasters will play their parts on an ever-more frightening world stage. Technology has changed. Today's victims often manage to communicate last words using their cell phones, while rescue teams use high technology, including robots, to defuse toxic threats. Mental health professionals are increasingly using the Internet to reach out to the frightened public, to educate other professionals, and to offer counseling (e.g., ISTSS, 2001; Levy et al., 2000). Catastrophes involving toxic substances cause long-term suffering and disability to populations who believe that they were affected. Health education is needed to inform the affected populations about which symptoms indicate serious disease and to appreciate the impact of stress on their symptoms (Barsky & Borus, 1999). When the media sensationalize the physical health effects, the population will be even more vulnerable to believing that they are sick and that their future, or their children's future, is in jeopardy. So long as government agencies and prominent officials offer competing advice and contradictory information about the exposure's effects, the public will be unable to grasp and understand what may happen to them and overinterpret every symptom as ensuing from the exposure. As this book shows, the "developmental" aspects of ecological disasters are complex and dynamic, and hence interventions must be multifaceted and dynamic. This book is the first step in describing the influences of various psychosocial factors. The future requires that effective intervention strategies be developed and tested so that in future similar situations, preventive strategies can be established before it is too late.

REFERENCES

Barsky, A. J., & Borus, J. F. (1999). Functional somatic syndromes. *Annals of Internal Medicine, 130,* 910–921.

Bertazzi, P. A. (1989). Industrial disasters and epidemiology. A review of recent experiences. *Scandinavian Journal of Work and Environmental Health, 15,* 85–100.

Bowman, M. L. (1999). Individual differences in posttraumatic distress: Problems with the DSM-IV model. *Canadian Journal of Psychiatry, 44,* 21–33.

Brady, K. T. (1997). Posttraumatic stress disorder and comorbidity: Recognizing the many faces of PTSD. *Journal of Clinical Psychiatry, 58* (Suppl. 9), 12–15.

Brewin, T. B. (1993). Radiation, Chernobyl and the media. *Medico-Legal Journal, 61,* 204–215.

Breznitz, S., & Eshel, Y. (1983). Life events: Stressful ordeal or valuable experience. In S. Breznitz (Ed.), *Stress in Israel* (pp. 228–261). New York: Van Nostrand Reinhold.

Bromet, E. J., Goldgaber, D., & Gluzman, S. (in press). Somatic symptoms in women 11 years after the Chornobyl accident: Prevalence and risk factors. *Environmental Health Perspectives.*

Chambless, D. L., Baker, M. J., Baucom, D. H., Beutler, L. E., Calhoun, K. S., & Crits-Christoph, P. (1998). Update on empirically validated therapies II. *Clinical Psychologist, 51,* 315–319.

Cwikel, J., Kacen, L., & Slonim-Nevo, V. (1993). Community consultation on stress management to Israeli social workers during the Gulf War. *Health and Social Work, 18,* 172–183.

Danieli, Y., Rodley, N. S., & Weisaeth, L. (1996). *International responses to traumatic stress.* Amityville, NY: Baywood.

Dart Center for Journalism & Trauma. (2000). University of Washington, School of communications. Available from http://www.dartcenter.org

Donabedian, A. (1980). *Exploration in quality assessment en monitoring* volume 1. *Definition of quality and approaches to its assessment.* Ann Arbor, MI: Health Administration Press, University of Michigan.

Emerit, I., Quastel, M., Goldsmith, J., Merkin, L., Levy, A., Cernjavski, L. et al. (1997). Clastogenic factors in the plasma of children exposed at Chernobyl. *Mutation Research, 373,* 47–54.

Green, B. L., & Lindy, J. D. (1994). Post-traumatic disorder in victims of disasters. *Psychiatric Clinics North America, 17*(2), 301–309.

Havenaar, J. M., De Wilde E. J., van den Bout, J., Drottz-Sjöberg, B. M., & van den Brink, W. (in press). Perception of risk and subjective health among victims of the Chernobyl disaster. *Social Science and Medicine.*

Havenaar, J. M., Rumyantzeva, G., Kasyanenko, A. P., Kaasjager, K., Westermann, A. M., van den Brink, W. et al. (1997). Health effects of the Chernobyl disaster: Illness or illness behaviour? A comparative general health survey in two former Soviet Regions. *Environmental Health Perspectives, 105* (Suppl. 6), 1533–1537.

International Society Traumatic Stress Studies (ISTSS). (2001). Available from www.istss.org

Kasperson, R. E., Renn, O., Slovic, P., Brown, H. S., Emel, J., Goble, R. et al. (1988). The social amplification of risk: A conceptual framework. *Risk Analysis, 3,* 177–191.

Keyes, L. (2001, October 10). Jewish counselors tap experience with Holocaust survivors in aftermath of terror. *The Forward.*

Kleber, R. J., Figley, C. R., & Gersons, B. P. R. (Eds.), (1995). *Beyond trauma: Cultural and societal dynamics.* New York: Plenum Press.

Lebedun, M., & Wilson, K. E. (1989). Planning and integrating disaster response. In R. Gist & B. Lubin (Eds.), *Psychosocial aspects of disaster* (pp. 268–279). New York: Wiley.

Levy, K., Aghababian, R. V., Hirsch, E. F., Screnci, D., Boshyan, A., Ricks, R. C. et al. (2000). An internet-based exercise as a component of an overall training program addressing medical aspects of radiation emergency management. *Prehospital Disaster Medicine, 15,* 18–25.

Øvretveit J. (1998). *Evaluating health interventions. An introduction to evaluation of treatments, services, policies and organisational interventions.* Buckingham: Open University Press.

Pennebaker, J. W. (1994). Psychological bases of symptom reporting: Perceptual and emotional aspects of chemical sensitivity. *Toxicology and Industrial Health, 10,* 497–511.

Shigematsu, I., Chikako, I., Kamada, N., Akiyama, M., & Sasaki, H. (1995). *Effects of A-bomb radiation on the human body.* Translated by B. Harrison. Tokyo: Harwood Academic Publishers.

Steingraber, S. (1998). *Living downstream: A scientist's personal investigation of cancer and the environment.* New York: Vintage Books.

Talbot, A., Manton, M., & Dunn, P. J. (1995). Debriefing the debriefers: An intervention strategy to assist psychologists after a crisis. In G. S. Everly, Jr. & J. M. Lating (Eds.), *Psychotraumatology: Key papers and core concepts in post-traumatic stress. Plenum series on stress and coping* (pp. 281–298). New York: Plenum Press.

Weinberg, H. S., Korol, A. B., Kirzher, V. M., Avivi, A. Fahima, T., Nevo, E. et al. (2001). Very high mutation rate in offspring of Chernobyl accident liquidators. *Proceedings of the Royal Society London B. Biological Sciences, 268*(1471), 1001–1005.

World Health Organization (WHO). (1992). *Psychosocial consequences of disasters—Prevention and management.* WHO/FHE/MNH/93. Geneva: Author.

Young, M. J., & Launer, M. K. (1991). Redefining Glasnost in the Soviet media: Their contexualization of Chernobyl. *Journal of Communication, 41,* 102–124.

Index

273